Oculoplastic Surgery
Second Edition

Editors

Clinton D. McCord, M.D., F.A.C.S.

Clinical Professor of Ophthalmology
Emory University
Director, Southeastern Oculoplastic Clinic
Piedmont Hospital
Atlanta, Georgia

Myron Tanenbaum, M.D.

Clinical Instructor
Bascom Palmer Eye Institute
University of Miami
School of Medicine
Miami, Florida

Raven Press ⬥ New York

Raven Press, 1185 Avenue of the Americas, New York, New York 10036

Made in the United States of America
9 8 7 6 5 4 3 2 1

International Standard Book Number 0–88167–257–2

The material contained in this volume was submitted as previously unpublished material, except in the instances in which credit has been given to the source from which some of the illustrative material was derived.

Great care has been taken to maintain the accuracy of the information contained in the volume. However, Raven Press cannot be held responsible for errors or for any consequences arising from the use of the information contained herein.

Materials appearing in this book prepared by individuals as part of their official duties as U.S. Government employees are not covered by the above-mentioned copyright.

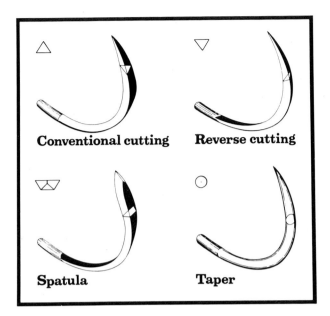

FIG. 2. Needle types used in oculoplastic surgery.

on a 4-0 chromic (Ethicon needle G-2) is excellent for suturing the mucosal flaps in a dacryocystorhinostomy.

Three types of needle holders are available. Most commonly used is a spring-type needle holder such as the Castroviejo. This is a general-purpose needle holder that can handle needles bearing 4-0 to 7-0 suture. Another type often used is a Kalt needle holder, which is a somewhat larger instrument and can also hold 4-0 to 7-0 sutures. The third type of needle holder is the Webster, which is the standard general plastic surgery needle holder. It is used in holding 4-0 to 6-0 sutures.

Plastic surgery forceps come with either toothed or smooth tips. Except in rare cases we confine our practice to the use of forceps with teeth; they are less traumatic than smooth forceps, which tend to crush tissues. Although there is a large variety of these available, we find the Bishop-Harmon forceps to be especially useful. ''Bishops'' come in two varieties, those with fine teeth and those with extra-delicate teeth. The fine-toothed Bishop-Harmon are good general-purpose forceps useful for handling most periocular tissues. We use the extra-delicate Bishop-Harmon forceps to gently hold thin skin flaps and other delicate tissues such as conjunctiva. The Lester forceps are similar to the Bishop-Harmon and also come in a fine and extra-fine variety. For handling especially large and heavy tissues, we use the Adson tissue forceps.

Whenever possible it is advantageous to use tiny, fine skin hooks to retract tissue flaps; this provides the least amount of tissue trauma. Especially useful is the Tyrell iris hook (Storz #E-548), which is very useful for retracting thin skin flaps.

It is very important to use scissors appropriate to the tissue being cut, because use of an incorrect instrument will increase tissue trauma and also ruin the instrument. For cutting tougher tissues, such as skin flaps in blepharoplasties and large skin muscle flaps, we prefer to use either round or pointed-tip baby Metzenbaum scissors. We find the Stevens tenotomy scissors and the Westcott spring-action scissors to be extremely useful for finer structures. These three provide a good variety and enable one to cut any tissue. Among other instruments (see Figs. 3, 4, and 5) our general purpose ophthalmic plastics tray includes:

1 Westcott scissors
1 fine stitch scissors
1 general utility scissors (Stevens type)
1 Webster or Kalt needle holder
1 small Metzenbaum scissors
1 Castroviejo needle holder
2 fine Tyrell skin hooks
2 Adson forceps
2 fine-toothed Bishop-Harmon forceps
2 extra-delicate-toothed Bishop-Harmon forceps
1 Desmarres retractor
2 Rake retractor
1 Castroviejo caliper
1 scalpel handle and #15 blade
2 protective scleral contact lenses

WOUND CLOSURE AND DRESSINGS

Once one has decided on the suture and instruments to be used to close a surgical wound, the next step is to inspect the wound and make certain that it is in optimal condition to be closed. The margins should be straight and sharp with no ragged tissue. Any necrotic or irregular tissues in the wound should be excised. During this procedure, the wound

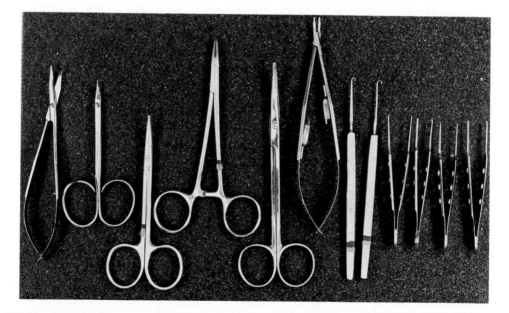

FIG. 3. Instruments used in oculoplastic surgery (*left to right*): Westcott scissors; Storz stitch scissors; Stevens scissors; 5″ plastic needle holder; Metzenbaum scissors; Castroviejo needle holder; skin hooks (2); Bishop-Harmon forceps with various size tips (4).

Preface to the Second Edition

As editors and authors of the Second Edition of *Oculoplastic Surgery,* our goal has been to fashion a cohesive, updated textbook not only reflecting surgical management principles of the contributors but also containing many surgical techniques of our own, as editors. All chapters from the first edition have been revised, and in some cases, extensively rewritten, with additional material added from our personal experience. New chapters have been added that cover Graves' disease, essential blepharospasm, and anatomy of the eyelids, orbit, and lacrimal apparatus. The chapters on the lacrimal system and on eyelid malpositions have been extensively revised. While a variety of surgical procedures may exist for a given oculoplastic problem, the editors present only those methods that are sound in principle because they have stood the test of time with experienced surgeons. We have specifically tried to avoid presenting a multitude of different surgical approaches, which can confuse the beginning surgeon. Details of surgical techniques and related material that are not emphasized in the current oculoplastic literature will make this text of interest to the surgeon with many years' experience.

Since the heart of the practice of oculoplastic surgery is surgical performance, the text and figures of the Second Edition describe all of the surgical procedures in detail to enable the reader to comfortably pursue a procedure after reading about it. In many areas of the text, line drawings are used in combination with photographs of the surgical procedures for further clarification.

We have intended this textbook to update, guide, and expand the skills of the surgeon interested in eyelid, lacrimal, and orbital surgery.

Clinton D. McCord, Jr.
Myron Tanenbaum

Preface to the First Edition

The single question asked most frequently by residents and ophthalmologists in general practice is, "What one book covers most oculoplastic problems that I may encounter and presents techniques that I can understand?" The second most frequently asked question is, "What are the best simple procedures that I can learn to allow me to handle specific straightforward eye plastic conditions?"

This manual attempts to respond to these questions, although many techniques and problem situations cannot be simplified to that level. Each oculoplastic subject is treated in a problem-solving manner that includes mode of presentation of the problem, differential diagnosis of the problem, the indicated surgical procedure or procedures, and complications that may be encountered.

The surgical techniques presented are those used by the authors and found to be "tried and true." Although some alternate procedures are shown, the reader is not confused with multiple procedures which he may not use or need. A bibliography of more elaborate or advanced surgical techniques and special clinical problems is provided at the end of each chapter for further reading.

Three chapters (8, 9, and 10) cover repair of full thickness eyelid defects, and require some special prefatory comments. This section emphasizes that the repair of all eyelid defects can be approached systematically, provided that certain basic reconstructive techniques are first learned. The chapters on upper lid and inner canthal defect repair and lower lid and lateral canthal defect repair describe the specific techniques that must be mastered and emphasize the surgical details of each technique. Following these two chapters is a section that considers a variety of defects that may be encountered and describes the application of the techniques used either singly or in combination to repair these defects.

This volume will provide a comprehensive understanding of the large majority of oculoplastic problems and surgical techniques and will be useful to ophthalmologists and all surgeons interested in this area.

Clinton D. McCord, Jr.

Contents

Contributors

Henry I. Baylis, M.D.
Division of Ophthalmic Plastic and
*   Reconstructive Surgery*
Jules Stein Eye Institute
University of California at Los Angeles
Los Angeles, California

Donald J. Bergin, M.D.
U.S. Army Medical Corps
Department of Ophthalmology
Letterman Army Medical Center
San Francisco, California

Craig E. Berris, M.D.
Department of Ophthalmology
University of California Medical School
Davis, California

Marcos T. Doxanas, M.D.
Department of Ophthalmic Plastic Surgery
Greater Baltimore Medical Center
Baltimore, Maryland

Robert M. Dryden, M.D.
Department of Ophthalmology
University of Arizona Medical School
Tucson, Arizona

Arthur S. Grove, Jr., M.D.
Department of Ophthalmology
Harvard Medical School; and
Massachusetts Eye and Ear Infirmary
Boston, Massachusetts

Gerard J. Hunter, M.D.
Department of Ophthalmology
University of Texas Medical School
Houston, Texas

Dwight R. Kulwin, M.D.
Department of Ophthalmology
University of Cincinnati Medical School; and
Cincinnati Veterans Administration Hospital
Cincinnati, Ohio

Clinton D. McCord, Jr., M.D.
Department of Ophthalmology
Emory University School of Medicine
Atlanta, Georgia

James L. Moses, M.D.
Department of Ophthalmology
Mount Carmel Medical Center
Ohio State University
Columbus, Ohio

William R. Nunery, M.D.
Department of Ophthalmology
Indiana University School of Medicine
Indianapolis, Indiana

John W. Shore, M.D.
U.S. Air Force Medical Corps
Department of Ophthalmology
Wilford Hall USAF Medical Center
San Antonio, Texas

Norman Shorr, M.D.
Division of Ophthalmic Plastic and
*   Reconstructive Surgery*
Jules Stein Eye Institute
University of California at Los Angeles
Los Angeles, California

Myron Tanenbaum, M.D.
Bascom Palmer Eye Institute
University of Miami
School of Medicine
Miami, Florida

Robert R. Waller, M.D.
Department of Ophthalmology
Mayo Clinic
Rochester, Minnesota

Ralph Wesley, M.D.
Ophthalmic Plastic and Reconstructive Surgery
Vanderbilt University Medical Center; and
Ophthalmic Service
Parkview Medical Center
Veterans Administration Medical Center
Nashville, Tennessee

Robert B. Wilkins, M.D.
Department of Ophthalmology
University of Texas Medical School
Houston, Texas

To Cissy, Monica, Bernard, and Beverly

We would like to thank Sandra J. Sidwell for many tireless hours of typing manuscripts.

Oculoplastic Surgery, 2nd edition, edited by
Clinton D. McCord, Jr., and Myron Tanenbaum.
Raven Press, New York © 1987.

Chapter 1

Skin and Tissue Techniques

*Robert B. Wilkins, **Dwight R. Kulwin, †Clinton D. McCord, Jr., and
‡Myron Tanenbaum

*Department of Ophthalmology, University of Texas Medical School, Houston, Texas 77025;
**Department of Ophthalmology, University of Cincinnati Medical School, and Cincinnati Veterans
Administration Hospital, Cincinnati, Ohio 45221; † Department of Ophthalmology, Emory University
School of Medicine, Atlanta, Georgia 30308; and ‡ Bascom Palmer Eye Institute, Department of
Ophthalmology, University of Miami School of Medicine, Miami, Florida 33101

BASIC PRINCIPLES

There is a wide variety of operations available to the ophthalmic plastic surgeon, and many different procedures may be used to treat each disease entity satisfactorily. However, certain basic principles and practices promote the best possible result regardless of the procedure used. Simply stated, these principles and practices result in gentle tissue handling, rapid and effective surgery, cosmetically acceptable scars, and good results. Throughout this chapter we will present those techniques we feel are most effective in achieving this goal. Gentle handling allows the healing of operative incisions as quickly as possible without hematomas and necrotic tissue caused by rough manipulation. Rapid, effective surgery allows as short a time in the operating room as possible. With continued exposure of tissues, especially mucous membranes and areas that are not normally exposed to the air, there is substantial drying and devitalization. This results in decreased viability and substantial tissue necrosis. In addition, bacterial colonization of exposed tissues is time related.

INCISIONS

All skin incisions will result in the formation of a scar. It is the surgeon's objective to minimize or disguise the inevitable scar. Skin incisions should be made as vertical as possible to eliminate beveling of the edges. A vertical incision results in the smallest possible scar and the most rapid healing of the epithelium. We prefer the disposable "super-sharp" blades (e.g., the Bard-Parker 15, the Martin Blade 15) for most skin incisions. The cutting action of these blades is very clean, and they are heavy enough to offer the surgeon excellent control of the cutting motion. A razor knife made from a broken razor blade is a suitable alternative.

1

Lidocaine 2% with 1:100,000 epinephrine and hyaluronidase (Wydase®) is infiltrated locally at least 10 min before making the skin incision. This mixture offers an excellent advantage in promoting hemostasis and is used even if the patient has been placed under general anesthesia. Wydase® promotes dissolution in a local injection so that tissue distortion does not occur. It is always helpful to outline a skin incision with methylene blue or a surgical marking pen before actually making the incision. To avoid beveling of the wound or irregular edges, the skin must be held taut. The optimal incision is made in a single, steady motion. Stopping and starting motions are to be avoided. It is helpful to cut from the lowest point ''up hill'' to the highest point, to avoid having blood obscure the surgical field. Forceps may be used to fixate tissues to facilitate making an incision. The Adson forceps is an excellent all-purpose toothed forceps for use on the periocular tissues. More delicate forceps can often tear the tissues if improperly used. Nontoothed forceps will cause crush injury to the skin and should be avoided. When excising skin, the straight Steven's scissors is an excellent tool.

Incisions should be placed in folds or wrinkles whenever possible. This will result in mild accentuation of a preexisting crease, rather than creation of a new scar. An upper eyelid incision in the upper lid crease is an example of this principle. An incision near the brow will be least conspicuous if placed at the infrabrow or suprabrow margins. If these locations are not suitable for the incision, one should at least try to keep the incision parallel to the lines of minimal skin tension (Fig. 1).

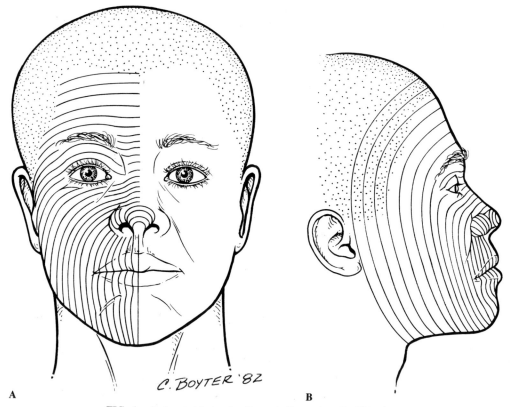

A   B

FIG. 1.   Relaxed skin tension lines. **A:** Front view. **B:** Side view.

WOUND HEALING

Because all surgery is based on the assumption that healing will occur at suture lines or over open areas, it is important to have an understanding of the process of wound healing.

The wound-healing process may be divided into four phases. First is the inflammatory phase, also called the latent or lag phase. This is followed by the fibroblastic phase and, third, the scar maturation phase. Another phase sometimes described is that of wound contraction. This phase occurs to varying degrees in all wound healing, but is most common in spontaneous healing such as that following untreated trauma.

The inflammatory phase begins immediately following any wounding, either traumatic or surgical. It prepares the wound for the subsequent fibroblastic and scar maturation phases. This first phase is often termed latent because during this phase no actual healing occurs. Rather, an environment is prepared for healing, and the necessary substances are gathered together so the healing process can proceed. Chemotactic substances attract leukocytes, macrophages, and other cells into the wound site to cleanse the wound area of debris, necrotic tissue, and bacteria.

Usually the inflammation subsides in 4 to 6 days. When the wound retains foreign material that cannot be absorbed and removed during the acute inflammatory phase, chronic inflammation results. Fibroblasts lay down collagen about the foreign substance and along with epithelioid and giant cells form recognizable granulomas that we see in eyelids about absorbable sutures. Fibrous capsules around nonabsorbable materials are also a source of chronic inflammation. We often see these fibrous capsules around implanted synthetic materials used in orbital work.

During the initial phase of healing, epithelial cells bridge the wound surface, providing a barrier to infection. The migration and proliferation of these epithelial cells begin at the wound margin within hours, and a well-sutured wound may be entirely covered at 24 hr. In superficial epidermal wounds (scratches or abrasions), epithelial migration and proliferation are the entire healing process.

The inflammatory phase overlaps the fibroblastic phase, because healing is a continuum, not a sequence of isolated events. During the inflammatory phase fibroblasts have proliferated and migrated into the wound area. They then start to produce increasing amounts of collagen; this hyperproduction continues for about 2 to 4 weeks, throughout the phase of fibroplasia. As the collagen production exceeds collagenolysis, a temporarily hypertrophied scar results. However, toward the end of the fibroblastic phase collagenase is produced, and finally equilibrium occurs between collagen production and collagen degradation. It is during the 2- to 4-week period constituting the second phase of healing, or fibroplasia, that the tensile strength of the wound increases most rapidly.

About 1 month after wounding, the fibroblasts begin to leave the wound; this disappearance marks the end of the fibroblastic phase and the beginning of the maturation phase. At this time the scar is hypertrophic, but during the maturation phase the water-soluble and randomly oriented collagen fibrils become organized and dehydrated, resulting in a scar of greater strength and less bulk. The maturation process continues for years, but the scar reaches maximum strength at about 10 to 12 weeks.

Wound contraction occurs concomitantly with the fibroblastic phase. It tends to restore the normal shape of the body by decreasing the size of an open wound through centripetal skin movement. The greatest contraction occurs when skin is only loosely attached to the underlying tissues. For example, minimal contraction occurs in a pretarsal skin defect, but contracture of the preseptal part of the eyelid is well known.

During the second phase of healing, myofibroblasts (specialized fibroblasts with contractile properties), capillary buds, and collagen cover wound surfaces as granulation tissue. It is the shortening of the myofibrils in these fibroblasts that provides the contractile force.

At the same time, the constant stretching of the surrounding tissues causes them to undergo intussusceptive growth. This results in increased skin area. The epidermis increases in volume by mitosis. Underneath this the total number of dermal elements (glands, follicles, and so forth) remains constant, but the elements are more widely spaced. The intervening volume is filled with newly synthesized collagen. This process can be seen readily in ophthalmologic procedures such as the Cutler-Beard reconstruction of the upper lid or when a lid defect is closed primarily. Gradually the taut skin returns to a more normal tension.

Contraction also occurs in well-sutured wounds, but primarily in the vertical dimension. Therefore, it is important at the end of surgery to have a slightly everted closure that will level out with time. Otherwise, a depressed scar may result.

SUTURING TECHNIQUES AND INSTRUMENTS

Before closing a wound, the surgeon must make several decisions. The type and size of suture must be determined, the correct needle must be selected, and the appropriate instruments should be picked.

Sutures may be classified as absorbable or nonabsorbable. The commonly used nonabsorbable sutures are silk, nylon, Prolene, and Supramid. The first three are used interchangeably, depending upon the surgeon's preference. Silk has the best tying characteristics and is the most pliable. Nylon and Prolene cause much less tissue reaction. As 4-0 and 5-0 sutures these three are useful for deep, permanent suturing. For skin closure, 6-0 sutures are used; 6-0 Prolene slides much better than the other two and is used for subcuticular wound closure. Supramid is a braided suture used to attach structures to periosteum and for frontalis suspension.

Commonly used absorbably sutures include Dexon and Vicryl, plain gut, and chromic gut. Dexon and Vicryl are synthetic materials. Catgut is a natural suture made from sheep intestine. It comes in a plain form, or it may be soaked in a chromic salt solution to coagulate the proteins, making it harder and less reactive. As a general rule, but with wide variance, plain gut is the most quickly absorbed suture and will retain its tensile strength for 4 to 7 days. Dexon and Vicryl retain their tensile strength for 15 to 30 days. Chromic gut tensile strength retention falls somewhere between these two groups. These absorption times are related to the fact that gut is the most irritating and causes the most tissue reaction, whereas Dexon and Vicryl are the least reactive.

Plain and chromic gut sutures are used in the closure of mucosal surfaces and for closing skin in uncooperative children in whom it would be quite difficult to remove permanent sutures. For deep suturing, 4-0 and 5-0 gut sutures are generally used; 6-0 and 7-0 are especially useful for skin and mucosal closures. Dexon and Vicryl have very similar characteristics, but Vicryl catches tissue more easily "with drag" as it is pulled through, and this tendency must be watched as one is suturing.

There are four needle types used in ophthalmic plastic surgery: cutting, reverse cutting, taper, and spatula (Fig. 2). These are often three-eighths circle needles and have a variety of diameters. We use the cutting needle for deep sutures. Either a taper or a reverse cutting needle may be used for skin closure, at the surgeon's discretion. The spatula needle is especially effective in suturing structures to the tarsal plate. The tiny half-circle needle

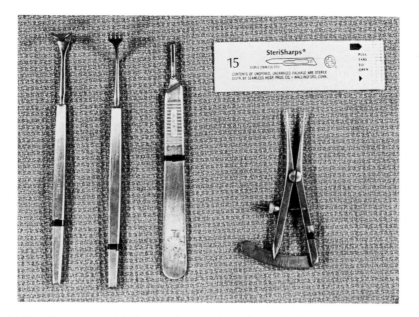

FIG. 4. Additional instruments useful in oculoplastic surgery (*left to right*): Desmarres lid retractor; four-pronged lacrimal retractor, Bard-Parker handle; Castroviejo caliper.

itself should be inspected and the various tissue layers identified. If a wound is traumatic or has been contaminated, we irrigate it copiously with neomycin in normal saline.

Surgical incisions and traumatic wounds should be closed in layers. This is extremely important to obtain a good functional and cosmetic result. All deep dead space should be eliminated, and the subcutaneous tissue should be closed so that the skin edges are in apposition, not overlapping. Thus, the skin sutures will serve merely to loosely approximate

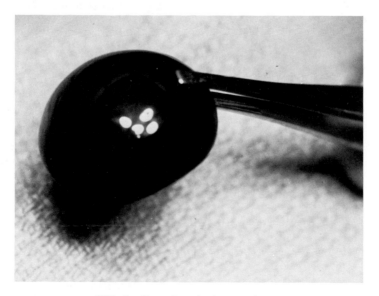

FIG. 5. Protective scleral contact lens.

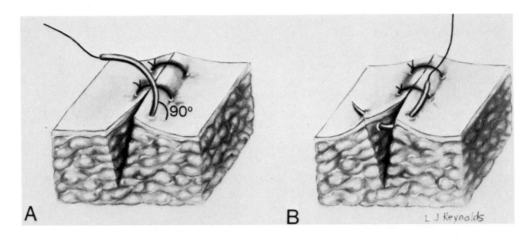

FIG. 6. Skin closure with eversion of wound edges. **A:** Needle introuduced vertically through skin and subcutaneous tissue of incision edge. **B:** Needle passed symmetrically out opposing incision edge.

the skin rather than to attempt to provide strength to the wound. If a wound is deeper than the subcutaneous tissue, we first close the deep tissues using interrupted sutures, usually 4-0 or 5-0 chromic or Dexon. Next the subcutaneous tissues are closed, using an inverted suturing technique so that the knot will lie at the base of the wound rather than just beneath the skin, where it would interrupt the integrity of the skin surface.

A key principle in wound closure is achieving good eversion of the skin edges (see Fig. 6). A prerequisite of good eversion of the skin edges, and thus eventual minimizing of scar formation, is adequate closure of the deep tissues. In cross-section a single everting stitch has a trapezoid configuration whereby more deep tissue is included than skin. When tied the skin edges are naturally forced outward. Tension-relieving sutures that can also produce skin edge eversion are the verticle mattress suture, the horizontal mattress suture, and the near-far/far-near suture (see Fig. 7). Because wounds contract vertically, margins should be slightly everted after skin closure. If this is not done, a depressed scar may result.

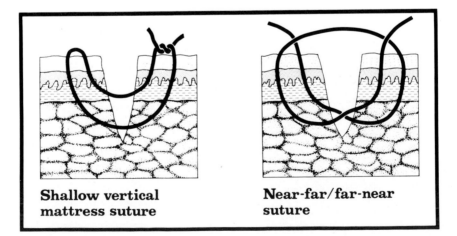

Shallow vertical mattress suture

Near-far/far-near suture

FIG. 7. Sutures that apply traction to large wounds.

We prefer to use 6-0 nylon or 7-0 silk to close skin incisions. Incisions of the eyelids that are parallel to the lines of minimal tension may also be closed using 6-0 Prolene running subcuticular suture. We have found that subcuticular closures in thicker skin such as the brow and forehead and in wound positions perpendicular to the lines of minimal tension tend to cause a more noticeable scar than an interrupted skin closure. As an alternative to interrupted closure, on occasion we will use a running suturing technique.

As a general rule, 6-0 silk skin sutures should be removed in 4 to 5 days; nylon and Prolene sutures can be left 6 to 7 days. We prefer to remove all skin sutures on the earliest possible day. If there is any evidence of wound margin gaping, or if there is any tension on the skin wound, we spread benzoin on the skin surface. After it dries we apply Steri-Strips across the wound and leave these on for another several days. If skin sutures are left in place longer than 3 to 4 days, their subsurface tract may become epithelialized, resulting in an inclusion cyst. This can be treated by inserting one blade of a pointed scissors and cutting, opening the cyst to the surface.

A large variety of special sutures has been described for wound closures. Of these we have found the near-far/far-near suture and the vertical mattress suture (see Fig. 7) to be especially valuable in closing the skin layers of a wound if there is some tension. The suture closest to the wound margin nicely approximates the wound edges, and the suture farthest away tends to remove tension from this margin so that it will leave as fine a scar as possible.

The postoperative dressing is an integral part of the operative procedure. It is the capstone ensuring a good surgical result. Our basic dressing is a single eyepatch with one or two pieces of tape. This dressing provides adequate protection of the wound but does not place any pressure on the suture line. If there is postoperative bleeding, this dressing is not tight enough to cause increased intraorbital pressure with resultant blindness caused by central retinal artery occlusion.

For blepharoplasties we place antibiotic ointment on the sutures, and then lay a single piece of an eyepatch liner over the incision. This holds the eyelid shut and provides sufficient coverage to protect the wound but does not insulate the surgical site from the ice used in the immediate postoperative phase to reduce swelling. It also allows one to spot the first evidence of postoperative bleeding.

For orbital surgery in the anophthalmic socket we advocate a completely opposite approach—that is, a firm pressure dressing. Since blindness is not a problem in these cases (such as enucleation, evisceration, and fornix reconstruction), pressure dressings can be used wth impunity. This is advantageous because it keeps swelling to a minimum. There is less suture tear-through and, we believe, a better postoperative result in general. Our usual pressure dressing begins with an eyepatch covered with adhesive tape. This is then covered with an Elastoplast dressing. Benzoin is used on the skin to improve tape adherence. We often use a head roll to add further pressure on the dressing. We leave the head roll in place for several days and the pressure dressing in place from 3 to 7 days.

HEMOSTASIS

Electrocautery is preferable to thermal cautery to obtain hemostasis of the surgical wound. We identify individual bleeding sites, grab them gently with small toothed forceps so that by stopping the bleeding with the forceps we have exactly isolated the bleeding site, and then briefly touch the electrocautery to the forceps. We prefer to use the unipolar Bovie. Wet-field and bipolar cautery are also excellent methods of obtaining hemostasis. The site to be coagulated should be free of any blood, because the presence of blood will diffuse the energy and diminish the coagulating effect.

In some wounds there is continuous oozing from many different sites. If gentle, prolonged pressure is not sufficient to stop this, three chemical approaches may be used to provide hemostasis. Cotton pledgets soaked in an anesthetic solution with epinephrine and placed on the wound for several minutes will cause vasoconstriction of the fine bleeders so that clotting can occur. If this is not successful, Gelfoam sponge soaked in thrombin can be placed on the wound and held with gentle pressure. This is an extremely effective way to create hemostasis, especially in a hole. If neither of these methods works, sprinkling Avitene® [Avicon (Alcon, Inc.) Fort Worth, Tx.] on the wound may be tried. This is expensive and should be used only as a last resort.

An excessive amount of bleeding may be encountered if a patient has been taking aspirin at the time of surgery. This is because aspirin is a potent inhibitor of platelet function. For this reason, we advise all of our preoperative patients not to take aspirin within 2 weeks of their surgery.

MANAGEMENT OF HYPERTROPHIC SCARS AND KELOIDS

Occasionally as a wound heals a hypertrophic scar or keloid develops. Hypertrophic scars involve only the tissue of the wound, whereas keloids are exuberant, tumor-like overgrowths of healing tissue that may invade the surrounding tissues. Gentle tissue manipulation will decrease the formation of such scars. One should attempt to close wounds with as little tension as possible, because the tension placed on a wound margin is in part responsible for hypertrophic scar development. In patients with a history of hypertrophic scars, especially those who have formed keloids in the past, 300 to 600 rads to the operative site immediately following surgery will diminish scar formation. Hypertrophic scars and keloids are most common in young adults and black patients.

Treatment of hypertrophic scars includes massage, topical steroid ointments, and steroid injections. Massage and kneading of the scar using cocoa butter throughout the postoperative period will soften the scar tissue. Biweekly injections of Triamcinolone® steroid suspension may be used for the treatment of hypertrophic scars or keloids. One-tenth ml of steroid suspension is injected with a 30-gauge needle on a tuberculin syringe. This should be followed by vigorous massage with cocoa butter. If injected intradermally, steroid suspensions may cause atrophy and depigmentation of the skin. This can be a disfiguring side effect in black patients. If one does not wish to inject the scar, topical Triamcinolone® 0.1% ointment may be messaged into the hypertrophic area.

For hypertrophic scars of the forehead, a 2-inch-wide strip of elastic may be worn as a headband. This provides continuous gentle pressure and is very effective in reducing the bulk of the scar.

It is of special interest to the oculoplastic surgeon that the eyelids do not seem to form keloids, even in patients with a history of prominent keloid formation. The explanation of this special eyelid privilege is not known at present.

SCAR REVISION

The previous sections dealt with optimal tissue handling techniques for minimizing scar formation. When faced with a scar, however, an individualized plan of attack must be formulated. The four basic methods of scar revision are: (1) dermabrasion, (2) excision with dermabrasion, (3) redirection (e.g., Z-plasty or W-plasty) and (4) excision with platform techniques. Careful explanation on the part of the physician will help the patient maintain realistic expectations. Scar revision is simply an attempt to replace an undesireable scar with a more desireable one. In general, surgical scar revision should not be attempted before 2 to 3 months of wound healing.

Dermabrasion is a true mainstay of scar revision. It is a technique much underutilized by ophthalmologists and other plastic surgeons. The scar and subcutaneous tissues are infiltrated with lidocaine 2% with 1:100,000 epinephrine and hyaluronidase. A fine rounded drill bit or burr, on a power-driven drill, is used to "sculpt" the scar and abrade the epidermal layer. This technique is excellent for smoothing the rough edges of a healed full-thickness skin graft. In this technique, the edges of the graft, the surface of the graft itself, and the surrounding skin is dermabraded to give a final uniform appearance.

Skin tension lines are of critical importance in scar formation and scar revision (see Fig. 1). If the scar parallels the relaxed skin tension lines, simple elliptical excision of skin, scar, and underlying dermis can be performed. The wound edges are undermined and direct closure can be achieved. Secondary dermabrasion can be utilized if necessary.

When an irregular scar or on that is perpendicular to skin tension lines is present, a redirection technique can be utilized for scar revision. Thus, in order to successfully redirect the original scar into a more favorable relationship with the relaxed skin tension lines, a thorough preoperative evaluation must be made.

Z-plasty techniques, either single or multiple, are the most common of the redirection procedures. They may be helpful in revision of eyelid scars, or even conjunctival scarring (e.g., symblepharon). The principle of the Z-plasty is to transpose two flaps of skin. This maneuver increases the length of the skin and the line parallel to the original scar while shortening the skin at right angles to the original scar. The result, however, will redirect the line of the scar toward the normal relaxed skin tension lines. The scar and surrounding tissues should be infiltrated with lidocaine 2% with 1:100,000 epinephrine and hyaluronidase at least 10 min before beginning the procedure. A Z-shaped incison is used to create two triangular flaps. The central limb of the Z is made parallel to the line of the scar. The arms of the Z are the same length as the central limb and at 60° to it. Creating longer arms of the Z-shaped incision will allow for greater lengthening in the direction of the original scar. After marking the skin, the incisions are made. The two triangular flaps must be undermined to allow for ready transposition. It is important to excise all traction bands and deep scar tissue in the bed of the original scar. Elevating triangular flaps of proper width and thickness will minimize the risk of vascular compromise. The final transposition of each triangular flap into its partner's bed will thus redirect the line of the original scar.

The W-plasty is a useful scar revision technique in thicker skin, such as that of the forehead, brow, or cheek. The W-plasty divides the scar into multiple small segments that are redirected from the line of the original scar. Unlike the transposition principle used in the Z-plasty, the W-plasty is a type of advancement flap. W-shaped, or zig-zag incisions are made perpendicular to the line of the scar. Short, acutely angulated incisions are made, undermined, and advanced to closure.

The dermal platform technique of scar revision may be used in patients prone to hypertrophic scar formation. A fusiform superficial excision of the cutaneous scar only is performed. The underlying subcutaneous traction bands and dermal scarring are not disturbed. The surrounding skin is undermined with shallow, sharp dissection and closed by advancement. The principle of this technique is to avoid restimulating dermal fibroblastic activity. Dermal platform scar revision is always used in conjunction with a later-stage cutaneous dermabrasion technique as discussed previously.

AUTOGENOUS GRAFTS AND THEIR APPLICATION

Knowledge of tissue grafting technique is an integral part of oculoplastic surgery. The surgeon must understand the indications for using tissue grafts, and be familiar with harvesting techniques. The optimal tissue graft would be cosmetically and functionally matched, have little or no shrinkage or absorption, and have a very low rate of infection or rejection. Under most circumstances autogenous tissue grafts can meet more of these criteria than can either homogenous tissue grafts (e.g., eye bank preserved sclera or preserved fascia lata) or alloplastic materials (e.g., Silastic implants or bone cement). The following sections discuss basic tissue harvesting techniques, including: full-thickness skin grafts, split-thickness skin grafts, ear cartilage grafts, mucous membrane and chondromucosal grafts, dermis fat grafts, fascia lata and temporalis fascia grafts, and bone grafts.

Skin Grafts

When there is insufficient tissue to close a wound primarily without tension, either a skin flap or a skin graft can be used to provide additional coverage and relieve the tension. If there is good blood supply and sufficient underlying soft tissue, a skin graft may be applied on the surface to provide wound coverage.

Full-Thickness Skin Grafts

A full-thickness skin graft contains both epidermal and dermal elements. The best match of skin color and thickness is usually obtained from the contralateral upper eyelid. If this skin is insufficient, the retroauricular region also provides a good match. Donor sites that are second choices because they do not provide as good a match are the supraclavicular regions, the inner arm, and the groin. All donor sites should be hairless to prevent trichiasis (Figs. 8 and 9).

When taking a full-thickness skin graft, one makes a template the shape and size of the graft needed and places the template on the donor site. Before anesthetic injection, a surgical marking pen is used to trace an outline of the template. A small amount of local anesthetic with epinephrine is used to diminish bleeding. The previously marked area is then incised, undermined, and excised freehand. One should try to remove as little subcutaneous tissue as possible along with the graft, but it is better to remove excess subcutaneous tissue than to buttonhole the graft.

The graft is then inverted and placed on a single thickness of cotton gauze over the finger. Scissors are used to excise all the subcutaneous elements so that the fine white color of the dermis with its associated rete pegs is visible. If one desires a little thinner full-thickness graft, the dermis can be partially excised in this same fashion.

The graft is sutured into place on the host site using interrupted 6-0 silk sutures after graft bed hemostasis is assured. If the graft is large, several tiny slits may be cut to drain any bleeding from the host site, preventing a hematoma from forming between graft and bed.

After the full-thickness skin graft has been sutured into place, it is covered with a

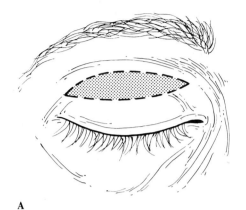

A

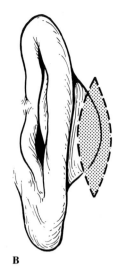

B

FIG. 8. Full thickness skin graft donor sites. **A:** upper eyelid. **B:** Retroauricular. **C:** Supraclavicular.

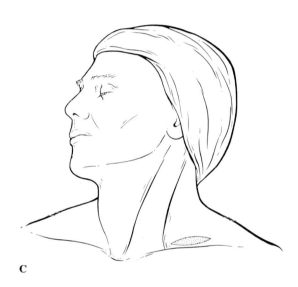

C

Telfa dressing. A sheet of softened dental wax is then molded over the Telfa dressing. The dental wax will conform to the shape of the tissue bed and prevent accumulation of fluids underneath the skin graft. A pressure dressing may be applied over the dental wax. The wound dressing and some of the sutures may be removed in 5 days. Antibiotic ointment is applied for several additional days, after which time the remaining skin sutures are removed.

Split-Thickness Skin Grafts

The split-thickness skin graft is comprised of epidermal elements only. It is harvested by a power-driven, mineral oil–lubricated dermatome. The mechanical dermatome shaves

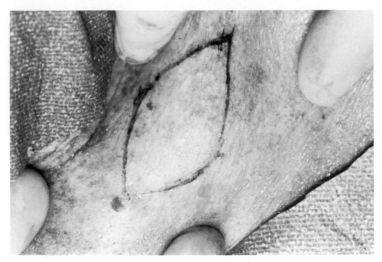

FIG. 9. Harvesting a full-thickness, supraclavicular skin graft. **A:** Ellipse marked on skin with methylene blue.

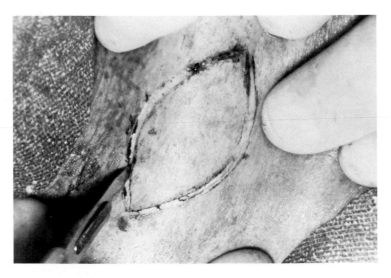

FIG. 9B. #15 blade skin incision.

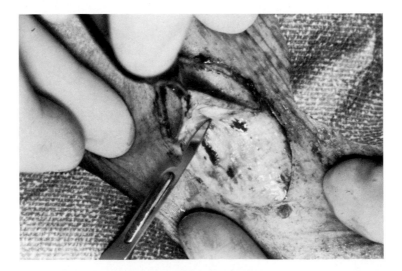

FIG. 9C. Sharp dissection to harvest full-thickness skin graft; tissues held under tension.

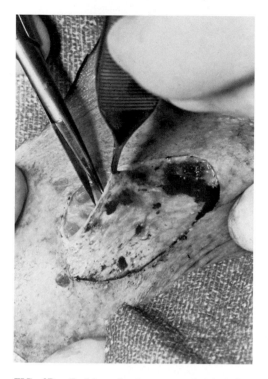

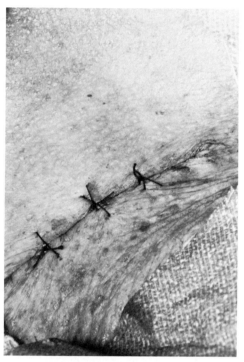

FIG. 9D. Excision of subcutaneous dermis before wound closure.

FIG. 9E. Preliminary closure of donor site with 4-0 silk retention sutures.

the split-thickness graft off of a donor site, often the anterior surface of the thigh. The graft is very thin, and it is important to lay the graft on a flat surface in order to maintain the proper orientation of the epidermis (Fig. 10).

In general, split-thickness skin grafts have a poor color match to normal eyelid skin. The tendency to contract also mitigates against their use in eyelid and periocular reconstruction.

Ear Cartilage Graft

Successful eyelid reconstruction necessitates restoration of both the anterior lamella and posterior lamella of the eyelid. Freshly harvested autogenous ear cartilage (Fig. 11) is an excellent material for reconstruction of the posterior eyelid lamella. To obtain the graft, the anterior and posterior subcutaneous tissues of the ear are first infiltrated with local anesthetic with epinephrine and hyaluronidase. Skin hooks are used to reflect the ear to expose the posterior surface. A curvilinear line is marked parallel to the edge of the helix. This line should be 4 mm from the edge of the helix to avoid causing an ear deformity. The skin incision is made and then careful dissection is performed down to the level of ear cartilage. The posterior surface of the cartilage when exposed is then marked with methylene blue or a marking pen. Again, it is important to remain 4 mm from the edge of the cartilage. A scalpel is used to carefully incise the cartilage and then a scissors is used to complete the incision through the full thickness of the cartilage. A periosteal elevator is helpful in reflecting perichondrium and subcutaneous tissues off of the anterior surface

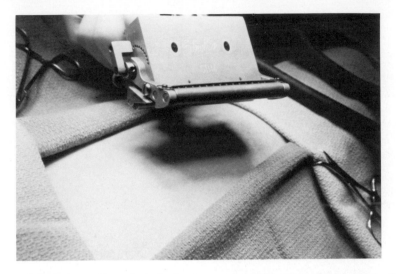

FIG. 10. Split-thickness skin graft. **A:** Stryker dermatome positioned over anterior surface of thigh.

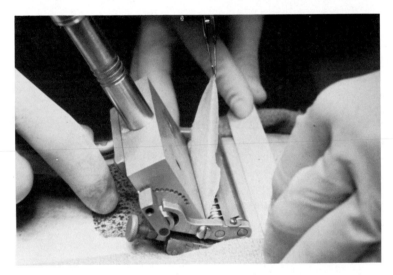

FIG. 10B. Harvesting split-thickness skin graft: mineral oil is used to lubricate skin and tongue blade is used to flatten skin in front of advancing dermatome.

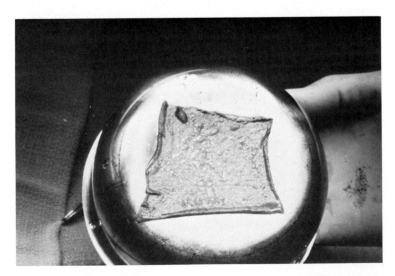

FIG. 10C. Harvested graft is spread out on a flat surface to maintain correct orientation of the epithelial layer.

of the cartilage. A scissors is then used to simply cut off the cartilage graft at its base. Hemostasis is achieved with electrocautery. Good closure can be achieved with either a subcuticular 4-0 Vicryl suture or a cutaneous silk suture closure. Cartilage may be stored in saline solution until needed later in the operation.

The larger ear cartilage grafts have a tendency to curl. Scoring one surface of the cartilage with a scalpel will help to flatten and relax the graft. When used for eyelid reconstruction, the concave surface of the cartilage should face the globe. Scoring a single surface of a cartilage graft with parallel lines will make that surface convex. Excess manipulation of these grafts is to be avoided because they are brittle.

To reiterate, cartilage is the material of choice for the reconstruction of the posterior eyelid lamella or when used as a spacer material in the treatment of eyelid diseases. The technique of harvesting ear cartilage is essential to oculoplastic and reconstructive surgery.

Mucous Membrane Grafts and Chondromucosal Grafts

When reconstructing the eyelid, one must maintain the posterior lamella. In many cases it is necessary to take a mucous membrane graft to reconstruct the mucosal portion of the posterior lamella. There is a ready supply of oral mucosa that can be grafted to the eyelid in these cases.

Mucosal grafts are handled in the same fashion as full-thickness skin grafts (Fig. 12). A template is made of the amount of the mucosa needed, and then the template is placed on the inner surface of the lower lip and roughly demarcated. If more is needed, additional grafts may be taken from the cheek and upper lip. The graft should be outlined in such a way as to avoid the margin of the lips, the gum, and Stensen's duct (approximate location opposing second upper molar). To diminish bleeding and obtain a dissection plane, the oral mucosa is infiltrated with lidocaine 2% with epinephrine 1:100,000 and hyaluronidase. The proposed graft is outlined with methylene blue and then an incision is made with a #15 blade. Because mucosal grafts tend to shrink, they are usually made slightly larger than the size of the template. A full-thickness graft is removed with sharp and blunt scissor dissection. The graft is then further thinned with a scissors. Because the tissue graft is harvested from a clearly nonsterile area, the oral cavity, we place the mucous membrane graft in a gentamicin solution, where it remains until needed later in the operation for either eyelid or socket reconstruction. No closure of the oral cavity donor site is necessary. Electrocautery is to be avoided because it only makes the recovery period more painful for the patient. A dry Gelfoam pad is placed over the donor site after harvesting the mucous membrane graft. This mucous membrane defect in the mouth will reepithelialize painlessly over several weeks. Split-thickness mucous membrane grafts can be harvested with a Castroviejo mucotome with a 0.3- to 0.5-mm. setting (Fig. 13).

When reconstruction of both the mucosa and its supporting elements is necessary, there is an alternative to a chondromucosal graft, that alternative being a two-stage procedure. In the first stage, an appropriate-sized ear cartilage graft is harvested in the usual fashion. This cartilage graft is then inserted in a submucosal pocket in the cheek of the patient. Several weeks must elapse for adequate vascularization of the cartilage and overlying mucous membrane graft to occur. After this occurs, a composite cartilage–mucous membrane graft can be harvested in the second stage of the procedure for use in eyelid reconstruction. Ear cartilage and oral cavity mucous membrane are preferable tissues to nasal cartilage and nasal mucosa in the patient who is a suitable candidate for a two-stage procedure.

For one-stage procedures using composite grafts, the oculoplastic surgeon must be familiar

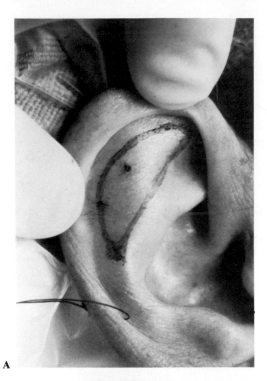

FIG. 11. Ear cartilage graft. **A:** Outline of graft site marked on anterior surface of ear—not for incision. **B:** Everted ear with methylene blue marking 4 mm from edge of helix for skin incision. **C:** Dissected skin and subcutaneous tissues expose posterior surface of ear cartilage. **D:** Reflected cartilage plate is grasped with forceps and incised at its base. **E:** Cartilage graft has been resected and good hemostasis achieved. **F:** Skin closure at donor site.

A

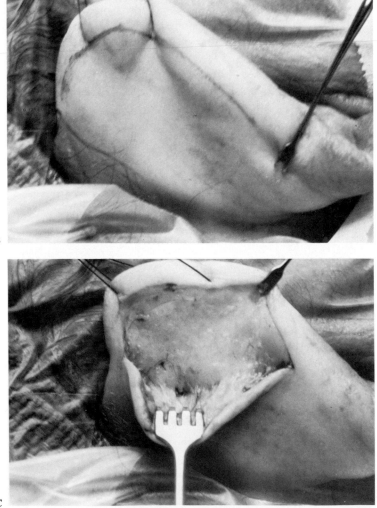

B

C

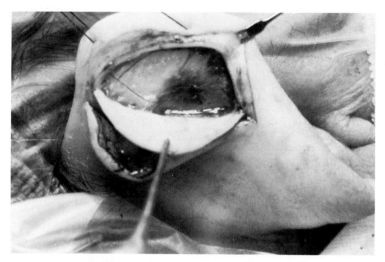

D

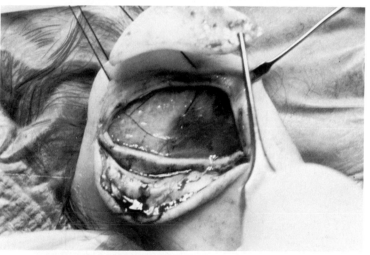

E

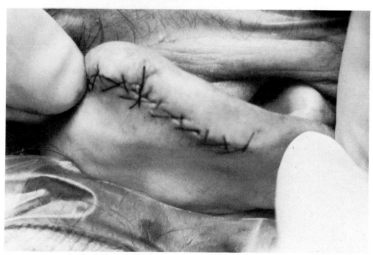

F

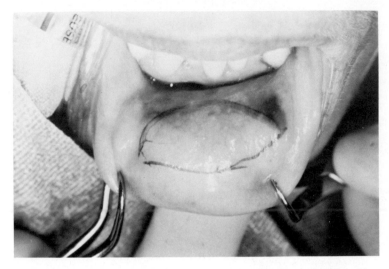

FIG. 12. Full-thickness mucous membrane graft. **A:** Lower lip is everted under tension with towel clips and marked with methylene blue.

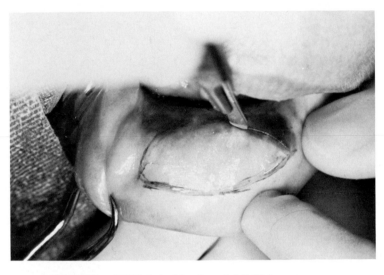

FIG. 12B. #15 blade incision through full-thickness mucosa.

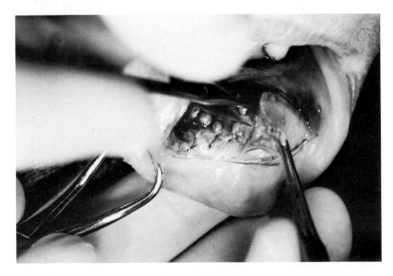

FIG. 12C. Sharp dissection with Westcott scissors to harvest graft.

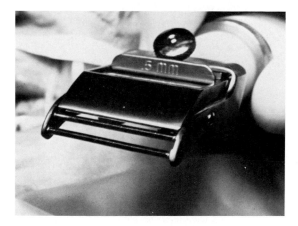

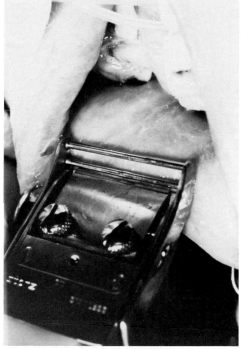

FIG. 13. Split-thickness mucous membrane graft. **A:** Castroviejo mucotome with a 0.5-mm spacer plate (shim). **B.** Mucotome positioned to shave the graft in an anterior-posterior direction with cheek held under tension.

with nasal chondromucosal harvesting techniques (Fig. 14). Injection of nasal mucous membrane with lidocaine and packing with 4% cocaine provides hemostasis.

A 4-0 silk retention suture is placed through the nasal ala and a flat, relaxing incision is made through the ala in the plane of the facial skin. Retraction of the nasal ala allows excellent exposure of the nasal septum. A rectangular strip of tissue, 10 mm × 5 mm, oriented parallel to the direction of the turbinates is outlined. The strip should include nasal mucosa and cartilage, but should not penetrate nasal mucosa on the opposite side of the cartilage. A peristeal elevator may be inserted to protect the contralateral mucosa. The graft is elevated with a razor knife or #64 Beaver blade. An angulated #66 Beaver blade or cottle knife is best for making the most posterior cut. A periosteal elevator can be used to dissect bluntly between cartilage and opposite mucosa, which is to be left behind in the donor site. The nasal ala is then resutured with interrupted 4-0 silk, and the naris is packed with petroleum jelly-impregnated gauze placed in the cut finger of a Latex surgical glove or in a fingercot. The cartilage is trimmed with an iris scissors or scalpel to approximately one-half the original width and thickness. The graft is sutured into place using interrupted 6-0 Vicryl sutures, making certain that the mucosal side is in correct alignment. Since this is a free graft, it is necessary to appose it with a skin flap containing its own blood supply rather than with another graft such as a skin graft.

Dermis-Fat Grafts

The autogenous composite dermis-fat graft has gained an important place in the management of the anophthalmic socket. Unlike free fat grafts, the composite dermis-fat graft is much more resistant to resorption. This graft serves as an excellent replacement of the

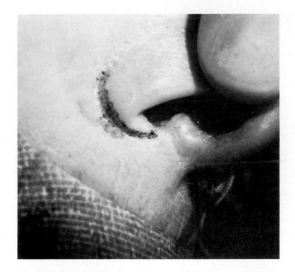

FIG. 14. Nasal chondromucosal graft. **A:** Nasal alar fold marked with methylene blue for incision.

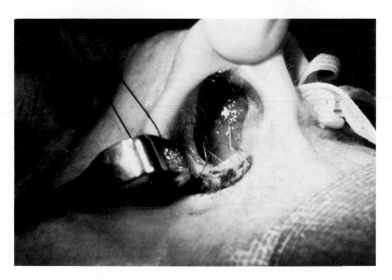

FIG. 14B. Incision is made and nostril retracted to expose septum.

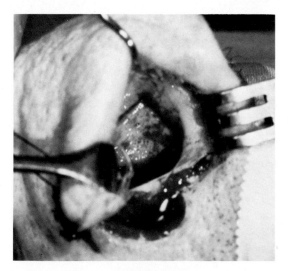

FIG. 14C. Incision is made through mucosa and nasal septal cartilage.

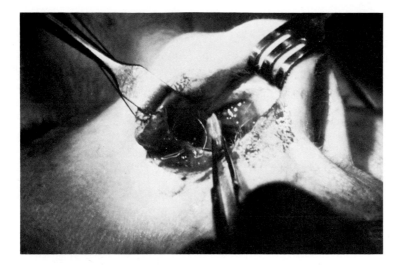

FIG. 14D. Graft is mobilized and further separated from opposite perichondrium with a periosteal elevator.

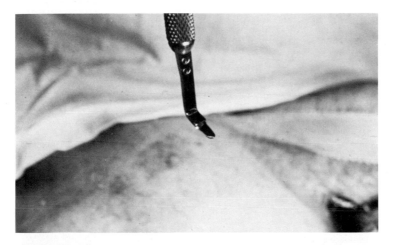

FIG. 14E. Angled Beaver blade (#66) used to excise distal end of composite graft.

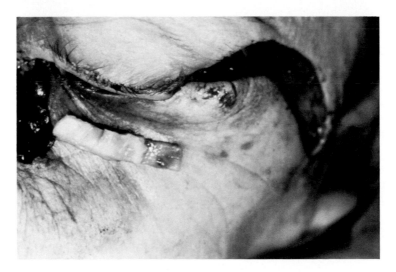

FIG. 14F. Harvested graft ready for use in eyelid reconstruction.

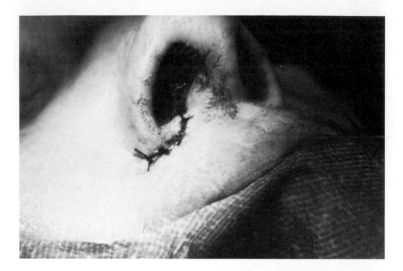

FIG. 14G.   Nasal alar incision is sutured closed.

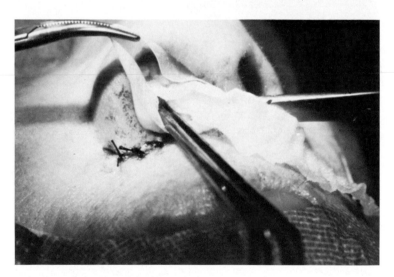

FIG. 14H.   Nare is packed with Vasoline gauze in fingercot packing.

extruding implant and is a natural socket expander in anophthalmic states with inadequate mucous membranes. The indications and use of this autogenous graft are discussed in detail in Chapter 15. The same technique for harvesting the composite graft may be used to simply harvest dermis. Autogenous dermis serves as an excellent tissue graft for facial soft tissue defects.

The best donor site is usually the patient's lower abdominal quadrant or flank. This graft can be harvested with the patient in the usual supine position (Fig. 15). This site is less prone to be tender, and is non–weight bearing, unlike the lateral portion of the thigh or buttock. The surgical site is locally infiltrated with lidocaine 2% with epinephrine 1:100,000 and hyaluronidase. An ellipse is next outlined on the skin. The ultimate diameter of the harvested dermis fat graft should not exceed 25 mm, and will usually be 20 mm or less.

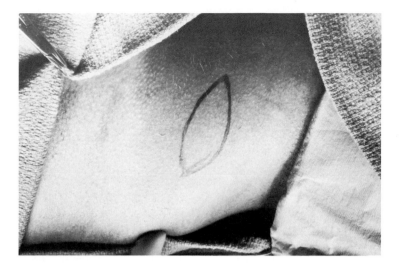

FIG. 15. Dermis-fat graft. **A:** Methylene blue outlines ellipse on area above iliac crest for incision.

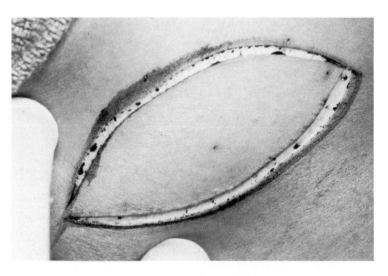

FIG. 15B. Skin incision has been made.

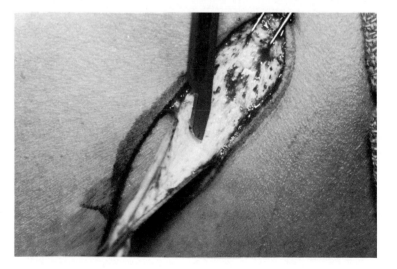

FIG. 15C. Tissues are held under tension and sharp blade dissection is used to excise epidermal layer from dermis.

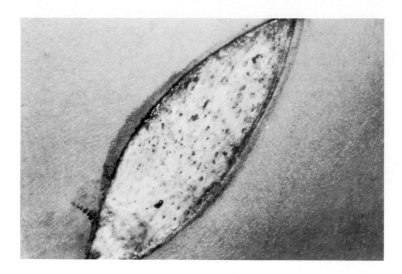

FIG. 15D. Exposed dermis.

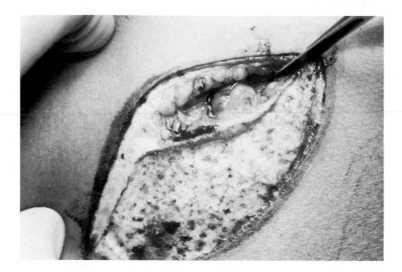

FIG. 15E. #15 blade incision through dermal layer into fat.

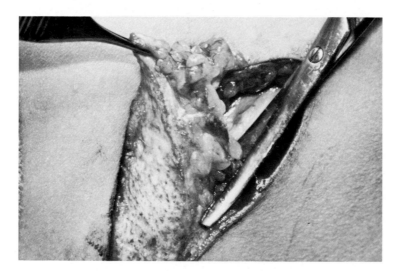

FIG. 15F. Excising composite dermis-fat graft.

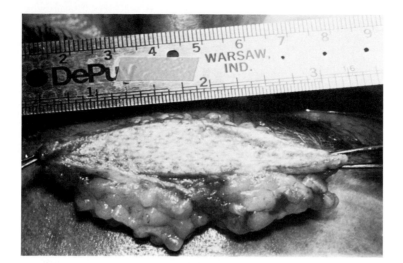

FIG. 15G. Harvesting free dermis-fat graft.

A skin incision is made with a #15 blade. The epidermal layer is then sharply dissected off of the dermis. This is important so as not to have epidermal inclusion cysts forming later on. The epidermis is best removed with the dermal tissue *in situ*. Holding the knife perpendicular to the dermal face, an incision is made through the dermis, following the outline of the ellipse. Holding the scalpel perpendicularly is important in harvesting an adequate-sized composite graft. Beveling of the blade will yield a conical-shaped graft with inadequate fatty tissue. The entire plug of dermis and fat is held up and excised at its base with a scissors. Electrocautery is necessary to achieve meticulous hemostasis. The composite graft is handled very gently and placed in physiologic saline solution until needed. Interrupted 3-0 chromic sutures with buried knots are used to close the fat layer. Interrupted 4-0 Prolene sutures with buried knots are used to meticulously close the dermis and subcutaneous tissues. It is this closure that will maintain the strength of the wound. Skin staples are used and provide excellent everting action of the skin edges. Ointments, a Telfa dressing, and a pressure bandage are applied for 1 week. In 1 week's time approximately staples are removed. We place all patients in whom autogenous tissue grafts are used on oral cephalosporins for 5 to 7 days.

Fascia Grafts

Obtaining fascia lata can be done by an orthopedist colleague, but the ophthalmic surgeon can save time and trouble by learning the procedure. Fascia is quite easy to obtain in the adult but can be somewhat difficult in the child with a short thigh. (Fig. 16).

A skin incision 3 to 4 cm in length should be made in the lower lateral thigh, safely above the knee joint and along an imaginary line between the head of the fibula and the anterior superior iliac crest. (Caution: The leg *must* be internally rotated to avoid making an improper incision. We prefer to have an operating room assistant rotate the foot internally during this part of the procedure.)

Dissection through skin and subcutaneous fat will reveal the glistening white fascia

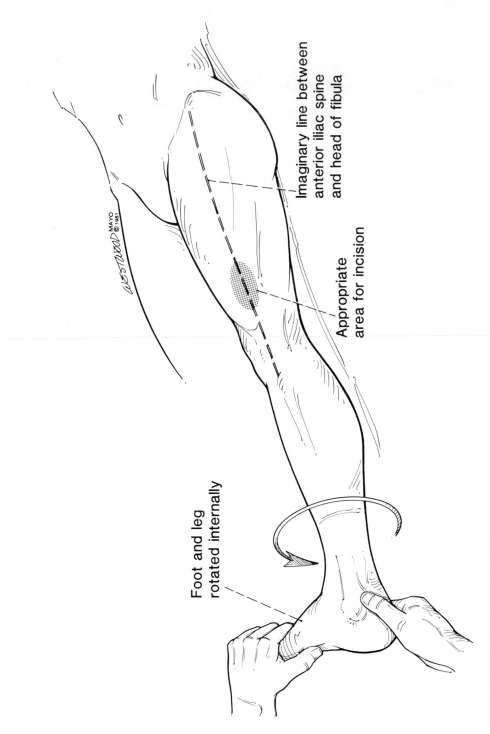

Imaginary line between
anterior iliac spine
and head of fibula

Appropriate
area for incision

Foot and leg
rotated internally

FIG. 16. Fascia lata skin graft. **A:** The skin incision, 3–4 cm in length, should be in the lower lateral thigh, safely above the knee joint and along an imaginary line between the head of the fibula and the anterior superior iliac crest.

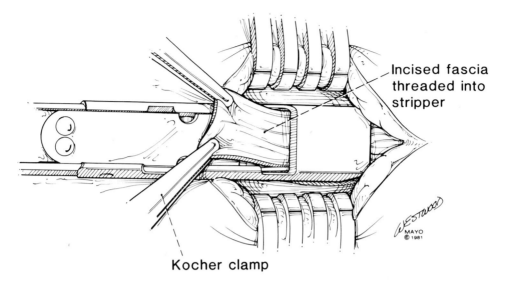

FIG. 16B. The fascia is threaded through the stripper mechanism, and fixed with two Kocher clamps (Crawford stripper).

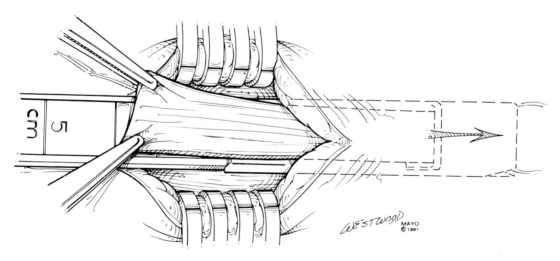

FIG. 16C. When the desired length of fascia is captured in the stripper (10 cm or more is usually desirable), the fascia is severed (Crawford stripper).

lata, which can be easily exposed using a sponge wrapped around the index finger and sometimes using forceps and scissors to clean away the loose areolar tissue. Using a scalpel, parallel incisions are made in the fascia 6 to 8 mm apart at the inferior-most aspect of the incision to initiate the dissection that will result in acquiring the fascia strips. Once parallel incisions have been made within the confines of the wound, several steps may then be taken to facilitate removal of fascia in the upper thigh. It is most helpful if the fascia stripper can be passed easily into the upper thigh without soft tissue obstruction. Release of soft tissue adhesions easily can be accomplished by passing a long, thin scissors between the fascia and subcutaneous fat as far as possible into the superior aspect of the wound, then opening the scissors as wide as possible during its slow removal from the wound. Similarly, soft adhesions posterior to the fascia adjacent to the muscle belly can be lysed by passing the scissors beneath the defect created in the fascia, then passing the scissors superiorly as far as possible. The fascia is then threaded through the stripper mechanism and fixed (we prefer two Kocher clamps) while the cutting portion of the stripper is passed into the upper thigh within the tunnel created by the scissors. When the desired length of fascia is captured in the stripper (10 cm or more is usually very desirable), the fascia is severed. Closure does not usually have to include closing the fascia defect; however, closure of subcutaneous tissue should be firm and tight with 4-0 Prolene. We use skin staples to achieve good eversion of the wound edges. Healing is rarely a problem and ambulation 12 to 24 hr after surgery is rarely, if ever, a problem. Skin staples are removed in approximately 10 days.

The fascia can be divided into the number of strips desired; usually strips 2 mm in width are quite satisfactory, but the width can be smaller or larger, if preferred. Before dividing the fascia, one should wipe away the connective tissue that is invariably present. The fascia should be free of connective tissue when used in the eyelid. Appropriate widths can be started with scissors as parellel as possible to the direction of the fiber, after which the fibers may be pulled apart with the fingers to attain the desired length for use. Fascial strips whose fibers are cut obliquely are to be avoided, because they are weaker and more prone to breakage.

Fascia lata can be harvested as a rectangular patch of tissue (Fig. 17). In this form it is useful as a patch graft or in socket reconstruction.

An alternate site from which to harvest fascia is that overlying the temporalis muscle (Fig. 18). It may be conveniently harvested in conjunction with certain brow and eyelid procedures, (e.g., reanimation procedures of the eyelids). If is a useful harvest site when broader pieces of fascia are necessary. The temporalis fascia covers the temporalis muscle, orginating on the superior arch of the temporalis fossa and inserting on the zygomatic arch. To harvest it, a 4-cm vertical incision is made through the scalp above the anterior to the ear. Ultimately, the scar will be hidden by the hairline. The temporalis fascia is exposed exactly as one would expose the fascia lata. The scalp edges are retracted and a #15 blade is used to outline the graft. In anophthalmic socket surgery, a graft to be used as a patch should be approximately 15 mm square. A graft of 50 mm × 25 mm would be needed to encapsulate a 16-mm sphere implant. Hemostasis is achieved with electrocautery. Either skin staples or 6-0 silk sutures are used to close the skin incision.

Bone Grafts

Autogenous iliac bone grafts may be used by the oculoplastic surgeon for reconstruction of the bony orbits. The rate of extrusion or infection is much lower with autogenous bone than with other alloplastic material (e.g., bone cement). Unlike the alloplastic material, however, a significant drawback of autogenous bone is the possibility of reabsorption of the graft. The technique presented here is the Tessier method of harvesting iliac bone, as modified by Wolfe and Kawamoto (Fig. 19). This method is not applicable to children less then 10 years old, in whom there is inadequate ossification of the iliac crest.

A folded towel is placed beneath the donor hip. Subcutaneous tissues are infiltrated with lidocaine 2% with 1:100,000 epinephrine and hyaluronidase. The skin is stretched superiorly up over the iliac crest so that the final scar will be hidden beneath the bathing suit line. A Curvilinear skin incision with a #15 blade is made along the iliac crest, from

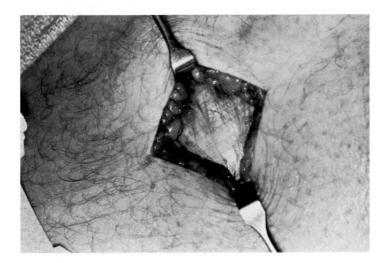

FIG. 17. Fascia lata rectangular patch graft. **A:** Skin incision and subcutaneous dissection exposes fascia lata.

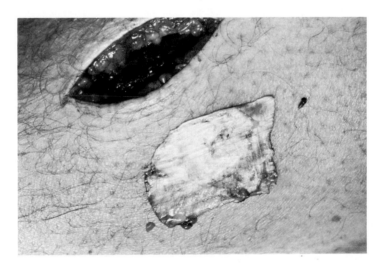

FIG. 17B. Rectangular patch graft of fascia lata has been harvested.

the anterior-superior spine running posteriorly and superiorly. A Bovie dissection is carried down through the muscle. A periosteal incision is made along the iliac crest. With a sharp osteotome, the outer ridge of the iliac crest is obliquely split. The inner and outer iliac crest fragments are reflected and remain attached to muscle and periosteum. The iliac spine is left intact. A periosteal elevator is used to reflect periosteum from the inner and outer surfaces of the ilium. Leaving intact a small area of bone next to the anterior superior iliac spine, an approximately 8 × 10-cm portion of bone is available for harvest with an osteotome. The two reflected fragments of iliac crest are then wired firmly to one another, and then wired to the anterior-superior spine. The subcutaneous tissues are closed with interrupted 4-0 Prolene sutures. A 6-0 silk suture is used to close the skin. A suction drain is left in the wound, and removed after 24 hr. Because the bone reconstitution is

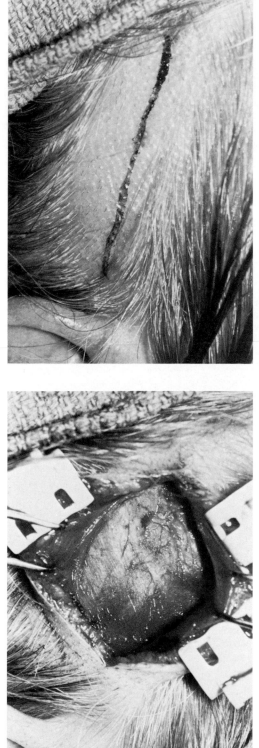

A

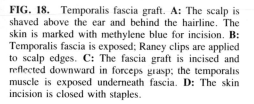

FIG. 18. Temporalis fascia graft. **A:** The scalp is shaved above the ear and behind the hairline. The skin is marked with methylene blue for incision. **B:** Temporalis fascia is exposed; Raney clips are applied to scalp edges. **C:** The fascia graft is incised and reflected downward in forceps grasp; the temporalis muscle is exposed underneath fascia. **D:** The skin incision is closed with staples.

B

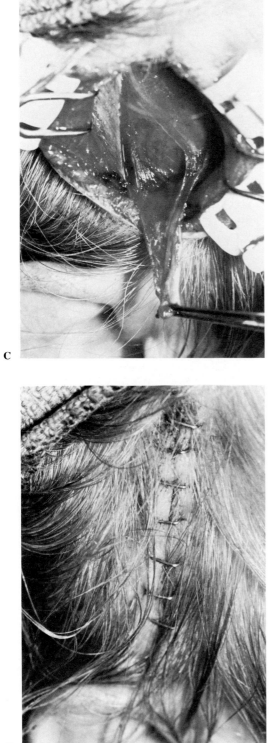

C

D

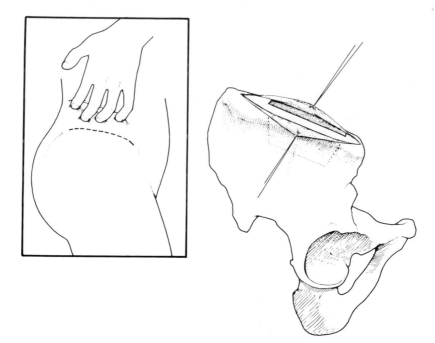

FIG. 19 Iliac bone graft. Skin from beneath the bathing suit line is pulled up over the iliac crest. The iliac crest is marked in methylene blue for incision. Bone drawing demonstrates periosteum opened with bone graft outlined.

quite solid, the patient can often ambulate a few days after surgery. In experienced hands, the complication rate for this technique is extremely low.

FLAPS

A flap is a segment of tissue that is transposed from one area of the body to another, while its base and original blood supply remain intact. With the exception of so-called free flaps, a transposed tissue flap is not dependent upon the recipient area for its nutrition. This fact makes the flap an ideal method of providing skin and soft tissue coverage for regions that have poor vascularization, or lack soft tissue. The most commonly used flaps in ophthalmic plastic surgery are skin flaps. Myocutaneous flaps contain skin and underlying muscle and soft tissue. Eyelid cutaneous flaps can be used to reconstruct the entire anterior lamella of the eyelid, and provide an adequate blood supply for a posterior lamellar graft in these cases.

Flaps are commonly categorized as either random or axial, depending on their blood supply. An axial flap is one that runs parallel to and contains an artery or arteriole. A random flap is dissected perpendicular to its main arterial supply. Because it has a poorer blood supply, the random flap can be no longer than four times its base. On the other hand, because it carries an artery its full length, an axial flap can have a much larger length-to-base ratio.

Free flaps involve the transfer of a composite free tissue graft with microvascular anastomoses at the recipient site. When harvesting a free tissue graft, it is necessary to include both an artery and a vein in the dissection of the flap. In turn, this artery and vein must

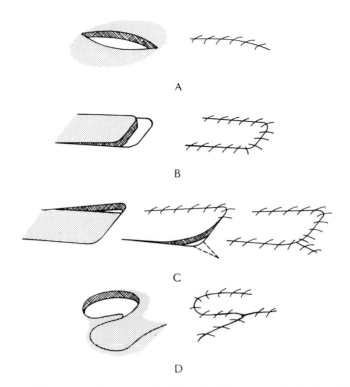

FIG. 20. Flaps useful in oculoplastic surgery. **A:** Sliding. **B:** Advancement. **C:** Rotation. **D:** Transposition.

be anastomosed to another artery and vein in the recipient bed. While not commonly used in oculoplastic surgery, microvascular surgery can be readily learned by the ophthalmologist already accustomed to microprocedures. Free flaps can be useful in the reconstruction of the exenterated orbit via microvascular anastomoses to the superficial temporal artery. Under certain circumstances, such as burn injuries or local radiation treatments, adjacent soft tissue structures such as temporalis muscle may have been lost.

Flaps may also be described according to shape, such as sliding, advancement, rotation, or transposition (Fig. 20). A sliding flap is an area that is undermined and then pulled forward on its underlying subcutaneous base so that the skin defect can be closed primarily. An advancement flap is a more complex sliding flap in which a three-sided skin flap is undermined and then advanced to cover an adjacent area. Examples of these are the lateral canthotomy and the Cutler-Beard upper eyelid reconstruction. The rotation flap is a segment of skin and subcutaneous tissue that is undermined and rotated into a defect. Examples of this are the Tenzel semicircle reconstruction and the Mustarde flap. The transposition flap is a flap moved from its donor site to another nonadjacent area. Examples of such flaps are the temporal forehead flap, the rhombic flap (Fig. 21), and the median forehead flap. Whereas sliding, advancement, and rotation flaps are usually random, a transposition flap is most often an axial flap.

HOMOGRAFTS

In all aspects of oculoplastic surgery, we have found autogenous fresh grafts to be far superior to either fresh homogenous or preserved homogenous grafts. The autogenous graft

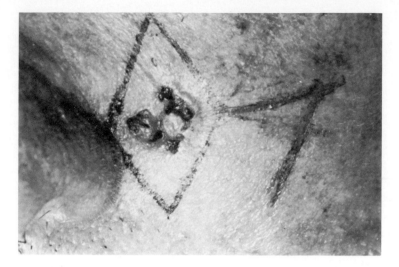

FIG. 21. Rhombic transposition flap. **A:** Basal cell carcinoma of nasojugal fold and rhombic flap are outlined with methylene blue for incision.

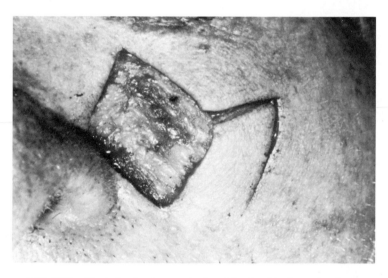

FIG. 21B. The lesion has been excised and the rhombic flap undermined.

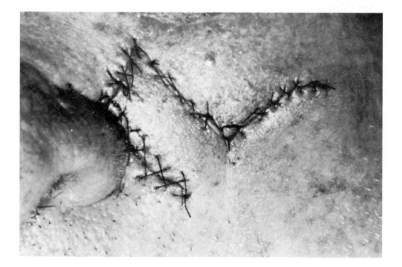

FIG. 21C. The rhombic flap is transposed and the remaining defects are closed by advancement, the wound is closed with everting sutures.

has the advantage of not inciting an immune reaction or foreign body reaction, not causing inflammation, not shrinking, and predictably surviving if an adequate blood supply is present. On the other hand, homogenous grafts create an immune reaction, cause additional inflammation, and may shrink or even be totally absorbed. In a socket with an extruding implant, socket contracture is already a significant problem. The additional inflammation caused by a fresh homogenous graft will worsen this contracture. Preserved homogenous grafts, such as preserved sclera, cause an even greater reaction.

Despite the above limitations, the surgeon should be aware of available homografts. The homografts most commonly used in oculoplastic surgery are sclera and fascia lata. Sclera is obtained from enucleated donor eyes. It is often stored in 70% alcohol, giving it a useful life of several months. We prefer to store sclera frozen in Polmyxin B–neomycin-gramicidin (Neosporin®) ophthalmic drops. Using this method, its useful life is 1 year. Some eye banks may use glycerin-preserved sclera. Frozen donor sclera needs merely to be defrosted prior to use. Alcohol-preserved sclera must be soaked in normal saline for 1 to 2 hr prior to insertion in the surgical wound, to dilute out the extremely irritating preservatives. Fresh homogenous sclera will cause less inflammatory reaction than the preserved sclera. Homografted fascia lata is available as a commercial preparation. It is more rapidly metabolized and thus loses its tensile strength more quickly than autogenous material. In above-knee amputees and very small children, homograft fascia lata must be used, because autogenous material is not available.

ALLOPLASTIC MATERIAL

A number of alloplastic materials are used in ophthalmic plastic surgery. We use the Teflon plates available from Storz (E-5608) in small, medium, and large sizes, both left and right, for orbital floor implants. They are shaped correctly, provide excellent support, and are nonreactive.

Supramid sheeting (Storz E-5602) comes in various thickness and is less rigid than the Teflon plates. For smaller floor fractures it provides adequate support. In medial wall fractures, where gravity does not push against the implant and little support is needed, it is an excellent choice to cover the fracture site.

Bone cement (Howmedica) is an excellent alloplastic material for reconstruction of the bony orbit. The strength of this material is attested to by the fact that it is used in total hip reconstruction. Bone cement polymer is prepared during the operative procedure. When a soft, doughy consistency is reached, the material is molded into the desired shape. While still soft, the material can be cut with a scissors or scalpel. Final sculpting of the bone cement can be accomplished with a power-driven dental burr. To expand orbital volume in the anophthalmic socket, it is placed between the periorbita and the floor or lateral wall of the orbit. It can be fixed to bone and can be shaped to match missing or deformed bone, as occurs in depressed orbital fractures and zygoma fractures.

Numerous alloplastic materials, including Silastic, methylmethacrylate, titanium, tantalum mesh, and glass, have been described for use as orbital implants in enucleated or eviscerated eyes. There does not exist an ideal alloplastic material for this purpose. Under most circumstances we prefer to use a methylmethacrylate or soft silicone sphere.

We give all patients with alloplastic implants a 5- to 7-day course of oral cephalosporin antibiotics.

PHOTOGRAPHY

Photographs are an integral part of the evaluation of all plastic surgery patients. Photographs serve as the best record of the patient's preoperative appearance, as an invaluable aid during surgery, as a teaching tool, and as a medical-legal adjunct. It is common for patients to forget or deny their initial appearance, and photographs serve as a helpful reminder. During surgery, we use photographs of the patient in much the same way as a retinal surgeon would refer to a detailed retinal drawing. It is helpful during the operation to recheck the photographs for such things as scars, creases, eyelid fat pads, and the level of the eyelids in reference to upper lid ptosis or lower lid retraction. No matter how routine an operation, it is wise to photograph all surgical candidates preoperatively.

A wide variety of cameras may be used to take satisfactory preoperative photographs. A good photographic system should be easy to use, be reliable, and rapidly yield high-quality results. For our purposes, a simple Polaroid camera with black and white film meets all of these criteria. Even those with no interest in photography can achieve excellent results. The surgeon can immediately review the photographic results, thus affording the opportunity to take more pictures as needed or at different camera angles or with different lighting. Black and white photographs yield much more detail and shadowing than do color photographs. Black and white photographs also reproduce very well for publication or for insurance forms.

An abundance of 35-mm camera systems are available with which to take color slides. Excellent but complex camera systems featuring multiple flash units secured to the camera by brackets are available. The surgeon must work out a photographic "system" in which the flash unit settings, f-stop settings, and camera focal lengths must be changed if one is photographing one eye versus both eyes versus the full face. The 35-mm camera system we use combines simplicity with excellent results. One such system is the medical Olympus camera setup featuring the Olympus OM-2 35-mm camera with an Olympus 232 electonic flash coupled with a Panagor 90-mm 1:1 Macro lens and a Prinz 62 #1 closeup lens. Light meter readings in the plane of the film are integrated with the camera's automatic flash, thus ensuring correct exposure with each photograph. The surgeon simply changes the magnification of each shot and then moves forward or backward to achieve perfect focus. Again, there are many excellent 35-mm camera systems; the oculoplastic surgeon must simply choose one and become adept at using it.

SELECTED BIBLIOGRAPHY

Wound Healing

1. Bryant, W. (1977): Wound healing. *CIBA Clin. Symp.*, 29:2–36.
2. Peacock, E., and Van Winkle, W. (1976): *Wound Repair*. Saunders, Philadelphia.
3. Wilkins, R., and Kulwin, D. (1976): Wound healing. *Ophthalmology*, 4:507–510.

Suturing Techniques, Instruments, and Dressings

1. Converse, J. (1977): *Reconstructive Plastic Surgery*. Saunders, Philadelphia.
2. Troutman, R. (1974): *Microsurgery of the Anterior Segment of the Eye*, Vol. 1. Mosby, St. Louis.

Management of Hypertrophic Scars

1. Ketchum, L., Robinson, D., and Masters, E. (1971): Follow-up on treatment of hypertrophic scars and keloids with triamcinolone. *Plast. Reconstr. Surg.*, 3:256–259.

Autogenous Grafts

1. Rudolph, R., Fisher, J., and Ninnemann, J. (1979): *Skin Grafting*. Little, Brown, Boston.
2. Baylis, H. I., Rosen, N., and Neuhaus, R. W. (1982): Obtaining auricular cartilage for reconstructive surgery. *Am. J. Ophthalmol.*, 93:709–712.
3. Wolfe, S. A., and Kawamoto, H. K. (1978): Taking the ilial-bone graft: A new technique. *J. Bone Joint Surg.*, 60A(3):411.
4. Smith, B., and Petrelli, R. (1978): Dermis-fat graft as a moveable implant within the muscle cone. *Am. J. Ophthalmol.*, 85:62–66.
5. Crawford, J. S. (1968): Fascia lata: Its nature and fate after implantation and its use in ophthalmic surgery. *Trans. Am. Ophthalmol. Soc.*, 66:673–745.

Flaps

1. Converse, J. (1977): *Reconstructive and Plastic Surgery*. Saunders, Philadelphia.
2. McGregor, I., and Morgan, G. (1973): Axial and random pattern flaps. *Br. J. Plast. Surg.*, 26:202–213.
3. Borges, A. (1981): The rhombic flap. *J. Plast. Reconstr. Surg.*, 67:458–466.
4. Kazanjian, V. H., and Roopenian, A. (1956): Median forehead flaps in the repair of defects of the nose and surrounding areas. *Trans. Am. Acad. Ophthalmol. Otoclaryngol.*, 60:557–566.
5. Anderson, R. L., and Edwards, J. J. (1979): Reconstruction by myocutaneous eyelid flaps. *Arch. Ophthalmol.*, 97:2358–2362.

Homografts

1. Flanagan, J. C. (1974): Eyebank sclera in oculoplastic surgery. *Ophthalmic Surg.*, 5(3):45–53.
2. Beyer, C. K., and Albert, D. M. (1981): The use and fate of fascia lata and sclera in ophthalmic plastic and reconstructive surgery. *Ophthalmology*, 88:869–886.

Oculoplastic Surgery, 2nd edition, edited by
Clinton D. McCord, Jr., and Myron Tanenbaum.
Raven Press, New York © 1987.

Chapter 2

Anatomy of the Eyelids, Lacrimal System, and Orbit

Donald J. Bergin

Department of Ophthalmology, Letterman Army Medical Center, San Francisco, California 94129

OSTEOLOGY

The orbits are pyramidal structures, 30 cm^3 in volume, that lie 25 mm from each other (Fig. 1). Frontal, sphenoid, maxillary, zygomatic, lacrimal, palatine, and ethmoid bones make up the orbit. At the entrance, the orbits are 40 mm in height and 35 mm in width. The orbital covering of periorbita is most firmly attached at the sutures. The roof of the orbit (Fig. 2) is formed principally by the frontal bone and by a smaller, posterior portion of the lesser wing of the sphenoid. The orbital lobe of the lacrimal gland is located in the lacrimal gland fossa, which appears as a depression in the anterior lateral roof. Nasally, about 5 mm behind the rim, the trochlea is attached to periorbita. The supraorbital nerve and artery are transmitted through a foramen 25% of the time, or, more commonly, though a notch. The frontal sinus (Fig. 3) lies above the medial to the orbits and drains into the anterior middle meatus via the nasofrontal duct.

The lateral orbital wall (Fig. 4), 47 mm in length, is formed by the zygoma and the greater wing of the sphenoid. The two lateral orbital walls form a 90° angle to each other. Zygomaticofacial (Fig. 1) and zygomaticotemporal foramina penetrate the zygomatic bone. The lateral orbital (Whitnall's) tubercle is about 10 mm below the zygomaticofrontal suture and 4 mm behind the anterior lateral orbital rim. The lateral canthal tendon, Whitnall's ligament, lateral retinaculum, and Lockwood's ligament attach here.

Each of the medial orbital walls (Fig. 5) are approximately 45 mm long, and they are parallel to each other. From front to back, the medial wall is formed by the frontal process of the maxilla, the lacrimal bone, the orbital plate of the ethmoid (lamina papyracea), and the lesser wing of the sphenoid. The anterior lacrimal crest is the attachment of the anterior crus of the medial canthal tendon. The lacrimal fossa contains the lacrimal sac and is bounded by anterior and posterior lacrimal crests, the latter being formed by the lacrimal bone. Anterior and posterior ethmoid foramina, lying at the frontoethmoidal suture, transmit

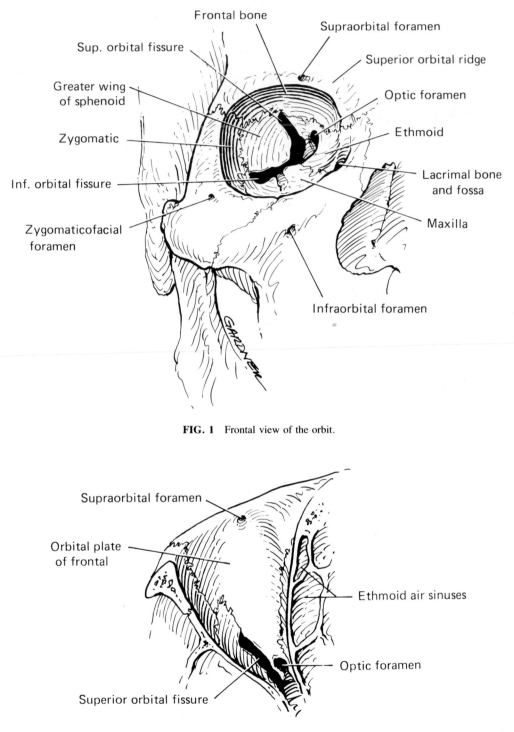

FIG. 1 Frontal view of the orbit.

FIG. 2 Orbital roof.

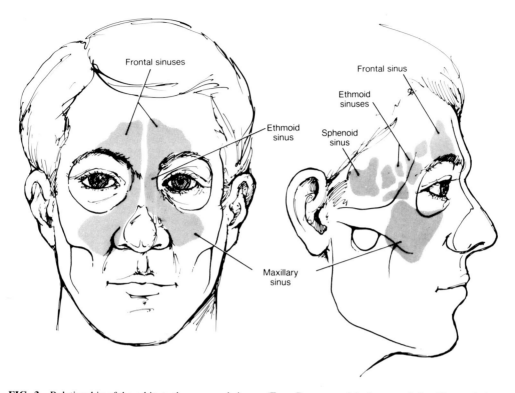

FIG. 3 Relationship of the orbits to the paranasal sinuses (From Doxanas and Anderson, ref. 9, with permission. © 1984, The Williams & Wilkins Co., Baltimore.)

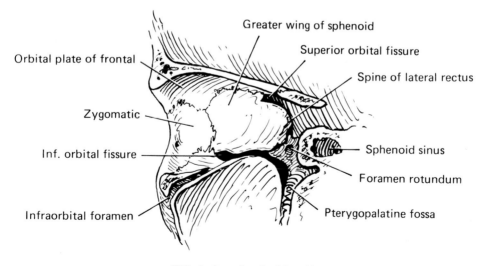

FIG. 4 Lateral wall of the orbit.

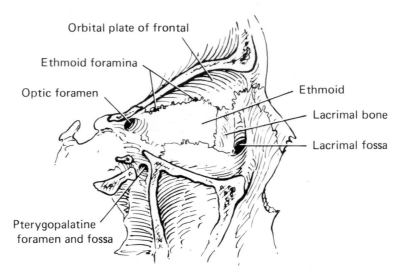

FIG. 5 Medial wall of the orbit.

the corresponding nerves and arteries. The average distance from anterior lacrimal crest to anterior ethmoid foramen is 24 mm, that between the ethmoid foramina 12 mm, and that from posterior ethmoid foramen to optic foramen 6 mm. Anterior and posterior ethmoid foramina lie at about the same horizontal level as the cribriform plate. The ethmoid sinus is medial to the orbit and extends anteriorly to the posterior lacrimal crest. However, air cells may extend anteriorly between the lacrimal fossa and nasal mucosa (Fig. 6). Anterior ethmoid air cells drain into the middle meatus, while posterior ethmoids drain into the superior meatus (Fig. 7).

The floor of the orbit (Fig. 8) is formed by the zygomatic, orbital plate of the maxilla and the orbital process of the palatine bone. Emptying into the middle meatus, the maxillary antrum lies below the orbital floor. The posterior wall of the maxillary antrum is 40 mm from the inferior orbital rim, and the optic foramen is about 50 mm. The orbital floor is thinner nasally and forms a triangle with the apex posterior. The infraorbital nerve and

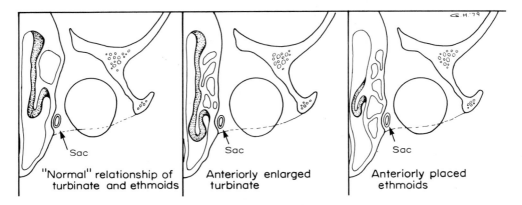

FIG. 6 Axial view of the normal relationship of lacrimal sac fossa, ethmoid air cells, and tip of the middle turbinate, with variations that may be encountered. (From McCord, ref. 19, with permission of Lippincott/Harper & Row.)

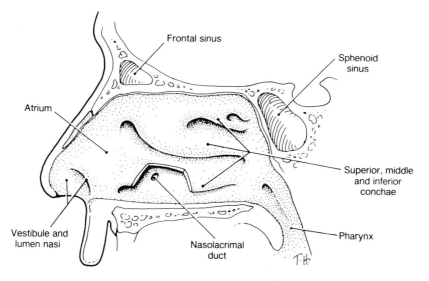

FIG. 7 The lateral wall of the nose. The nasolacrimal duct enters the nose beneath the inferior turbinate. (From Doxanas and Anderson, ref. 9, with permission. © 1984, The Williams & Wilkins Co., Baltimore.)

artery pass through the infraorbital groove, canal, and foramen. Four millimeters in diameter, the infraorbital foramen is 8 mm below the inferior orbital rim.

The optic foramen (Fig. 1) in the lesser wing of the sphenoid transmits the optic nerve, the ophthalmic artery, and the sympathetic nerve fibers to the orbit. The posterior ethmoids and sphenoid sinus form the medial wall of the optic canal. The superior orbital fissure is bounded by the greater and lesser wings of the sphenoid. The annulus zinnii is a fibrous ring continuous with the periorbita, which includes the optic foramen and the central superior orbital fissure. The superior and inferior divisions of the third nerve, nasociliary nerve,

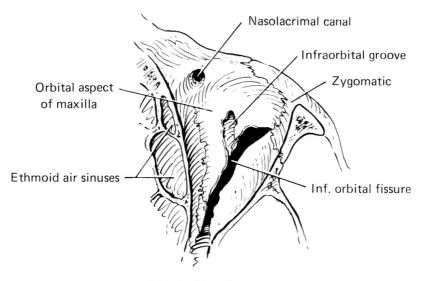

FIG. 8. Floor of the orbit.

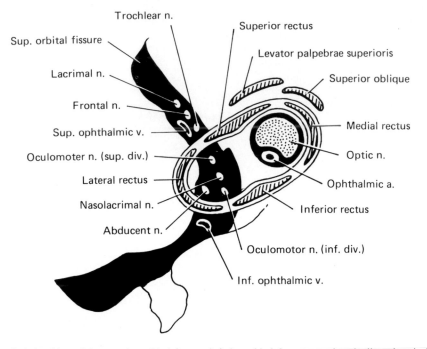

FIG. 9. Relationships of the superior orbital fissure, inferior orbital fissure, annulus zinnii, and optic foramen and their contents.

and sixth nerve enter the orbit through the superior orbital fissure in the annulus zinnii (Fig. 9). The superior ophthalmic vein, lacrimal nerve, frontal nerve, trochlear nerve, and inferior ophthalmic vein all lie in the fissure outside the annulus. The inferior orbital fissure (Fig. 1) separates maxillary and palatine bones from the greater wing of the sphenoid and zygoma. It connects the orbit with the sphenopalatine (pterygoid) fossa. The maxillary division of the trigeminal nerve (before it becomes the infraorbital nerve) and venous connections between the inferior ophthalmic vein and pterygoid plexus, pass through the inferior fissure. The inferior orbital fissure extends within 15 mm of the inferior orbital rim.

BLOOD SUPPLY

Internal and external carotid arteries supply blood to the orbit. The two terminal branches of the external carotid artery are the maxillary and the superficial temporal arteries. The infraorbital artery (Fig. 10) is a continuation of the maxillary artery and traverses the inferior orbital fissure, pterygopalatine fossa, infraorbital groove and canal, and infraorbital foramen to supply blood to the lower eyelid. Transverse facial, zygomaticofacial, and frontal arteries branch from the superficial temporal artery to the lateral orbit and forehead.

Dorsal nasal, supratrochlear, supraorbital, and lacrimal arteries are the contribution of the internal carotid artery to the eyelid surface vascular system. The dorsal nasal and supratrochlear arteries are terminal branches of the ophthalmic artery (Fig. 11). After arising from the ophthalmic artery laterally, close to the optic foramen, the lacrimal artery gives off a branch that passes through the superior orbital fissure and anastamoses with the

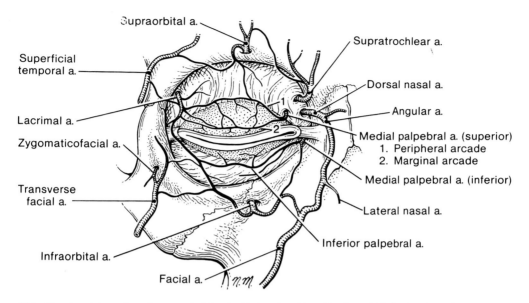

FIG. 10. Arterial supply to the upper facial and orbital region. (From Bergin and McCord, ref. 8, with permission of Lippincott/Harper & Row.)

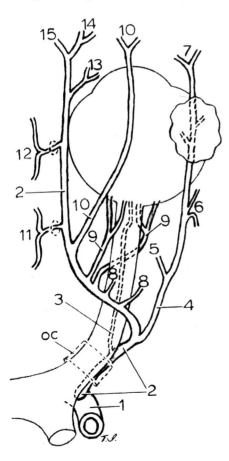

FIG. 11. Vascular supply to the orbit: 1, internal carotid artery; 2, ophthalmic artery; 3, central artery of the retina; 4, lacrimal artery; 5, muscular branches of lacrimal artery; 6, zygomatic branches of lacrimal artery; 7, lateral palpebral arteries; 8, muscular branches; 9, posterior ciliary arteries (long and short); 10, supraorbital artery; 11, posterior ethmoid artery; 12, anterior ethmoid artery; 13, medial palpebral arteries; 14, frontal artery; 15, dorsal nasal artery; OC, optic canal.

middle meningeal artery. The lacrimal artery proceeds anteriorly along the superior border of the lateral rectus to the lacrimal gland.

Superior and inferior palpebral arteries connect laterally with the lacrimal artery and medially with the superior and inferior medial palpebral arteries. Medial palpebral arteries arise from the ophthalmic artery temporal to the trochlea, just before traversing the orbital septum. The superior palpebral artery consists of a peripheral arcade, which is located between Müller's muscle and the levator aponeurosis at the upper border of the tarsus, and a marginal arcade, just above the lash follicles in the pretarsal space (Fig. 12). The inferior palpebral artery travels along the inferior border of the tarsus in the pretarsal space.

The ophthalmic artery (Fig. 11) is the first intracranial branch of the internal carotid after its exits the cavernous sinus. It lies beneath the optic nerve and, with its surrounding sympathetic fibers, enters the orbit through the optic foramen. It runs temporally and upward between the ciliary ganglion and the optic nerve. The central retinal artery is the first branch of the ophthalmic artery, arising below the optic nerve and perforating the nerve 8 to 15 mm from the globe. The ophthalmic artery passes over the nerve and becomes two long and six to eight short posterior ciliary arteries, the lacrimal artery, and the anterior and posterior ethmoid arteries. Each rectus muscle is supplied by two small arterial branches, with the exception of the lateral rectus, which receives one. These arteries enter the muscles posteriorly. The inferior oblique artery runs along the lateral border of the inferior rectus muscle to the corresponding muscle.

The supraorbital vein (Fig. 13) runs below the orbicularis oculi muscle and pierces it medially, coursing on the frontalis muscle to communicate with frontal branches of the

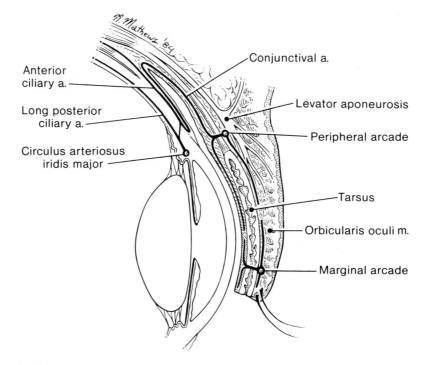

FIG. 12. Arterial supply to the upper eyelid. (From Bergin and McCord, ref. 8, with permission of Lippincott/Harper & Row.)

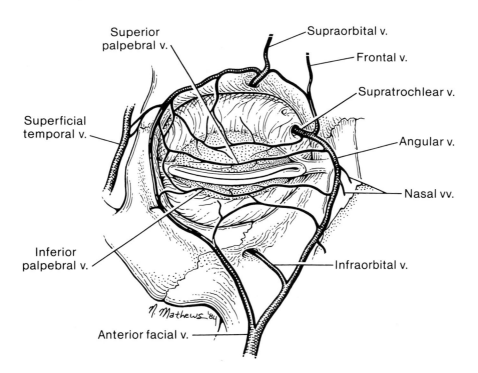

Superior palpebral v.

Supraorbital v.

Frontal v.

Supratrochlear v.

Superficial temporal v.

Angular v.

Nasal vv.

Inferior palpebral v.

Infraorbital v.

Anterior facial v.

η. Mathews '84

FIG. 13. Veins of the upper facial and orbital region. (From Bergin and McCord, ref. 8, with permission of Lippincott/Harper & Row.)

superficial temporal vein. The angular vein lies temporal to the angular artery over the insertion of the medial canthal tendon, 8 mm from the medial commissure. A confluence of angular, supraorbital, and supratrochlear veins forms the superior ophthalmic vein. The superior ophthalmic vein then passes posteriolaterally, piercing the muscle cone in the midorbit. It then receives the venous drainage from the globe and, traveling along the lateral border of the superior rectus, exits the superior orbital fissure above the annulus zinnii on its way to the cavernous sinus. The inferior ophthalmic vein drains the floor and inferiomedial orbit to the pterygoid plexus (through the inferior orbital fissure) and superior ophthalmic vein.

There are no identifiable lymphatic vessels or nodes as such in the orbit. Medial lymphatics of the eyelids and conjunctiva follow the anterior facial vein to the submandibular lymph nodes (Fig. 14). The lateral group drains the remainder of the lids to the superficial parotid lymph nodes anterior to the ear (Fig. 14).

INNERVATION

Trigeminal Nerve

The ophthalmic (V_1), maxillary (V_2), and mandibular (V_3) nerves are the three divisions of the trigeminal nerve (Fig. 15). The ophthalmic division traverses the cavernous sinus in its lateral wall and enters the orbit through the superior orbital fissure. Here it divides into the frontal, nasociliary, and lacrimal nerves. Frontal and lacrimal nerves lie in the

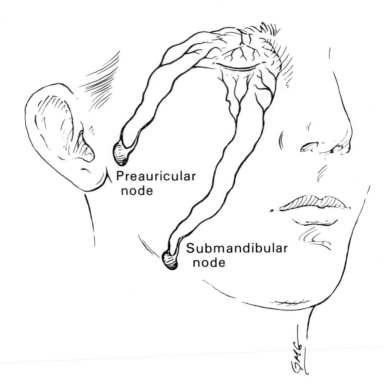

FIG. 14. Lymphatic drainage from the eyelids.

superior orbital fissure above the annulus zinii (Fig. 9). The nasociliary nerve provides sensory branches to the ciliary ganglion lateral to the optic nerve. It gives off the two long posterior ciliary nerves and then runs forward superionasally with the ophthalmic artery, giving off the anterior and posterior ethmoidal nerves. The infratrochlear nerve, the terminal branch of the nasociliary nerve, supplies the side and tip of the nose, medial conjunctiva, caruncle, and lacrimal sac (Figs. 16 and 17). The lacrimal nerve courses along the superior border of the lateral rectus muscle to the lacrimal gland (Fig. 18). It pierces the orbital septum and innervates the skin and conjunctiva of the lateral part of the upper eyelid (Figs. 16 and 17). The frontal nerve, the largest of the three divisions of the ophthalmic nerve, runs directly forward between the periorbita and levator palpebrae superioris. Centrally in the orbit, it divides into the supraorbital and supratrochlear nerves (Fig. 15). Proceeding anteriorly above the trochlea, the supratrochlear nerve innervates the skin of the glabella, forehead, medial upper eyelid, and medial conjunctiva. The supraorbital nerve exits the orbit in the supraorbital notch or foramen. It provides sensory innervation to the skin and conjunctiva of the upper eyelid and scalp.

The maxillary nerve (Fig. 19) passes forward in the lower lateral wall of the cavernous sinus and exits the middle fossa via the foramen rotundum. It crosses the pterygopalatine fossa and enters the orbit in the inferior orbital fissure. In the posterior orbit, it becomes the infraorbital nerve, and lies in the infraorbital groove. Continuing in the infraorbital canal, it emerges through the infraorbital canal. The nasal, labial, and palpebral branches carry sensation to the skin of the nose, upper and lower eyelids, and face. The zygomatic

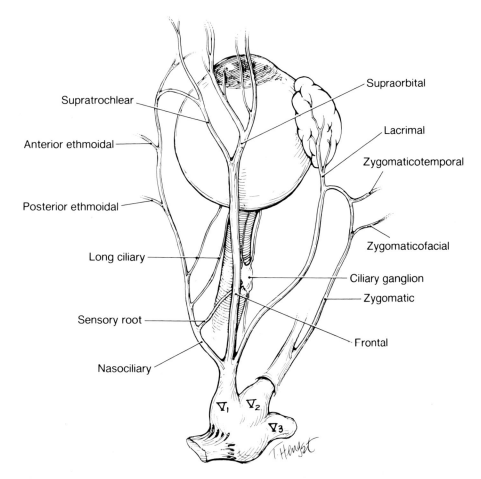

FIG. 15. Trigeminal nerve viewed from above. (From Doxanas and Anderson, ref. 9, with permission. © 1984, The Williams & Wilkins Co., Baltimore.)

nerve branches from the maxillary nerve in the pterygopalatine fossa. It enters the orbit in the inferior orbital fissure and divides into the zygomaticofacial and zygomaticotemporal nerves. The latter runs along the lateral orbital wall and traverses the zygomaticotemporal foramen posterior to the anterior, lateral orbital rim to supply sensation to the anterior temporal region. In the inferior lateral orbit, posterior to the orbital rim, the zygomaticofacial nerve exits its foramen to innvervate the malar eminence.

Ciliary Ganglion

The ciliary ganglion, about 2 mm in cross-section and 10 mm from the orbital apex, lies between the optic nerve and lateral rectus. Parasympathetic pulillomotor and accommodative fibers from the inferior oblique nerve synapse here. The sensory root from the nasociliary nerve and sympathetic vasomotor and dilator fibers pass through the ciliary ganglion. These fibers, along with the tertiary parasympathetic fibers, then travel to the globe via the 10 to 20 short ciliary nerves that pierce the sclera around the optic nerve.

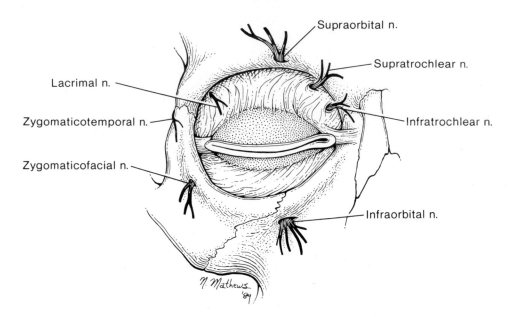

FIG. 16. Sensory nerves of the eyelids. (From Bergin and McCord, ref. 8, with permission of Lippincott/Harper & Row.)

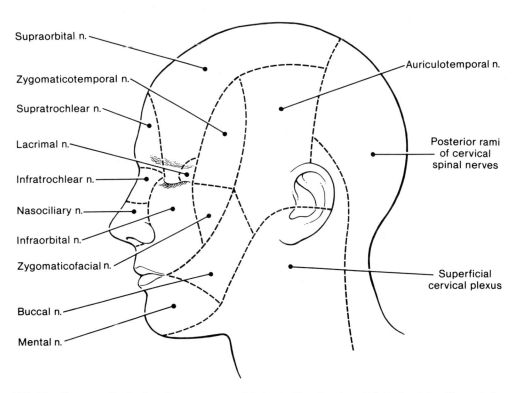

FIG. 17. Cutaneous distribution of sensory nerves of the head. (From Bergin and McCord, ref. 8, with permission of Lippincott/Harper & Row.)

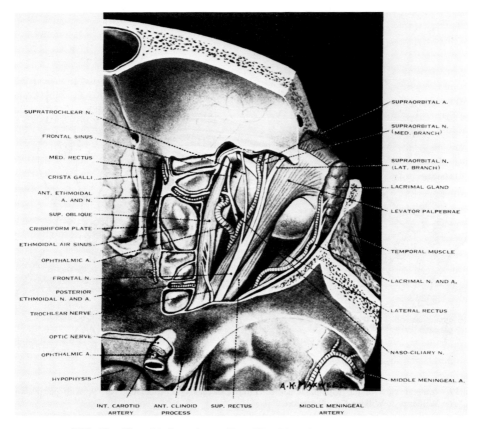

FIG. 18. The orbit from above. (From Warwick, ref. 26, with permission.)

Seventh Nerve

The facial nerve, originating in the pons, emerges from the stylomastoid foramen. It runs in the substance of the parotid gland (Fig. 20) and posterior to the ramus of the mandible, and divides into superior temporofacial and inferior cervicofacial branches (Fig. 21). The temporofacial nerve divides into the temporal, zygomatic, and buccal nerves; the cervicofacial nerve divides into the buccal, mandibular, and cervical nerves. However, there are major variations in the branching and anastomosis pattern of the facial nerve (Fig. 22). The muscles of facial expression are innervated on their deep surfaces by the facial nerve.

FOREHEAD AND TEMPORAL REGION

The eyebrows extend over the superior orbital rim, and consist of four layers: skin, muscle, fat, and galea. The skin of the brow is much thicker than orbital skin. There are four muscles of the brow: frontalis, procerus, corrugator superciliaris, and orbicularis oculi (Figs. 23 and 24). The frontalis muscle is a paired subcutaneous muscle that inserts into the skin of the brow. The procerus muscle is continuous with the frontalis and inserts into the nasal bones. Inserting subcutaneously in the glabellar region, it pulls inferiorly and is

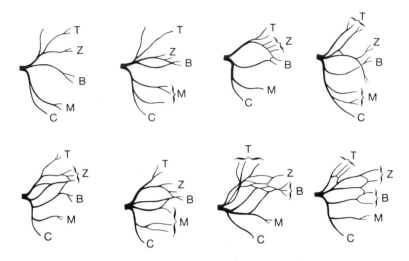

FIG. 22. Eight major types of branching and anastamoses of the facial nerve. The temporal (T), zygomatic (Z), buccal (B), mandibular (M), and cervical (C) branches are shown (From McCormack, Cauldwell, and Anson, ref. 21, with permission.)

temporal branch of the facial nerve lies on the periosteum of the zygomatic bone about 3 cm anterior to the external auditory meatus. This nerve innervates the frontalis, currugator, and procerus muscles on their undersurface. The temporalis muscle fills the temporal fossa, originating at the temporal line and inserting on the coronoid process and anterior surface of the ramus. The motor branch of the mandibular division of the fifth cranial nerve innervates the temporalis muscle on its inner inferior surface. The temporalis muscle closes the jaws.

EYELIDS

Eyelids are the protective covering of the eye. They consist of an anterior lamella of skin and orbicularis muscle and a posterior lamella of tarsus and conjunctive (Fig. 25).

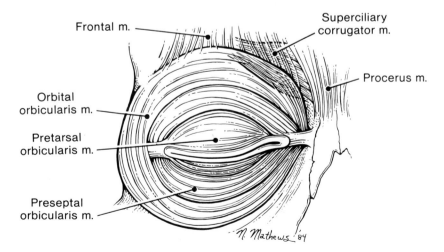

FIG. 23. Facial muscles of the orbital region. (From Bergin and McCord, ref. 8, with permission of Lippincott/Harper & Row.)

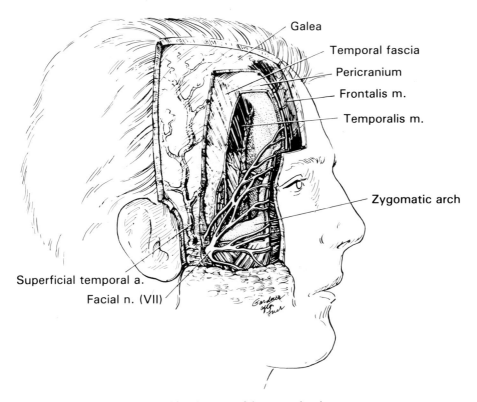

FIG. 24. Anatomy of the temporal region.

The normal palpebral fissure is 9 to 10 mm vertically when the lids are open, and 30 mm horizontally.

The orbicularis oculi is a subcutaneous muscle that serves as the sphincter of the eyelids. It spreads over the eyelids and out onto the forehead, temple, and cheeks. The muscle is divided into an orbital and palpebral portion. The latter is further divided into preseptal and pretarsal parts (Fig. 23). Pertarsal muscle is attached laterally to Whitnall's tubercle by the lateral canthal tendon (lateral palpebral ligament) (Fig. 26). This is not so much a ligament as a band of connective tissue attached medially to the tarsi. Medially, the pretarsal orbicularis forms two heads that pass superficial and deep to the canaliculi. The anterior pretarsal orbicularis muscle forms the anterior crus of the medial canthal tendon that inserts into the frontal process of the maxillary one. The posterior pretarsal orbicularis inserts into the posterior lacrimal crest (Horner's muscle) (Fig. 27). A small strip of pretarsal orbicularis at the lid margin is referred to as Riolan's muscle. The preseptal muscle forms the horizontal raphe laterally and also medially inserts into the anterior crus of the medial canthal tendon (Fig. 27). Jones' muscle forms a deep insertion of the preseptal orbicularis into the lacrimal diaphragm of the tear sac (Fig. 27). The orbital orbicularis attaches medially to the medial canthal tendon, the nasal part of the frontal bone, and along the inferiomedial orbital margin. The orbital portion of the orbicularis completes an ellipse around the orbit without interruption at the lateral canthus. The superciliaris muscle is sometimes described in the literature, and comprises the superomedial peripheral fibers of the orbital orbicularis. Anderson (4) described a superior supporting branch of the anterior medial canthal tendon that inserts into the periosteum of the frontal bone.

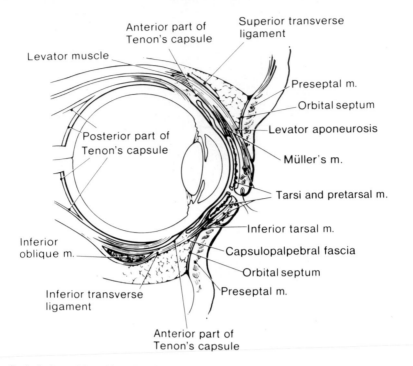

Anterior part of
Tenon's capsule

Superior transverse
ligament

Levator muscle

Preseptal m.

Orbital septum

Levator aponeurosis

Müller's m.

Posterior part of
Tenon's capsule

Tarsi and pretarsal m.

Inferior tarsal m.

Inferior
oblique m.

Capsulopalpebral fascia

Orbital septum

Preseptal m.

Inferior transverse
ligament

Anterior part of
Tenon's capsule

FIG. 25. Sagittal view of the orbit and eyelid structures. (From McCord, ref. 20, with permission of Lippincott/ Harper & Row.)

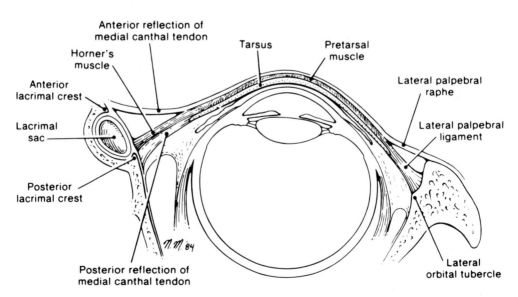

Anterior reflection of
medial canthal tendon

Tarsus

Pretarsal
muscle

Horner's
muscle

Anterior
lacrimal crest

Lateral palpebral
raphe

Lacrimal
sac

Lateral palpebral
ligament

Posterior
lacrimal crest

Posterior reflection of
medial canthal tendon

Lateral
orbital tubercle

FIG. 26. Horizontal section through the orbit depicting the medial and lateral attachments of the orbicularis oculi muscle. (From Bergin and McCord, ref. 8, with permission of Lippincott/Harper & Row.)

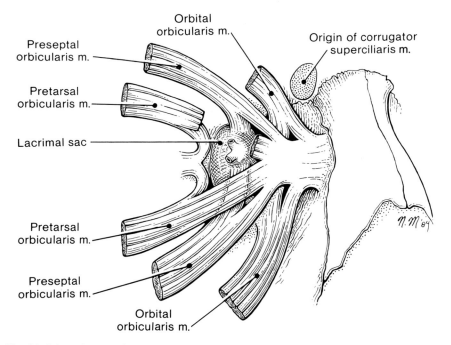

Preseptal
orbicularis m.

Pretarsal
orbicularis m.

Lacrimal sac

Pretarsal
orbicularis m.

Preseptal
orbicularis m.

Orbital
orbicularis m.

Orbital
orbicularis m.

Origin of corrugator
superciliaris m.

FIG. 27. Medial attachments of the orbicularis oculi muscle. (From Bergin and McCord, ref. 8, with permission of Lippincott/Harper & Row.)

The orbital septum forms the anterior border of the orbit, confining the orbital fat. The orbital septum (septum orbitale) (Fig. 28) is a fibrous sheath beneath the orbicularis muscle. It is formed at the orbital rims as the arcus marginalis, which is a thickening of the periosteum. Medially, it inserts at the posterior lacrimal crest and laterally, just anterior to Whitnall's tubercle. Nasally, the orbital septum is thinnest. In caucasians the orbital septum inserts approximately 10 mm above the superior border of the tarsus into the levator aponeurosis (Fig. 29). In orientals, the orbital septum inserts inferiorly onto the levator aponeurosis over the tarsus, allowing the anterior orbital fat to extend to the anterior tarsal space. The inferior extension of the orbital fat prevents the levator aponeurosis fibers from fanning out to the subcutaneous tissue to form the eyelid crease. In the lower eyelid the septum inserts into the inferior border of the tarsus.

The anterior extension of the extraconal orbital fat lies immediately posterior to the orbital septum. In the upper lid there are two fat pockets (Fig. 30). The preaponeurotic fat pad is bordered posteriorly by the levator aponeurosis, medially by the trochlea, and temporally by the orbital lobe of the lacrimal gland. The nasal fat pad, lying beneath the trochlea, is whitish in color as is the nasal fat pad in the lower eyelid. In the lower eyelid, there are three fat pads (Fig. 30). The nasal fat pad is separated posteriorly from the medial fat pad by the inferior oblique muscle (Fig. 31).

The tarsi are dense, fibrous tissue that form the skeleton of the eyelids. They are about 25 mm in length, 1 mm in thickness, and 10 mm and 4 mm in height vertically in the upper and lower eyelids, respectively.

The levator palpebrae superioris muscle originates above the annulus zinnii in the periorbita. It is innervated in the inner posterior one-third by the superior division of the third nerve

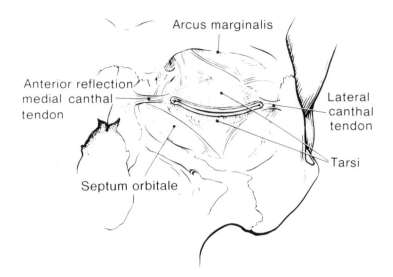

FIG. 28. Frontal view of the eyelids and orbit. The skin and protractor muscle layers have been removed. (From McCord, ref. 20, with permission of Lippincott/Harper & Row.)

after the nerve passes through the superior rectus muscle. The levator muscle extends anteriorly for 40 mm and becomes tendinous at Whitnall's ligament. The tendon fans out medially and laterally to the orbital retinacula. Anteriorly, the levator aponeurosis fuses with the orbital septum above the superior border of the tarsus and sends fibrous strands between the orbicularis oculi muscle septa to the skin, forming the supratarsal eyelid crease. The levator aponeurosis inserts into the anterior lower 7 to 8 mm of the tarsus.

The superior transverse (Whitnall's) ligament (Fig. 31) is a band of condensed fascial sheath of the levator muscle approximately 14 to 20 mm above the superior border of the

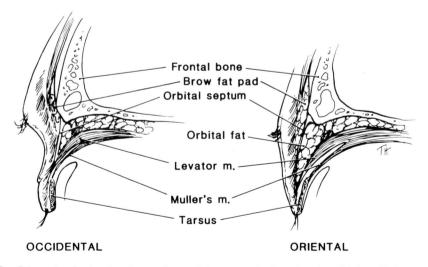

FIG. 29. Schematic of oriental and caucasion eyelid anatomy. In the oriental eyelid the orbital septum fuses with levator aponeurosis below the superior tarsal border. (From Doxanas and Anderson, ref. 9, with permission. © 1984, The Williams & Wilkins Co., Baltimore.)

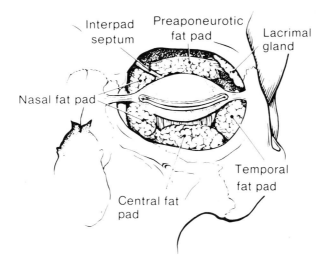

FIG. 30. Frontal view of the eyelids and orbit. The musculocutaneous layer and orbital septum have been removed, showing the orbital fat pad distribution. (From McCord, ref. 20, with permission of Lippincott/Harper & Row.)

tarsus. It extends from the fascia of the trochlea and reflected superior oblique tendon to the capsule of the lacrimal gland, continuing on to the lateral orbital retinaculum. It functions to convert the anterior posterior pulling force of the levator muscle to a superior inferior direction, which raises and lowers the eyelid.

The sympathetic (Müller's) smooth muscle of the eyelid forms at terminal striated muscle fibers of the levator palpebrae superioris. It lies posterior to the aponeurosis, is firmly

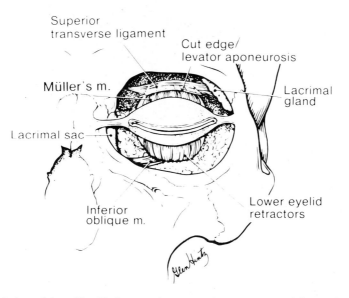

FIG. 31. Frontal view of the orbit with the musculocutaneous layer, septum, and fatty pads removed. (From McCord, ref. 20, with permission of Lippincott/Harper & Row.)

adherent to the conjunctiva, and is attached by a 1-mm tendon to the superior border of the tarsus.

The structures of the lower eyelid are analogous to those of the upper eyelid (Fig. 32). The capsulopalpebral fascia is analogous to the levator. It is formed by the capsulopalpebral head of the inferior rectus muscle. Shortly past this origin, the first fibers of the inferior tarsal muscle begin. A few fine fascial strands extend from the inferior rectus muscle through the orbital fat to the periorbita of the floor. The capsulopalpebral head splits around and fuses with the sheath of the inferior oblique muscle. Anterior to the inferior oblique muscle, the two heads fuse to form Lockwood's ligament (analogous to Whitnall's). The capsulopalpebral fascia is anterior to Lockwood's ligament. Its superior portion sends strands to the inferior fornix and becomes Tenon's fascia, extending onto the globe. The inferior part fuses anteriorly with the orbital septum. Inferior tarsal muscle fibers extend to about 2.5 mm below the inferior tarsal border. Five millimeters below the inferior tarsal border, the capsulopalpebral fascia fuses with the orbital septum. The fusion of the inferior tarsal muscle, capsulopalpebral fascia, and orbital septum inserts into the anterior and inferior surface and base of the tarsus. Some of the capsulopalpebral fibers extend through the orbicularis to the eyelid skin and form a lower eyelid crease.

The lateral retinaculum (Fig. 33) is formed by the lateral horn of the levator aponeurosis, lateral canthal tendon, inferior suspensory ligament (Lockwood's), Whitnall's ligament (via the intralacrimal gland fibrous septae), and check ligaments of the lateral rectus muscle. The lateral retinaculum inserts into the lateral orbital tubercle. The medial retinaculum (Fig. 33) is attached to the periorbita just behind the posterior lacrimal crest. It consists of the medial end of Lockwood's ligament, medial horn of the levator aponeurosis, check

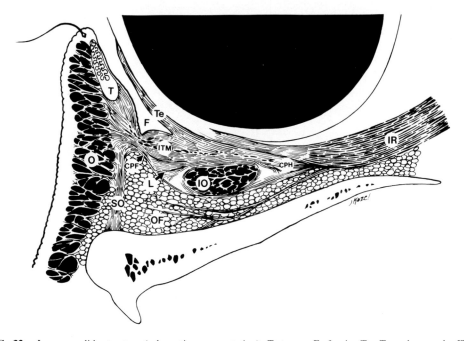

FIG. 32. Lower eyelid retractors (schematic representation). T, tarsus; F, fornix; Te, Tenon's capsule; ITM, inferior tarsal muscle; CPH, capsulopalpebral head; IR, inferior rectus; O, orbicularis oculi muscle; CPF, capsulopalpebral fascia; L, Lockwood's ligament; IO, inferior oblique muscle; SO, orbital septum; OF, orbital fat. (From Hawes and Dortzbach, ref. 12, with permission.)

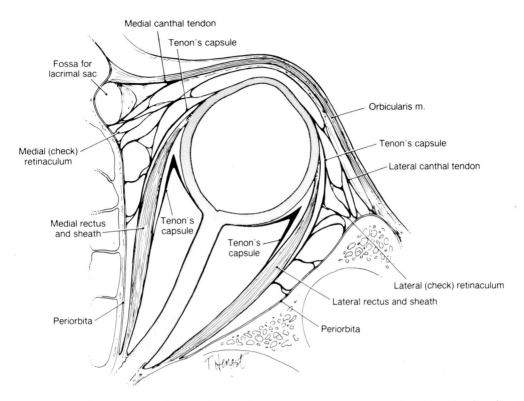

FIG. 33. Horizontal section of the orbit illustrating the contribution to the medial and lateral retinacula. (From Doxanas and Anderson, ref. 9, with permission. ©1984, The Williams & Wilkins Co., Baltimore.)

ligaments of the medial rectus muscle, Whitnall's ligament, deep heads of pretarsal orbicularis, and orbital septum.

LACRIMAL SYSTEM

The lacrimal system consists of secretory, distributional, and excretory components. The lacrimal gland (Fig. 34) is an excretory gland that functions as the main aqueous secretor. It is located in the anterior superolateral quadrant of the orbit in the lacrimal fossa. The ligament of Soemmering consists of loose connective tissue that extends from the stroma of the gland to the periorbita of the orbital roof to suspend the lacrimal gland. The main suspension for the lacrimal gland, however, comes from Whitall's ligament and the lateral levator aponeurosis. The latter also separates the orbital and palperbral lobes of the lacrimal glands. The orbital lobe of the lacrimal gland is twice the size of the palperbral lobe. The orbital lobe secretory ducts run through the palpebral lobe and about 12 ductules empty into the superior cul-de-sac, approximately 5 mm above the superiolateral border of the tarsus. The lacrimal nerve supplies sensory innervation to the lacrimal gland. The reflex afferent pathway is provided by the trigeminal nerve. The efferent pathway follows a complicated route. Nerve fibers originate in the lacrimal nucleus of the pons and travel in the pons as the nervus intermedius. These fibers exit the cerbellopontine angle between the motor root of the facial nerve and the acoustic nerve. After entering the internal auditory canal and passing through the geniculate ganglion, they become the greater superficial

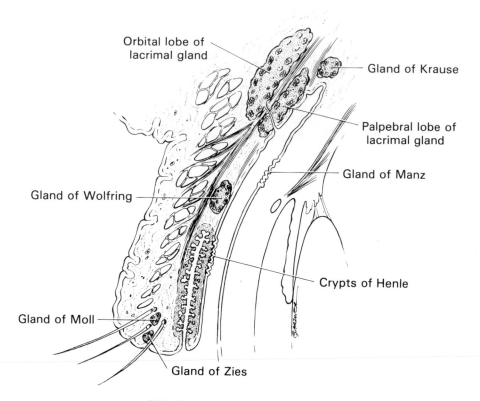

Orbital lobe of
lacrimal gland

Gland of Krause

Palpebral lobe of
lacrimal gland

Gland of Manz

Gland of Wolfring

Crypts of Henle

Gland of Moll

Gland of Zies

FIG. 34. Lacrimal secretory apparatus.

petrosal nerve running along the petrous ridge. Sympathetic fibers from the internal carotid artery join the greater superficial petrosal nerve to form the Vidian nerve. Parasympathetic fibers synapse in the sphenopalatine ganglion. Teritiary axons travel via the maxillary, zygomatic, zygomaticotemporal, and lacrimal nerves to provide secretomotor fibers for the lacrimal gland.

The accessory glands of Wolfring are located at the tarsal border, while the glands of Krause are in the conjunctival fornices (Fig. 34). These glands, having no efferent nerve supply, are believed to be responsible for basic lacrimal secretion. The main lacrimal gland accounts for reflex and basic secretion.

Aqueous secretors form the central layer of the tear film, 7 microns in thickness. The goblet cells of the conjunctiva produce mucin, forming a thin mucous lining that contributes to the wettability of the corneal epithelial surface. The meibomian glands, about 20 per eyelid, and to a smaller degree the pilosebaceous glands of Zeis and apocrine glands of Moll (Fig. 34), produce the oily surface layer, which is 0.1 microns in thickness. This layer helps to prevent evaporation of the tear film. The eyelids distribute the tear film during blinking.

The lacrimal excretory system consists of the canaliculi, lacrimal sac, and nasolacrimal duct (Fig. 35). Puncta are located medially at the mucocutaneous junction of the eyelids and are apposed to the globe. The superior punctum, 5 mm from the medial commissure, is slightly nasal to the inferior punctum. The initial portion of the canaliculi is vertical and 2 mm in length. This portion is joined at the ampulla to the 8-mm horizontal canaliculus. A common canaliculus is usually formed by the superior and inferior canaliculi before

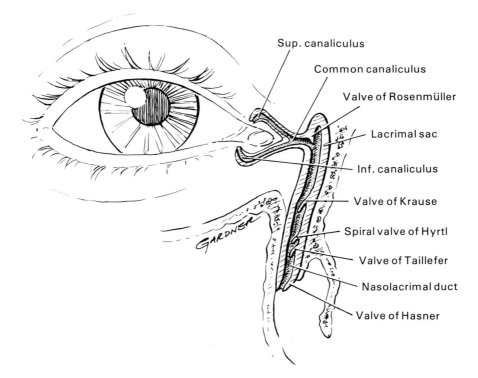

FIG. 35. Lacrimal drainage system, including valves.

entering the lateral wall of the tear sac at the interal common punctum. The common canaliculus is located directly below the anterior crus of the medial canthal tendon. At the common canaliculo–tear sac junction is the valve of Rosenmueller (Fig. 35), which prevents the reflux of tears. The anterior lacrimal crest is formed by the frontal process of the maxillary bone, while the posterior lacrimal crest is part of the lacrimal bone. An extension of the periorbita ensheathes the lacrimal sac in the lacrimal sac fossa, forming the lacrimal diaphragm. The lacrimal sac fundus extends 4 mm above medial canthal tendon, and the sac extends 10 mm down to the maxillary nasolacrimal duct. Passing in an inferior, lateral, and posterior direction, the 12-mm long nasolacrimal duct empties into the inferior meatus. A mucosal fold, the valve of Hasner, covers this ostium, which is about 40 mm from the anterior opening of the nose and 15 mm above the nasal floor. In infants about 20 to 25 mm and in adults 30 to 35 separate the valve of Hasner from the puncta.

The lacrimal pump (Figs. 36 and 37) depends on the deep head of the preseptal orbicularis (Jones' muscle), superficial and deep heads of the pretarsal orbicularis (Horner's muscle), and lacrimal diaphragm. When the eyelids are open, tears collect medially in the palpebral fissure and the puncta and canaliculi are open (Fig. 37A). The tear sac is collapsed. Blinking results in medial movement of the canaliculi and closure of the puncta, lateral canaliculi, and ampulla. Tears are milked medially. Simultaneously, the deep preseptal tendon expands the lacrimal diaphragm, creating a negative pressure (Fig. 37B). This action facilitates the movement of tears from the canaliculi to the tear sac. As the lid reopens, the lacrimal diaphragm returns to its normal position, pushing tears into the nasolacrimal duct. Tears are allowed to collect as the canaliculi, ampulla, and puncta reopen (Fig. 37C).

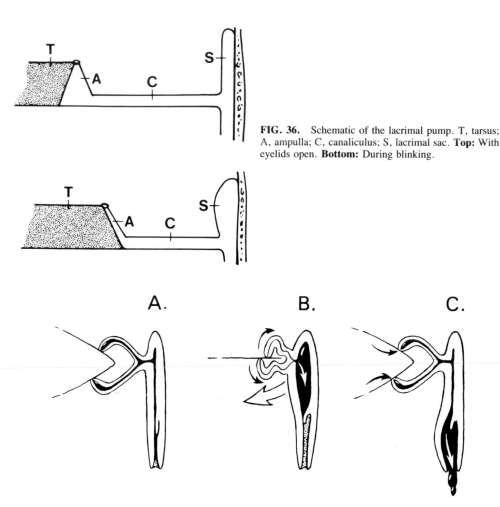

FIG. 36. Schematic of the lacrimal pump. T, tarsus; A, ampulla; C, canaliculus; S, lacrimal sac. **Top:** With eyelids open. **Bottom:** During blinking.

FIG. 37. Lacrimal drainage system and the lacrimal pump. **A:** With eyelids open. **B:** During blinking. **C:** Reopening of lids.

CONNECTIVE TISSUE SYSTEM

Tenon's capsule (Fig. 38) serves as a barrier between the globe and other structures of the orbit. This fibroelastic tissue surrounds the eye and extraocular muscles in the anterior orbit. Tenon's capsule fuses with the conjunctiva at the limbus and extends posteriorly to the optic nerve. Posterior to the equator of the globe, four rectus muscles penetrate Tenon's capsule. Lateral to the inferior rectus muscle, the inferior oblique muscle pierces Tenon's capsules. Three to 4 mm nasally to the medial border of the superior rectus muscle and 4 mm from its insertion, the superior oblique passes through Tenon's capsule.

A connective tissue system of septa with enclosed fat attaches the globe to the periorbita in the anterior orbit (Fig. 39). In addition, the connective tissue septa connect the extraocular muscles to Tenon's capsule. In the anterior orbit, well-developed fascial sheaths form an intermuscular septum. More posteriorly, the orbital connective tissue is less well defined.

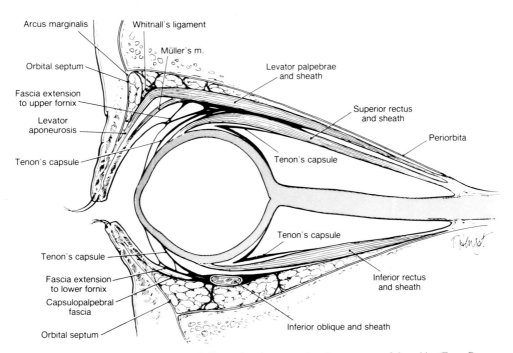

Arcus marginalis
Whitnall's ligament
Müller's m.
Orbital septum
Levator palpebrae and sheath
Fascia extension to upper fornix
Superior rectus and sheath
Levator aponeurosis
Periorbita
Tenon's capsule
Tenon's capsule
Tenon's capsule
Tenon's capsule
Inferior rectus and sheath
Fascia extension to lower fornix
Capsulopalpebral fascia
Orbital septum
Inferior oblique and sheath

FIG. 38. Sagittal section through the orbit illustrating the connective tissue system of the orbit. (From Doxanas and Anderson, ref. 9, with permission. © 1984, The Williams & Wilkins Co., Baltimore.)

EXTRAOCULAR MUSCLES

The rectus muscles originate from the annulus zinnii at the orbital apex (Fig. 9). The lateral rectus muscle arises from the posterior lateral orbital wall at the spina recti lateralis. All the extraocular muscles are approximately 40 mm in length and proceed anterior in the orbit to tendinous insertions on the globe. These tendons range in width from 9.2 mm for the lateral rectus muscle to 10.6 mm for the superior rectus muscle. The spiral of Tillaux refers to the distance from the limbus to the extraocular muscle insertions: 5.5 mm to the medial rectus, 6.5 mm to the inferior rectus, 6.9 mm to the lateral rectus, and 7.7 mm to the superior rectus. These insertions attach to sclera at about the level of the ora serrata. The sclera is thinnest (0.3 mm) immediately posterior to the muscle insertions. Superior and inferior muscular branches of the ophthalmic artery vascularize the rectus muscles. An inferior branch supplies the media rectus, inferior rectus, and inferior oblique muscles. A superior branch vascularizes the other ocular muscles.

With the expection of the inferior oblique muscle, the extraocular muscles are innervated in the posterior one-third of the muscle (Fig. 40). After passing through the annulus zinnii, the superior ramus of the third nerve provides motor innervation to the superior rectus and levator muscles. Also passing through the annulus zinnii, the inferior ramus of the third nerve supplies the inferior rectus, medial rectus, and inferior oblique muscles. The inferior oblique nerve courses anteriorly along the lateral border of the inferior rectus muscle to the midportion of the inferior oblique muscle. Laterally, in the annulus zinnii, the abducens nerve enters the orbit to innervate the lateral rectus muscle. Outside the

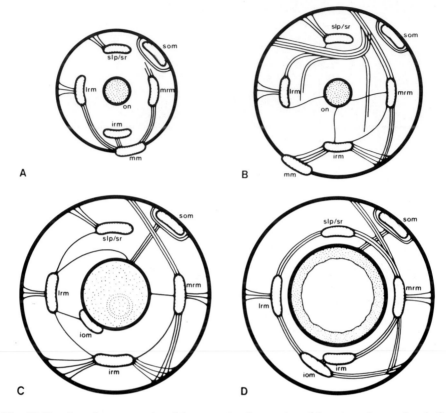

FIG. 39. Highly schematic representation of the connective tissue system of the extraocular muscles. **A:** Coronal section near the orbital apex. **B:** Coronal section near the posterior portion of the globe. **C:** Coronal section lying just anterior to the posterior portion of the globe. **D:** Coronal section near the equator of the oblique muscle. irm, inferior rectus muscle; mm, Muller's muscle; lrm, lateral rectus muscle; mrm, medial rectus muscle; som, superior oblique muscles; slp/sr, superior levator palpebra/superior rectus muscle; on, optic nerve. (From Koornneef, ref. 17, with permission.)

annulus zinnii, in the superior orbital fissure, the trochlear nerve enters the orbit. It enters the superior oblique muscle at the superiolateral edge.

Superiomedial to the annulus, the superior oblique muscle orginates at the frontoethmoid suture (Fig. 9). Ten to 15 mm from the anterior orbital margin, the superior oblique muscle becomes tendinous. Passing through the cartilaginous ring formed by the trochlea, the tendon proceeds posterotemporally under the superior rectus to insert in the globe near the superior temporal vortex vein. Slightly posterior and lateral to the nasolacrimal duct on the orbital plate of the maxilla, the inferior oblique muscle originates. It proceeds posteriolaterally and is firmly attached to the inferior rectus by a fusion of their fascial sheaths. A 1- to 2-mm tendon connects the inferior oblique muscle to the globe near the macula.

OPTIC NERVE

The optic nerve, which is approximately 50 mm long (Fig. 41), extends from the globe to the optic chiasm. There are four parts to the optic nerve: intraocular (1 mm), intraorbital

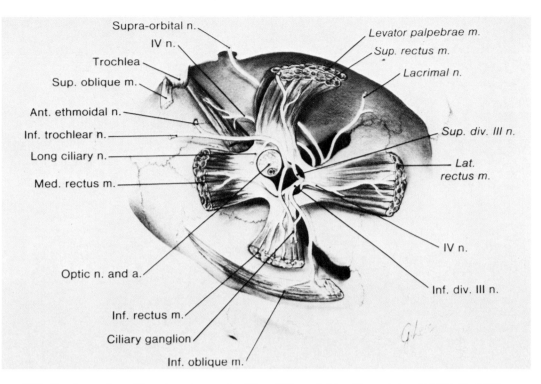

FIG. 40. Innervation of the extraocular muscles. (From Miller, ref. 23, with permission. © 1982, The Williams & Wilkins Co., Baltimore.)

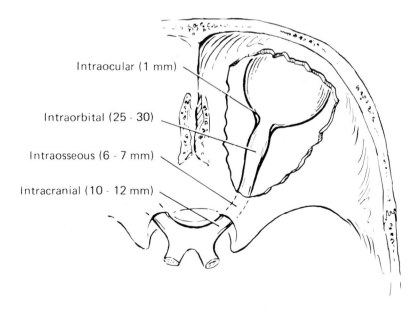

FIG. 41. Optic nerve viewed from above illustrating its four parts.

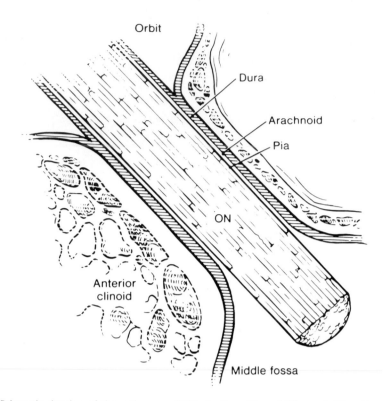

FIG. 42. Schematic drawing of the optic nerve (ON) sheaths. (From Miller, ref. 23, with permission. © 1982, The Williams & Wilkins Co., Baltimore.)

(30 mm), intraosseous (6 mm), and intracranial (10 mm). At the optic disc, the nonmyelinated optic nerve is 1.5 mm in diameter. After traversing the lamina cribrosa and Tenon's capsule, the optic nerve becomes myelinated and 4 mm in diameter. The orbital portion of optic nerve is 10 mm longer than the distance from the globe to the orbital apex. Pia, arachnoid, and dura surround the optic nerve. The dura fuses anteriorly with the sclera and posteriorly with the periorbita of the optic foramen. Eight to 15 mm from the eye, the dura is pierced by the central retinal artery. In the optic canal the dura is fused with the periosteum (Fig. 42). Below the frontal lobe of the brain, the optic nerve extends to the optic chiasm.

BIBLIOGRAPHY

1. Ahl, N. C., and Hill, H. C. (1982): Horner's muscle and the lacrimal system. *Arch. Ophthalmol.*, 100:488–493.
2. Anderson, R. L., and Beard, C. (1977). The levator aponeurosis. Attachments and their clinical significance. *Arch. Ophthalmol.*, 95:1437–1441.
3. Anderson, R. L., and Dixon, R. S. (1979): The role of Whitnall's ligament in ptosis surgery. *Arch. Ophthalmol.*, 97:705–707.
4. Anderson, R. L. (1977): Medial canthal tendon branches out. *Arch. Ophthalmol.*, 95:2051–2052.
5. Beard, C. (1981): *Ptosis*, 3rd ed. Mosby, St. Louis.
6. Beard, C. (1985): Mueller's superior tarsal muscle: Anatomy, physiology and clinical significance. *Ann. Plast. Surg.*, 14:324–333.
7. Beard, C., and Quickert, M. (1977): *Anatomy of the Orbit.* Aesculapius, Birmingham, Alabama.
8. Bergin, D., and McCord, C. D. (1985): Anatomy relevant to blepharospasm. In: *Advances in Ophthalmic Plastic and Reconstructive Surgery—Blepharospasm,* edited by S. Bosniak. Harper & Row, Philadelphia.

9. Doxanas, M. T., and Anderson, R. L. (1984): *Clinical Orbital Anatomy.* Williams & Wilkins, Baltimore.
10. Doxanas, M. T., and Anderson, R. L. (1984): Oriental eyelids: An anatomic study. *Arch. Ophthalmol.,* 102:1232–1235.
11. Goss, C. M. (1959): *Gray's Anatomy of the Human Body,* 27th ed. Lea & Febiger, Philadelphia.
12. Hawes, M. J., and Dortzbach, R. K. (1982): The microscopic anatomy of the lower eyelid retractors. *Arch. Ophthalmol.,* 100:1313–1318.
13. Hollinshead, W. H. (1982): *Anatomy for Surgeons: Vol. 1, The Head and Neck,* 3rd ed. Harper & Row, New York.
14. Jakobiec, F. A., and Iwamota, T. (1983): Ocular adnexa: Introduction to lids, conjunctiva, and orbit. In: *Biomedical Foundations of Ophthalmology,* edited by T. D. Duane and E. A. Jaeger. Harper & Row, Philadelphia.
15. Jones, I., and Jakobiec, F. (1985): Patient examination and introduction to orbital diseases. In: *Clinical Ophthalmology,* Vol. 2 edited by T. D. Duane and E. A. Jager. Harper & Row, Philadelphia.
16. Jones, L. T., Reeh, M., and Wirtschafter, J. D. (1970): *Ophthalmic Anatomy.* American Academy of Ophthalmology and Otolaryngology, Rochester, Minnesota.
17. Koornneef, L. (1979): Orbital septa: Anatomy and function. *Ophthalmology,* 86:876–880.
18. Lemke, B. N., and Stasior, O. G. (1982): The anatomy of eyebrow ptosis. *Arch. Ophthalmol.,* 100:981–986.
19. McCord, C. D. (1980): The lacrimal drainage system. In: *Clinical Ophthalmology,* edited by T. D. Duane and E. A. Jaeger. Harper & Row, Philadelphia.
20. McCord, C. D. (1983): Surgery of the eyelids. In: *Clinical Ophthalmology,* Vol. 5l, edited by T. D. Duane and E. A. Jaeger. Harper & Row, Philadelphia.
21. McCormack, L. J., Cauldwell, E. W., and Anson, B. J. (1945): The surgical anatomy of the facial nerve with specific reference to the parotid gland. *Surg. Gyencol. Obstet.* 80:620.
22. McMinn, R. M. H., Hutchings, R. T., and Logan, B. M. (1981): *Color Atlas of Head and Neck Anatomy.* Year Book, Chicago.
23. Miller, N. R. (1982): *Walsh and Hoyt's Clinical Neuro-ophthalmology,* 4th ed., Vol. 1. Williams & Wilkins, Baltimore.
24. Putterman, A. M., and Urist, M. J. (1974): Surgicial anatomy of the orbital septum. *Ann. Ophthalmol.,* 6:290–294.
25. Stewart, W. B. (ed.) (1984): *Ophthalmic Plastic and Reconstructive Surgery.* American Academy of Ophthalmology, San Francisco.
26. Warwick, R. (1976): *Eugene Wolff's Anatomy of the Eye and Orbit,* 7th ed. Saunders,, Philadelphia.
27. Wesley, R. E., McCord, C. D., Jones, N. A. (1980): Height of the tarsus of the lower eyelid. *Am. J. Ophthalmol.,* 90:102–105.
28. Zide, B. M., Jelks, G. W. (1985): *Surgical Anatomy of the Orbit.* Raven Press, New York.

Oculoplastic Surgery, 2nd edition, edited by
Clinton D. McCord, Jr., and Myron Tanenbaum.
Raven Press, New York © 1987.

Chapter 3

Reconstruction of the Upper Eyelid and Medial Canthus

*Clinton D. McCord, Jr. and **Ralph Wesley

*Department of Ophthalmology, Emory University School of Medicine, Atlanta, Georgia 30308;
and **Ophthalmic Plastic and Reconstructive Surgery, Vanderbilt University Medical Center, and
Ophthalmic Section, Veterans Administration Medical Center, Nashville, Tennessee 37203*

This chapter will introduce descriptions of nine upper lid reconstructive techniques:

1. Direct closure of full thickness eyelid defects with lateral cantholysis.
2. Tenzel rotational flap for moderate upper lid defects.
3. Cutler-Beard or bridge flap technique of upper lid reconstruction for more extensive defects.
4. Sliding tarsal flap technique for isolated medial and lateral defects.
5. Split-level grafts.
6. Pedicle flap from the lower lid margin to reconstruct the upper lid margin, including lashes.
7. Full-thickness composite graft from the opposite eyelid to reconstruct the margin.
8. The median forehead flap technique.
9. The temporal forehead flap (Fricke flap).

The above techniques can be grouped into those utilizing *adjacent tissue* to repair the eyelid defects (direct closure of Tenzel flap and sliding tarsal flap), those utilizing the *opposing eyelid* tissue (Cutler-Beard technique or pedicle graft from the lower lid), and those utilizing *remote tissue,* when no adjacent or opposing eyelid tissue is available (split-level graft, composite graft from the opposing eyelid, median forehead flap, and temporal forehead flap).

The upper eyelid defects encountered by the surgeon most often are those caused traumatically or created by the removal of eyelid tumors. Less commonly encountered defects are those caused by congenital colobomas and loss of tissue from irradiation, burns, or inflammatory conditions such as herpes zoster. In general, upper eyelid defects should be reconstructed immediately, although patients who exhibit a firm Bell's phenomenon and tear film may tolerate an upper eyelid defect temporarily. Medial canthal defects occur most commonly following excision of skin cancer, and we will describe alternate modes of reconstruction: natural granulation, full-thickness skin graft, and glabellar flaps. The importance of medial canthal fixation of lid remnants or flaps in this area to the posterior reflection of the medial canthal tendon will be emphasized.

UPPER EYELID RECONSTRUCTION

Direct Closure

Upper eyelid defects, encountered from tumor, trauma, or congenital malformation, that are as large as one-third of the lid can be closed directly in younger patients. The increased laxity of tissues in older persons may allow direct closure of defects of up to one-half of the upper lid or more with the use of lateral cantholysis to allow approximation of the lid margin. Postoperatively these lids will appear tight and ptotic, but over the next several weeks the lid will undergo relaxation and possible intussusceptive growth to provide a normal appearance and opening of the upper lid. Direct closure minimizes discontinuity of the lashes and avoids multiple-staged procedures. The most important part of direct closure is reapproximation of the tarsal plate, in which the residual edges of the tarsus or "skeleton" of the upper eyelid are sutured together in as exact an approximation as possible. Use of the operating microscope or magnifying loupes facilitates this closure. In traumatic cases an irregular or traumatized tarsus should be trimmed perpendicularly for the full vertical height of the tarsus to help this reapproximation. With tumor removal these vertical incisions can be made electively (Fig. 1, left). The hesitation on the part of many surgeons

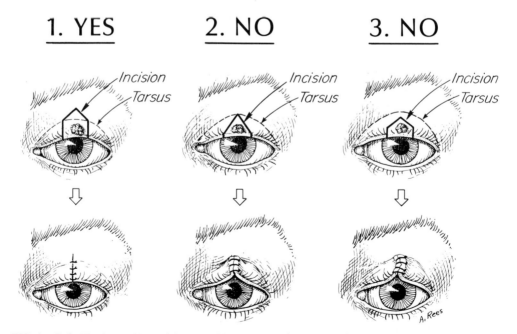

FIG. 1.   Left: Elective incisions of the upper lid or revisions of traumatic defects should extend in a perpendicular fashion from the lid margin to the superior border of the tarsus to allow even wound closure. **Middle:** An incision made to the superior tarsus border but in an angulated manner results in a lid notch. **Right:** A perpendicular incision not extending to the superior border of the tarsus results in buckling of the upper lid.

to perform a full vertical excision of a tarsal segment extending to the superior tarsal border before closure will result in notching (Fig. 1, middle) or buckling of the upper lid (Fig. 1, right) with an abnormal lid contour. The margin will not close evenly if a superior bridge of tarsus is left.

Technique

The wound edges are formed perpendicular to the lid margin (Fig. 2A). Before closure of the tarsal plate proper, an initial lid margin suture of 6–0 silk is passed through the gray line (mucocutaneous junction) and pulled, temporarily, to determine if the margin can be brought together directly with a moderate amount of tension on the eyelid. This suture must pass exactly through the gray lines of each wound edge with bites equidistant from the wound on each side of the defect. If the eyelid tension is excessive with the trial suture, lateral cantholysis must be performed. A #15 Bard-Parker blade is used to make an incision horizontally at the lateral canthus through the skin down to the orbital rim. Sharp Westcott scissors are used to detach the upper limb of the lateral canthal tendon from the bony orbital rim in a nibbling manner to obtain the desired amount of laxity. With larger defects the entire upper lateral canthal tendon must be severed to allow the edges of the upper lid defect to close without undue tension.

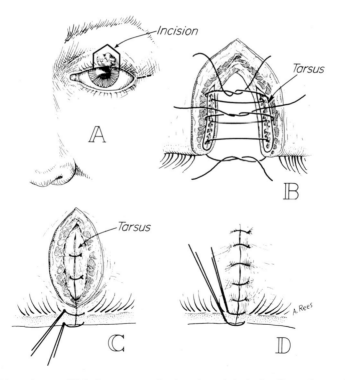

FIG. 2. **A:** Excision of upper lid lesion may require lateral cantholysis for direct closure. **B:** Lid margin suture of 6–0 silk is placed deep enough to include tarsus; 7–0 silk sutures are placed half-thickness through tarsus with knots buried on the anterior surface of the tarsus. **C:** Additional lid margin sutures in place; 7–0 silk sutures tied. **D:** Skin closure with interrupted 7–0 silk sutures. Lid margin sutures are left long, coated with ointment, and draped over the lid surface to prevent corneal irritation.

The vertical cut edges of the tarsal plate are now closed using three 7–0 silk sutures on an Ethicon G-7 needle placed half-thickness through the tarsus so that the knots are buried on the anterior surface of the tarsus (Figs. 2B and 2C). The separation of the orbicularis muscle from the tarsal plate, before the sutures are passed, ensures that only the tarsus is included in this initial part of the layered closure. Absorbable sutures such as Vicryl and Dexon can be used, but the ease of tying 7–0 silk is unequaled. The small silk sutures have caused no tissue reaction when left permanently and maintain approximation of the lid margin. Two sutures of 6–0 silk are then placed in the eyelid margin itself approximating the lash line and the posterior edge of the eyelid. These are tied separately and left long so that they can be draped anteriorly over the lid surface. They are coated with ointment so that they will not rub against the cornea. The skin is then closed using interrupted or running 7–0 silk sutures (Fig. 2D). Ointment is placed on the skin edges daily. Sutures can be removed 7 days later under normal healing conditions.

The tight postoperative appearance after closure of larger defects will resolve in subsequent months, and with relaxation of the tissues the lid will develop good mobility and cosmetic appearance. The necessity of sharp, vertical margins in the surgically created defects and the careful aproximation of the tarsal plate so that an even upper lid contour will be produced cannot be overemphasized. In problem cases, an additional step may be used at the time of closure to prevent notching. A reversed Frost suture may be placed at the suture line, creating downward traction on the upper lid in this area for 1 week to provide additional protection from retraction along the suture line.

Traumatic Defects

In most cases of acute full-thickness eyelid laceration, the tarsus and wound edges can be closed directly. If the lid margin is torn in an irregular manner, or if bits of the eyelid margin are missing, a lid notch can be avoided by revising each side of the tarsal wound with a vertical excision of approximately 1 mm of tarsus on each side of the lid margin to the superior tarsal border. A minimum of upper eyelid skin should be excised in ''freshening'' the wound. Closure is then carried out as we have described.

Tenzel Rotational Flap for Upper Lid Reconstruction

Central upper lid defects of up to 40% of the original lid margin can be closed in the upper lid by a semicircular flap rotated into the lid defect area as described by Tenzel (1) for upper and lower lid defects of a similar type (Fig. 3). The upper lid defect should first be fashioned so that the tarsal edges are perfectly perpendicular to the lid margin as described under the section on direct closure. An inferior arching semicircular line is drawn with Methylene blue at the lateral canthus. The diameter of the flap is approximately 20 mm, and it extends inferiorly and temporally to the lateral extension of the hairline. The musculocutaneous flap incision is made with a #15 Bard-Parker blade and the needle cutting Bovie is used to cut through the muscle fibers for hemostasis. A lateral canthotomy incision is made beneath the semicircular skin incision and dissection is carried out to the lateral orbital rim. The superior ramus of the lateral canthal tendon is cut and the upper lid mobilized completely at the lateral aspect, detaching it from the lateral orbital rim. Care should be taken to preserve the inferior ramus of the lateral canthal tendon. The flap is then undermined and rotated inward. The edge of the flap is advanced to the medial edge of the defect and repaired with layered closure as described in the direct closure

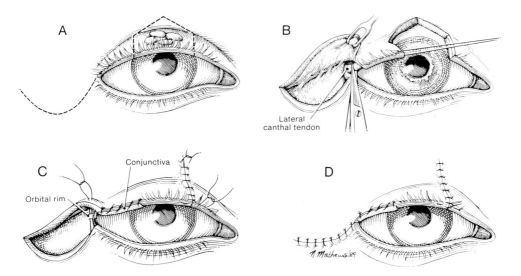

FIG. 3. Tenzel rotational flap for upper lid reconstruction. **A:** Methylene blue outlines the incision lines of the upper lid lesion and the semicircular flap, which curves inferiorly and temporally. **B:** The semicircular flap is elevated and undermined. The superior ramus of the lateral canthal tendon is cut and the lateral portion of the upper lid is advanced medially. **C:** The eyelid defect has been closed. Conjunctiva is undermined and advanced to line the inner surface of the rotational flap. The rotational flap is sutured to the inner periosteum of the lateral orbital rim with fixation to the inferior ramus of the lateral canthal tendon. **D:** Final closure.

section. Lateral lid support is obtained and canthal formation is accomplished by suturing the edge of the flap to the inner periosteum of the lateral orbital rim with fixation to the inferior ramus. This step of lateral canthal fixation is necessary to allow the new upper lid to curve inward and follow the contour of the globe. Conjunctiva can be undermined and advanced to the edge of the flap margin and sutured with a 7–0 silk running marginal suture. The lateral incision is closed directly with mattress sutures and standard skin closure. If a dog ear is encountered because of unequal edges, a small triangle may have to be excised temporally.

Cutler-Beard Flap Using Ear Cartilage

The Cutler-Beard (2), or bridge flap (3), technique is used to reconstruct larger full-thickness eyelid defects, including total loss of the upper lid, by borrowing a full-thickness flap from the opposing normal lower lid. A full-thickness flap of skin, muscle, and conjunctiva is developed beneath the lower lid margin (Fig. 4A) and advanced into the defect. The incision to create the flap is made 4 to 5 mm below the lower lid margin to reserve the vascular supply and prevent necrosis of the remaining bridge of the lower lid margin. Because this flap, replacing the upper lid, contains little or no tarsus (4), we have modified the original Cutler-Beard procedure (5) by inserting ear cartilage between the skin, muscle, and conjunctiva, to be used as a tarsal replacement in reconstructing a more stable upper lid.

Technique

The upper lid defect is created in a rectangular fashion (Fig. 4A), with adequate excision of the tumor mass or, in traumatic and congenital defects, by "freshening" the epithelialized

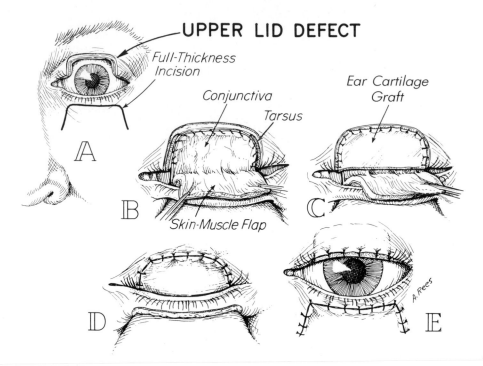

FIG. 4. A: Outline of full-thickness flap of tissue from lower lid, 4–5 mm below lower lid margin, to be advanced into rectangularly shaped upper lid defect. **B:** Conjunctiva separated from musculocutaneous flap and sutured to conjunctiva of defect with running 6–0 plain gut. **C:** Ear cartilage trimmed to appropriate size and sutured with interrupted 7–0 silk sutures to tarsal remnants medially and laterally (or to medial and lateral canthal tendons) and remnants of levator aponeurosis superiorly. **D:** Musculocutaneous flap sutured into defect with interrupted 7–0 silk suture. **E:** Six to 8 weeks later, after flap is separated, conjunctiva is rotated so that lid margin consists of keratinized mucous membrane rather than skin.

border. If the defect includes the entire upper lid, the lateral borders will contain no tarsal plates but rather the medial or lateral canthal tendons. The flap of tissue to be used from the lower lid should be approximately the same width as the upper lid defect. In very lax upper lids the flap of tissue from the lower lid may be narrower, because the upper lid edges may stretch to reduce the size of the defect.

A horizontal full-thickness incision is made in the lower lid 5 mm below the margin (just below the base of the tarsus and the marginal artery) using a #15 Bard-Parker blade, with a corneal protector or lid plate between the lower lid and globe for protection. At the end of the horizontal incision, full-thickness incisions with a #15 Bard-Parker blade are carried vertically downward to the lowest aspect of the inferior fornix on the conjunctival side of the flap. The skin is undermined over the malar eminence. Once the flap is incised, contraction of the orbicularis muscle and elastic tissue gives the appearance that inadequate horizontal dimension has been prepared; however, this will stretch to fit the defect in the closure to be described.

The flap is then put on a stretch with skin hooks, and sharp Westcott scissors are used to dissect the conjunctival layer of the flap from the musculocutaneous layer. Some relaxing incisions in the capsulopalpebral fascia may be needed. This flap of conjunctiva is pulled up under the bridge of the lower lid margin. The conjunctival layer of the flap is sutured to the conjunctiva of the upper lid defect with a running 6–0 plain gut suture (Fig. 4B).

An autogenous ear cartilage graft is harvested as described in Chapter 1. It is fashioned to fit the upper lid defect. Ear cartilage is then sutured with interrupted 7–0 silk medially and laterally to the tarsal remnants (medial or lateral canthal tendons if all the tarsus has been excised) and superiorly to the cut edge of the levator aponeurosis. If this has been excised the cartilage should be attached to the levator muscle itself.

Finally, the musculocutaneous flap from the lower lid (shown in Fig. 4C) is advanced under the bridge of the lid margin and sutured into the skin edges of the upper lid defect with interrupted 7–0 silk (Fig. 4D). Additional undermining of the skin flap may be necessary to allow this flap to advance into place. The orbicularis muscle in this flap of tissue will fit the shape of the defect without undue tension as the skin is closed. The cartilage graft has now been interposed in a sandwich manner between the flap of conjunctiva and the musculocutaneous layer from the lower lid (Fig. 5).

Separation of the flap is carefully carried out 8 weeks later. Premature separation may result in shrinkage. The flap should be left longer in cases of irradiated tissue or alkaline burns. Methylene blue is used to mark the incision to separate the flap approximately 2 mm below the desired position of the new upper lid margin. The assistant provides downward retraction on the bridge, and a grooved director is placed under the flap so that a knife can be used to make an incision through the skin. Stevens scissors are used to make the incision full thickness. One to 2 mm of keratinized skin and muscle is trimmed, leaving 2 mm of extra conjunctiva to rotate anteriorly over the lid margin so that the lid margin will be composed of mucous membrane rather than keratinized epithelium (Fig. 4E). Failure to "overcorrect" the amount of mucous membrane on the lid margin can result in corneal erosion from keratinized (skin) epithelium or trichiasis of hairs of the skin.

Attention is then directed to the lower lid, where the inferior aspect of the lower lid margin bridge is deepithelialized. The lower lid conjunctiva can be left open. The lower lid skin edges are closed with running 7–0 silk. The lower aspects of the cheek incision

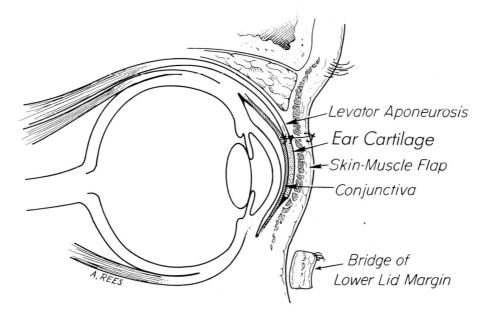

FIG. 5. Cross-section of Cutler-Beard flap showing cartilage graft between conjunctival layer and musculocutaneous layer of lower lid flap. Flap is attached superiorly with 7–0 silk sutures to levator aponeurosis.

may need to be undermined and dog ears excised to promote smooth closure and prevent lower lid malposition. Full-thickness mattress sutures of 4–0 silk can be used to form a lid fold at the time the bridge flap is separated. All sutures are removed 1 week after separation of the flap. Edema is usually present in the upper lid for 4 to 5 weeks and then the reconstructed eyelid resumes a more normal appearance, with a stable lid margin and good vertical mobility.

If cartilage or eyebank sclera is not available for a tarsal replacement, the flap from the lower lid (Fig. 4A) is sutured into the defect in two interrupted layers as originally described by Cutler and Beard (2) in the manner we have described, omitting the placement of eyebank sclera or cartilage.

Pitfalls of Cutler-Beard Bridge Flap

The absence of lashes from the reconstructed segment is best treated with artificial lashes rather than lash grafts. Although hair-bearing grafts can be placed, they generally have a poor appearance. Should a notch develop where the reconstructed segment meets the lid margin, revision can be accomplished by excising the notch, followed by direct closure. Corneal irritation from trichiasis of skin hairs can be eliminated with application of lid cryotherapy. A shortened upper lid with resultant lagophthalmos can be prevented by suturing upper lid remnants as far down on the advanced flap as possible to include the greatest amount of musculocutaneous flap in the reconstructed defect. Consequently, when the flap is finally separated, the upper lid will have a greater vertical dimension.

Sliding Tarsal Flap

Isolated medial or lateral defects of the upper lid (Fig. 6A) too large to close with direct closure in many cases can be reconstructed without borrowing from the lower lid, as in the Cutler-Beard technique. This is accomplished by horizontally sliding a section of tarsus from the remaining lid segment into the defect and covering the external surface with a skin graft.

Technique

To reconstruct the defect shown in Fig. 6A, the lid remnant is everted over a Desmarres retractor. A horizontal incision is made in the tarsal plate with a #15 Bard-Parker blade 4 mm above the lid margin and approximately the width of the defect (Fig. 6B). An additional relaxing incision is then made vertically in the tarsus with a #15 Bard-Parker blade to the superior border of the tarsus and into the upper fornix.

This tarsal-conjunctival flap is horizontally moved into the defect. One edge is attached to the periosteum or remnants of the lateral canthal tendon inside the orbital rim with a permanent suture such as 4–0 silky II Polydek. A half-circle ME-2 needle makes this placement easier. The superior border of the tarsal flap is sutured to the cut edges of the levator aponeurosis. The edge of the tarsal flap next to the remaining upper lid margin is anchored to the margin with a 4–0 silk suture (Fig. 6D). The suture is placed at half-tarsal thickness so as not to be exposed on the undersurface of the lid, to prevent corneal irritation.

A full-thickness graft from the retroauricular area is placed over this tarsoconjunctival flap and sutured into place with interrupted 7–0 silk (Fig. 6E). The eyelids are closed

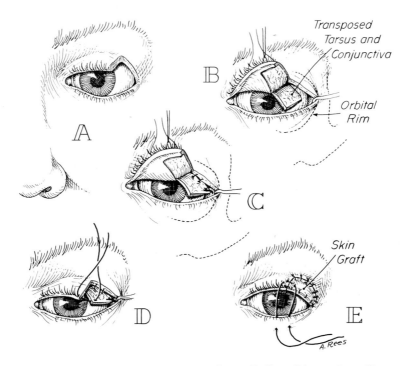

FIG. 6. **A:** Lateral upper lid defect too large for direct closure. **B:** Upper lid everted over Desmarres retractor and tarsal-conjunctival flap to prepare to fill internal aspect of defect. **C:** Tarsoconjunctival flap moved horizontally to fill defect. Edge of flap attached inside orbital rim to remnants of lateral canthal tendon or periosteum. Lateral edge of flap attached to remnants of levator aponeurosis. **D:** Placement of lid margin suture half-thickness through tarsus and tarso conjunctival flap avoids corneal irritation. **E:** Lid margin approximated and skin graft in place.

with 4–0 silk mattress sutures that are placed over cotton bolsters. These are left in place for 1 week before removal. Dressing of the graft is important. Telfa is placed directly over the graft, then dental baseplate Truwax is softened in hot water. Fashioned to the appropriate contour, and applied over the Telfa. Finally a moderate pressure dressing of eyepads is placed over the wound. Eyelid closure sutures immobilize the lid and prevent shrinkage; the dressing keeps gentle pressure to ensure better grafting results from the full-thickness graft.

Defects in the upper lid occuring at the inner canthus are repaired similary, sliding a tarsoconjunctival flap into the defect in a horizontal manner and covering the surface with a full-thickness posterior auricular graft. It is important that fixation of the sliding flap at the inner canthus be made to the posterior reflection of the canthal tendon. If the flap is fixed too anteriorly, the resultant lid will not follow the contour of the globe and separation of the lid from the globe will occur.

Loss of upper lid lashes is more conspicuous nasally than temporally, and in appropriate cases with nasal defects a vertical incision is made at the lateral canthus and the lid segment containing ashes is moved close to the nasal defect. The resulting temporal defect is then reconstructed as described previously.

The full-thickness skin graft over the area of the defect should be sutured carefully to the newly created lid margin or tarsus and conjunctiva, but should not be rotated underneath the margin, which would result in irritation of the cornea by the keratinized epithelium. Failure to use an intermarginal traction suture or a reverse Frost suture at the junction of the flap and eyelid margin can result in shrinkage of the graft and notching of that area of the upper eyelid.

Split-Level Eyelid Grafts for Vertical Full-Thickness Defects

A defect of full thickness vertical shortening of the upper eyelid with an intact lid margin is usually caused by cicatricial changes following burns, trauma, irradiation, or severe inflammation, such as herpes zoster. Brown and Beard (6) have developed a method to correct full-thickness defects of this type in the upper lid using split-level full-thickness eyelid grafts of skin and mucous membrane. Each graft is furnished a vascularized bed. In this method postauricular skin is used for the anterior lamella; buccal mucous membrane (or nasal chondromucosa) is used for the posterior lamella. The upper lid is split (Fig. 7A) and separated (Fig. 7B) so that the two grafts are laced at different levels in the eyelid, with each graft resting on its own vascular bed to ensure survival (Fig. 7C). Because this technique is usually employed with severely cicatrized upper lids, the grafts may undergo some shrinkage. The addition of a few millimeters' vertical lengthening with this procedure, however, may add an adequate margin of corneal protection to eliminate exposure in cases of reduced tear film or diseased corneas.

Technique

The vertically shortened upper lid (Fig. 8A) is everted if possible over a Desmarres retractor, and a horizontal incision is made through the tarsal surface approximately 5 mm above the eyelid margin (Fig. 8B). The retractor is removed, the lid is pulled downward with a 4–0 silk mattress suture through the margin, and a horizontal skin incision is made

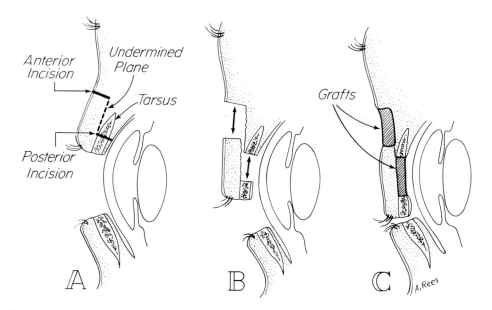

FIG. 7. Brown-Beard split-level grafts. **A:** Skin incision approximately 5 mm above superior tarsal border is joined to tarsal incision 5 mm above eyelid margin. **B:** Connecting the incisions allows vertical lengthening. **C:** External skin graft and internal mucous membrane grafts rest on individual vascular bed.

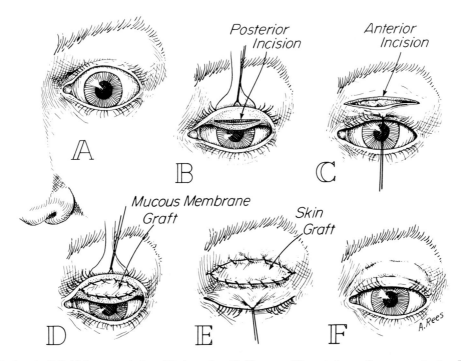

FIG. 8. A: Full-thickness vertical eyelid shortening. **B:** Upper eyelid everted over Desmarres retractor. Full-thickness tarsal incision made 5 mm above lid margin. **C:** Skin incision made approximately 5 mm above upper tarsal border (incisions are connected and lid lengthened). **D:** Position of mucous membrane graft. **E:** Position of skin graft. **F:** Final results, showing vertical full-thickness eyelid lengthening.

across the upper lid above the superior edge of the tarsal border (Fig. 8C) with a #15 Bard-Parker blade. If eversion of the upper lid is not possible because of rigidity, the external skin incision is made first; after retraction of the skin edge the second transtarsal incision is made. Sharp Westcott scissors are used to undermine the skin both superiorly and inferiorly, releasing any traction bands holding the eyelid in the retracted position.

The lower edge of the skin incision is then joined with the upper edge of the tarsal incision (see Figs. 7A and 7B). With the upper lid everted over a Desmarres retractor a full-thickness buccal mucous membrane or chondromucosal graft is sutured into the posterior incisions between the cut edges of the tarsal conjunctiva with a continuous 6–0 plain gut suture (Fig. 8D). With the lid retracted downward a retroauricular full-thickness skin graft is placed into the anterior incision with either interrupted or running 7–0 silk sutures (Fig. 8E). The pattern of graft placement may be revised if new mucous membrane is needed on the lid margin.

Margin sutures of 4–0 silk are used to perform a temporary tarsorrhaphy for 1 week to keep the lid stretched and prevent retraction. The skin graft is stented with Telfa, dental wax, and eyepads as mentioned in the section on sliding tarsal grafts. The graft is immobilized until all sutures are removed 1 week postoperatively (Fig. 8F).

An alternative method of suturing the mucous membrane graft in place on the undersurface of the lid is to utilize through-and-through mattress sutures of 4–0 silk, which are brought through the lid and tied externally.

Pedicle Flap from Lower Lid Margin to Upper Lid

The technique of rotating a pedicle flap from the lower lid margin to the upper lid is a modification of Mustarde's technique for total upper lid reconstruction (7). This modification is thought to be useful in cases in which an abnormal margin is encountered that resists reconstruction by conventional methods, or the patient simply wishes to have intact lashes in the upper lid. In this technique, the margin of the lower lid is transferred to the upper lid in a two-staged procedure with placement of the pedicle into the upper lid during the first stage and separation of the pedicle and revision of the lower lid during the second stage.

A full-thickness pedicle taken from the central portion of the lower lid margin is developed as shown in Fig. 9. It is important to outline the pedicle in the central portion of the lower lid because it makes subsequent closure of the lower lid defect easier in the second stage. It is possible to outline the pedicle closer to the canthal angles if the upper lid defect is off midline; however, it should be emphasized that closure of the lower lid defect is much easier if the pedicle is rotated from the central portion of the lower lid. Care is taken after developing the pedicle to ensure that the marginal artery is included, and this means including the entire tarsus of the lower lid in the pedicle flap. The vertical width of the tarsal plate in the lower lid averages 3.8 mm in most people (4), and the peripheral arcade is approximately at the base of the tarsus, so a flap at least 5 mm in height should

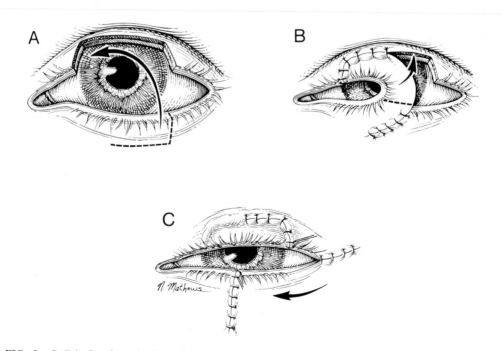

FIG. 9. Pedicle flap from the lower lid margin to the upper lid. **A:** Methylene blue outlines the lower lid pedicle flap, which corresponds to a size necessary to close the upper lid defect. **B:** The lower lid pedicle flap is elevated and rotated into the upper lid defect. Interrupted upper lid tarsal–to–lower lid tarsal sutures secure the flap. The *dotted line* demonstrates the future separation line of the pedicle flap at its base. **C:** Final closure following the second-stage procedure where the lower lid pedicle flap is separated from its base. A slanting wedge excision of skin and muscle at the base of the flap allows for avoidance of dog ears during lower lid closure. Cantholysis may be performed if tension is encountered during lower lid closure.

be designed. It can be rectangular and it does not have to be elliptical as in Mustarde's original technique. The end of the flap is then rotated and margin-to-margin attachment is made from the flap and lower lid margin to the upper lid. Some kinking may be encountered, but if the peripheral arcade from the lower lid is intact, good blood supply will ensue. It is impossible to suture the flap entirely in position in the upper lid, but the end of the flap and the edge must be approximated to establish blood supply in the upper lid. This is done with multiple sutures of 7–0 silk. Care is taken not to cauterize vessels because this may compromise the flap. A pressure bandage is not applied but rather a shield, so as to avoid any compression until the flap gains its blood supply. The flap will stay pink, and in about a 4- to 6-week period should gain its own blood supply on a firm basis so that it can be severed from the lower lid.

The second stage of the pedicle flap is the separation of the base of the flap from the lower lid, its rotation to the upper lid defect, and closure of the lower lid. A slanting wedge is designed encompassing the base of the flap in the lower lid. This is excised full thickness and the lower lid is then closed in a manner described under direct closure of full-thickness lower lid defects in Chapter 4. As stated previously, this oblique, slanting musculocutaneous wedge precludes in most cases the need for much dog ear correction in the lower lid closure. If marked tension is encountered, a cantholysis should be performed to close the lower lid. In most cases the resulting lower lid shows a reduction in the number of lashes, but if closure is accomplished in a precise manner the resulting contour is excellent. The defect in the upper lid commonly has to be modified to accept the full flap. Some additional tarsus may be trimmed from the upper lid so that the flap can be incorporated in an even manner.

When the flap is rotated in position, initially and over the next few weeks it may seem that too much tissue is present. As weeks go by, however, there will be a tendency for some shrinkage, and although revisional excision may be necessary, it should be delayed as long as possible to allow this shrinkage to take place. In most cases the result is quite excellent as far as restoring the contour of the lid. The lashes, although somewhat shorter than normal upper lid lashes, appear to be quite excellent from a cosmetic standpoint. This procedure is the penultimate corrective procedure for margin defects including lashes, but does require some skill on the part of the surgeon and patience on the part of the patient.

Composite Grafting for Upper Lid Defects

An alternative technique of upper lid reconstruction that may be used when precise margin reconstruction is necessary or when other methods cannot be used is the full-thickness composite graft from the opposite eyelid. Full-thickness sections of the upper and sometimes lower eyelid are harvested from the opposite side. Closure of these areas is performed as previously described. The musculocutaneous layer is removed from the graft down to a level just above the lashes. The donor graft may then be covered with a skin-muscle flap (8) in the recipient area for maximum vascularization (Fig. 10). Minimal cautery must be used, and meticulous suturing of the graft under minimum tension is necessary for a good take. Even though the soft tissue take is excellent with good margin restoration, in many cases (approximately 50%) the lashes will not be retained. Although in most cases it is not necessary, the skin excised from the donor graft may be used to supplement the recipient upper lid skin (Fig. 10). Putterman (9) has described this technique well, and Beyer-Machule et al. (10) have described the use of two composite grafts in tandem.

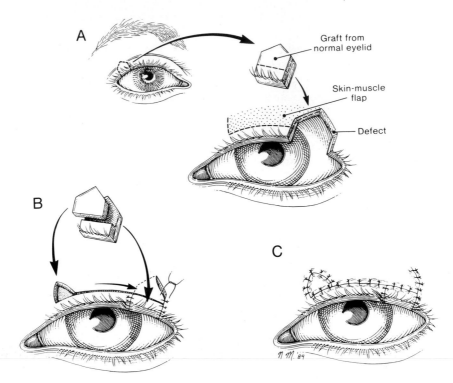

FIG. 10. Full-thickness composite eyelid graft for upper lid defects. **A:** A full-thickness composite graft is harvested from the normal upper eyelid corresponding to a size necessary to close the defect in the opposite upper lid. The donor site is closed directly (see Fig. 2). **B:** The musculocutaneous layer is excised from the composite graft down to a level close to the lashes. The graft is sutured into the upper lid defect with interrupted sutures. A musculocutaneous flap, previously undermined, is rotated to cover the composite graft and provide direct vascularization. **C:** Final closure of upper lid defect with composite graft in place and closure of the musculocutaneous rotational flap.

Median Forehead Flap

This technique, although rarely used, is needed with massive tissue loss of the upper eyelid when tissue cannot be borrowed from the lower lid or adjacent areas to reconstruct the defect. This technique is used to reconstruct an upper eyelid when no other technique is available (11).

A flap of vertically oriented skin is outlined with methylene blue (Fig. 11A), ideally so that the length does not exceed 5 times the width. The flap is incised and elevated. The surrounding tissue is extensively undermined in the forehead area to allow the flap to rotate into the defect (Fig. 11B) and to allow direct closure of the donor site. The vertical donor site incision is closed with subcutaneous 5–0 plain gut sutures or spanning 4–0 silk mattress sutures in interrupted fashion; 6–0 nylon sutures are used for skin closure. The undersurface of this flap, which opposes the globe, must be lined with a free buccal mucous membrane graft, a nasal chondromucosal graft, or remnants of the conjunctiva from the lower fornices, which can be advanced upward. The free grafts in most cases will "take" on a well-vascularized flap. A free graft of mucous membrane may be placed in the forehead area in an additional stage and allowed to "take" prior to transposition of the flap (12)

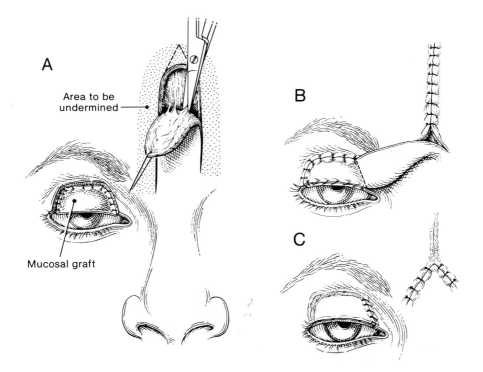

FIG. 11. Median forehead flap. **A:** A free full-thickness mucous membrane graft has been sutured in place in the upper lid defect. The median forehead cutaneous flap is elevated, with generous undermining of the surrounding area. **B:** The flap is sutured into the upper lid defect and the donor site closed by direct advancement. **C:** Final closure following the second-stage procedure where the flap is separated from its base.

(Fig. 11B). The ideal lining of the flap is conjunctiva from the lower lid or fornix, if available.

The forehead flap is attached to the levator aponeurosis or remnants of the levator muscle with 6–0 silk mattress sutures through the flap to give the appropriate vertical mobility to the upper lid. Laterally the tip of the flap is attached with 4–0 silky II Polydek sutures to the remnants of the lateral canthal tendon. The graft of mucous membrane is carefully rotated around the lid margin and sutured in place with running 7–0 silk to ensure that mucous membrane, rather than keratinized epithelium, will be in contact with the cornea. If the undersurface of the forehead flap has been lined with conjunctiva from the lower lid, it can be separated in 2 weeks, leaving enough conjunctiva to cover the lower margin of the forehead flap, which becomes the new upper eyelid margin.

Eight weeks later the base of the flap is separated and the base of the pedicle replaced into the donor (glabellar) area to prevent a narrowing of the eyebrows. The remaining donor incisions are closed with interrupted 6–0 nylon sutures (Fig. 11C).

A flap of sufficient width should be prepared to provide adequate vertical width of the resulting upper lid. With some contraction occurring during the postoperative period, vertical shortening is generally more of a problem than excessive length of the upper lid. Excess bulk tissue can be trimmed later if necessary. The lid will appear tight for many weeks before the levator muscle begins to provide vertical mobility. The resultant eyelid skin is thicker than normal and may be "thinned" cautiously at a later date.

Temporal Forehead (Fricke) Flap

An additional technique used to supply tissue to the upper lid and sometimes lower lid when no adjacent tissue or tissue from the opposing eyelid is available is the transposition of a temporally based flap from the suprabrow area. Many times this flap can be a true axial flap in that the superficial branch of the temporal artery can be included within the flap (13).

The temporal forehead flap provides tissue for the upper lid and lateral canthal area and is suited for large defects in that area; however, it does introduce skin of a much greater thickness than is normally found in the upper lid area and should be reserved as a ''last resort'' procedure. In many cases the flap is a bridge of tissue that spans normal skin and requires a second revisional procedure.

Methylene blue is used to outline the design of the flap above the brow as seen in Fig. 12. The flap is designed so that it is based temporally, and the base of the flap should angle as close as possible to the lateral canthus for good transposition. Incisions are then made through the skin down to the subbrow fatty pad. Very little muscle is included in this flap, so it is mainly a cutaneous flap. Undermining should be carried out temporally; however, one must remember that the superficial branch of the temporal nerve supplying the brow is in this area, and only subcutaneous undermining should be carried out. The flap is then transposed into the upper lid or canthal defect, with closure of the original site of the flap performed with deep and cutaneous sutures. The flap is anchored into position in the recipient skin. If there is a full-thickness defect present the flap must have a mucous membrane lining, which can be derived either by bringing down existing mucous membrane in the upper fornix and suturing it to the undersurface of the flap, or by using a buccal mucous membrane graft to line the portion of the flap that will oppose the cornea (12). Care must be taken to attach the upper lid retractors to the flap to establish movement.

In 6 to 8 weeks the flap can be trimmed at its temporal aspect if there is a pedicle present. If the defect extended in a way that a complete transposition was possible, no revision is needed. The thicker skin in many cases provides adequate movement but produces

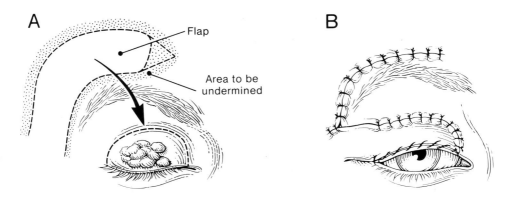

FIG. 12. Temporal forehead (Fricke) flap. **A:** The temporal forehead flap is outlined in Methylene blue with its base as close as possible to the lateral canthus. **B:** Final position of the flap when transposed into the upper lid defect. Note that the flap must be lined with mucous membrane if the lid defect is full thickness. The temporal forehead donor site has been closed directly.

a tethering effect on the lid. It can be thinned down and crease formation can be obtained. The resulting lid is functional but far from normal.

MEDIAL CANTHAL RECONSTRUCTION

The most common defects of the medial canthal region are encountered following excision of skin tumors. In any of the procedures that are used in medial canthal reconstruction— natural granulation, full-thickness skin graft, and glabellar flap—the edge of the lid remnants must be attached to the posterior reflection of the medial canthal tendon (not the anterior reflection) to restore the direction of the normal canthal angle. A permanent suture such as 4–0 silky II Polydek is used to obtain the desired posteriorly directed pull to the medial canthal angle. Attachment to the posterior reflection of the medial canthal tendon is necessary not only to create a normal appearance but also to facilitate the later placement of a Jones tube, which requires a normal medial canthal angle to function properly.

Defects in the medial canthal area that are diamond shaped, as shown in Fig. 13A, are most easily closed, and surgically created defects should be fashioned in this manner if possible. A strong permanent suture such as 4–0 silky II Polydek is placed through the tarsal remnants of each upper and lower lid and then attached to the posterior reflection of the medial canthal tendon. The half-circle ME–2 needle facilitates the placement of this suture.

With a defect such as that shown in Fig. 13A, the lid defect remnants are first pulled

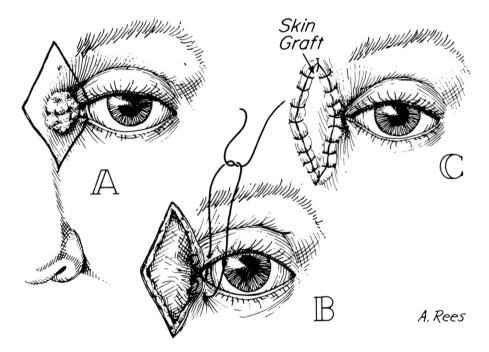

FIG. 13. **A:** Medial canthal defects should be diamond shaped if possible. **B:** Permanent sutures are used to attach upper and lower lid remnants to the posterior medial canthal tendon. **C:** Tying deep sutures reduces size of defect shown in B. **D:** Full-thickness skin graft in place. (Smaller, diamond-shaped defects can be closed directly without skin graft.)

over and attached with a permanent suture to the tarsal plate and to the posterior reflection of the medial canthal tendon. The remaining skin defect, shown in Fig. 13B, can be closed by any of three methods:

1. The defect can be allowed to granulate spontaneously over several weeks with daily dressing changes (14).
2. A full-thickness posterior auricular skin graft can be sutured in place with interrupted 7–0 silk as shown in Fig. 13C, with a dressing of Telfa, molded dental wax, and eyepads placed over this to stent the graft. Sutures are removed 1 week postoperatively.
3. A glabellar forehead flap can be used for immediate reconstruction. The flap is drawn with methylene blue (see Fig. 14A) and incised with a #15 Bard–Parker blade. The flap and skin around the area are extensively undermined to allow the flap to rotate into the defect, as well as to permit closure of the donor site (Fig. 14B). A small triangle may need to be excised for the flap to fit the defect. This may cause some postoperative narrowing of distance between the eyebrows.

The use of direct closure, full-thickness skin graft, or closure by granulation in the medial canthal defects tends to leave a normal concavity and contour to the medial canthal area. The glabellar flap tends to fill this area, giving less concavity, and may require additional debulking.

Unless clear margins are obtained with frozen sections in the removal of skin malignancies, defects in the medial canthal region should be allowed to granulate rather than receive full-thickness grafts or flaps in order to allow inspection and rebiopsy for tumor recurrence. Only after clear edges and deep margins are obtained should a medial canthal defect be

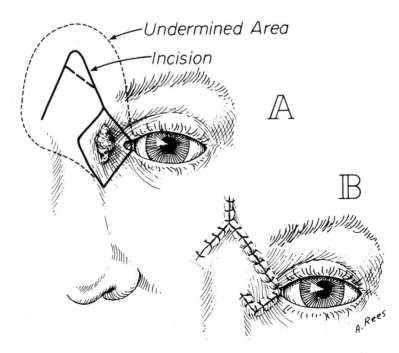

FIG. 14. **A:** Closure of medial canthal defect with glabellar flap requires wide undermining. Tip of flap is usually excised. **B:** Flap is rotated and sewn into defect.

covered with a flap or full-thickness graft (15). Covering unsuspected residual tumor with a flap or graft can allow the tumor to extend insidiously into the orbit.

ACKNOWLEDGMENT

Some of the illustrations for this chapter were prepared by Ms. Ann Rees, Department of Medical Illustration, Veteran's Administration Medical Center, Nashville, Tennessee.

REFERENCES

1. Tenzel, R. R. (1975): Reconstruction of the central one half of an eyelid. *Arch. Ophthalmol.*, 93:125–126.
2. Cutler, N., and Beard, C. (1955): A method for partial and total upper lid reconstruction. *Am. J. Ophthalmol.*, 39:1–7.
3. Smith, B., and Obear, M. F. (1966): Bridge flap technique for reconstruction of large upper lid defects. *Plast. Reconstr. Surg.*, 38:45–48.
4. Wesley, R. E., and McCord, C. D., Jr. (1980): Height of the lower tarsus of the lower eyelid. *Am. J. Ophthalmol.*, 90:102–105.
5. Wesley, R. E., and McCord, C. D., Jr. (1980): Transplantation of eyebank sclera in the Cutler-Beard method of upper eyelid reconstruction. *Ophthalmology*, 87:1022–1028.
6. Brown, B. Z., and Beard, C. (1979): Split level full thickness eyelid graft. *Am. J. Ophthalmol.*, 87:388–392.
7. Mustarde, J. C. (1982): Eyelid reconstruction. *Orbit*, 1:33–43.
8. Anderson, R. L., and Edwards, J. J. (1979): Reconstruction by myocutaneous eyelid flaps. *Arch. Ophthalmol.*, 97:2358–2362.
9. Putterman, A. M. (1978): Viable composite grafting in eyelid reconstruction. *Am. J. Ophthalmol.*, 85:237–241.
10. Beyer-Machule, C. K., Shapiro, A., and Smith, B. (1985): Double composite lid reconstruction: A new method of upper and lower lid reconstruction. *Ophthalmic Plast. Reconstr. Surg.* 1:97–102.
11. Kazanjian, V. H., and Roopenian, A. (1956): Median forehead flaps in the repair of defects of the nose and surrounding areas. *Trans. Am. Acad. Ophthalmol. Otolaryngol.*, 60:557–566.
12. Smith, B. C., and Nesi, F. A. (1979): Upper lid reconstruction: A new technique for the use of mucous membrane lined pedicle flaps. *Ophthalmic Surg.*, 10:17–19.
13. Krupp, S., Daverio, P., and Brupbacher, J. P. (1983): Island flaps for face and neck repair. *Facial Plast. Surg.* 1:37–50.
14. Fox, S. A., and Beard, C. (1964): Spontaneous lid repair. *Am. J. Ophthalmol.*, 58:947–952.
15. Chalfin, J., and Putterman, A. M. (1979): Frozen section control in the surgery of basal cell carcinoma of the eyelid. *Am. J. Ophthalmol.*, 87:802–809.

Oculoplastic Surgery, 2nd edition, edited by
Clinton D. McCord, Jr., and Myron Tanenbaum.
Raven Press, New York © 1987.

Chapter 4

Reconstruction of the Lower Eyelid and Outer Canthus

* Clinton D. McCord, Jr. and ** William R. Nunery

** Department of Ophthalmology, Emory University School of Medicine, Atlanta, Georgia 30308;
and ** Department of Ophthalmology, Indiana University School of Medicine,
Indianapolis, Indiana 46202*

This chapter deals with full-thickness tissue loss of the lower eyelid, lateral canthal area, and lacrimal canaliculi. Before one decides on a specific reconstruction procedure, the patient's age and elasticity of tissue must be taken into account. The elderly patient's skin has a laxity allowing the lid substance to stretch and reduce the defect size. The young person's skin, on the other hand, is less able to stretch and reduce the size of large defects. When considering any reconstructive procedure, we must bear in mind that functionally the lower lid consists of eyelid margin, skin covering, mucosal backing, and a rigid support supplied anatomically by the tarsal plate. Adequate reconstruction must deal with all these components to achieve an acceptable functional and cosmetic result. The following procedures should be mastered singly or in combination to close a variety of lower lid defects. Although the literature is replete with alternative procedures that have value in some situations, these are the standard procedures that should be in every ophthalmic plastic surgeon's repertoire.

LOWER EYELID RECONSTRUCTION

Direct Closure

As in the upper lid, the most commonly used of all reconstructive procedures in the lower lid is direct, end-to-end closure of the lid margin (Fig. 1). Although this relatively simple maneuver should be considered in the initial evaluation of most lower lid defects, it has its greatest usefulness in central eyelid defects affecting less than 40% of the original lid margin. In a younger patient with greater tissue elasticity, it may be practical to close only a wound of 30% or less of the lid margin with simple direct closure. In borderline cases, the added relaxation of a lateral cantholysis may provide sufficient relaxation to allow closure.

93

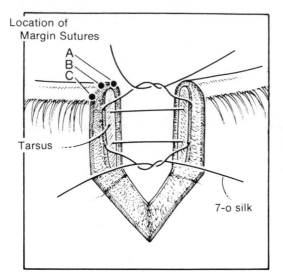

FIG. 1. Direct closure of eyelid defect showing placement of tarsal sutures and location of margin sutures. **A:** Posterior lid margin. **B:** Grey line of lid margin. **C:** Anterior lid margin.

A pair of skin hooks or fine-toothed forceps should be used to grasp and reapproximate the margins of the defect. This will provide a good estimate of the adequacy of direct closure. The borders of the tarsus must be squared with a scalpel to create perfectly perpendicular defect margins, from the lid margin to a level below the tarsus (Fig. 1). The tissue below the tarsus can be either cut into a wedge, creating a hexagonal configuration of lid defect, or left in a rectangular shape, with the excess tissue pucker excised more precisely after the tarsus has been reapproximated (Fig. 2).

A single 6–0 silk untied suture placed through the lash margin on either side of the defect will draw the wound together and provide sufficient retraction to allow closure of the tarsus. Two or three interrupted 7–0 silk sutures are placed through the tarsus in a

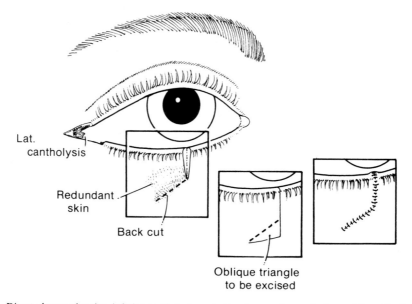

FIG. 2. Direct closure showing inferior cantholysis and skin closure. *Insets* depict excision of redundant skin tag.

vertical line. Conjunctiva should not be included in these sutures. Closure of the tarsus is the most important aspect of the lid repair, and great care should be taken to reapproximate the perpendicular edges precisely. Although larger caliber silk should not be buried in the lid, 7–0 silk can be left permanently with no ill effects to the tissue.

Attention is then turned to the lid margin. The 6–0 retention suture is removed and three interrupted 6–0 silk sutures are placed: one at the mucosal-epidermal margin, one at the gray line, and one at the lash margin (points A, B, and C, respectively, in Fig. 1). The ends of these sutures are left long and later brought down over the skin to avoid corneal irritation (Fig. 3).

Dog-eared redundant skin, which commonly occurs at the inferior limits of the skin defect, is excised next. This is best accomplished by making a full-thickness oblique skin cut with straight scissors, in a line parallel to the skin lines of the cheek (see insets, Fig. 2). Skin medial to this incision is draped in an overlapping manner, marked with methylene blue, and excised. This excises an oblique triangle of tissue parallel to the skin lines, rather than an equilateral triangle excised in the standard vertical orientation. The skin defect is then closed with 7–0 silk suture. Vertical mattress sutures provide for maximal wound edge eversion and alignment of the epithelium. At this point, conjunctiva will have been well approximated and need not be sutured.

If a lateral cantholysis is needed to reduce tension on the wound edges, this is done by making a horizontal incision at the lateral canthal angle, and extending approximately 5 mm on the skin surface. Sharp dissection is carried down to the periosteum of the lateral orbital rim, and the lower arm of the lateral canthal tendon is severed from the rim. Increased laxity will be noted immediately in the lower lid. The lateral margin of the wound can then be mobilized nasally to close the lid margin defect (see Fig. 2). The skin is then closed at the lateral canthus.

Because the main support to the eyelid repair consists of the nonabsorbable silk tarsal sutures, all external sutures, including margin sutures, may be removed in 5 to 7 days.

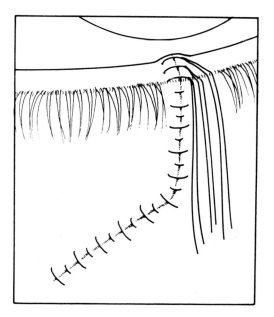

FIG. 3. Final appearance of direct eyelid closure.

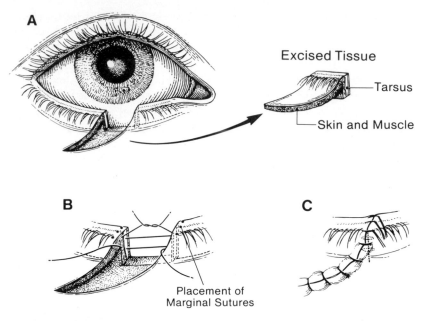

FIG. 4. Oblique skin excision with full-thickness resection of lower lid. **A:** An oblique excision of the skin muscle layer is performed with full-thickness resection of the lower lid. **B:** silk tarsal sutures are placed; diagram indicates location of marginal sutures. **C:** Final closure of the lid margin and musculocutaneous layer. The initial slanted excision of the musculocutaneous layer has avoided a dog ear.

Alternate Oblique Skin Excision

A slanting of the external musculocutaneous layer excision can be performed in the lower lid to avoid a dog ear, which is common with lower lid closure. By slanting the incision temporally, as shown in Fig. 4, the tension and length of the upper and lower edge remain more comparable, thereby avoiding a dog ear. This has become our standard usage in lower lid full-thickness resection.

Tenzel Lateral Rotational Flap

Central or lateral lower lid defects of 40% to 60% of the original lid margin can be closed by a lateral, semicircular miniflap rotated into the lid defect (1). The lower lid defect must first be fashioned so that the tarsal edges are perfectly perpendicular to the lid margin. The tissue beneath the tarsal defect is excised in a triangular manner as described in the section on direct closure. A superior arching line is drawn with methylene blue, beginning at the lateral canthus (Fig. 5A). The diameter of the flap is approximately 20 mm and it extends superiorly and temporally to the lateral extension of the brow line.

The musculocutaneous flap incision is made with a #15 Bard-Parker blade, and a lateral canthotomy incision is made beneath the semicircular skin incision. Dissection is carried down to the lateral orbital rim. The inferior ramus of the lateral canthal tendon is cut to mobilize completely the lateral aspect of the lid. Care should be taken to preserve the superior ramus of the lateral canthal tendon. The semicircular flap is thoroughly undermined and rotated inwardly (see composite of steps in Fig. 5B).

The lateral lid tissue is advanced to the medial edge of the defect and fixated in the manner described under direct closure. The lateral lid support must be recovered by suturing dermis of flap tissue to the inner periosteum of the superior inner aspect of the lateral orbital rim (Fig. 5C). This step of lateral canthal fixation is necessary for support to prevent lateral sagging of the lid.

Conjunctiva is then undermined, advanced to the skin edge of the lid margin, and sutured with 7–0 silk running marginal sutures. The lateral incision is closed directly with mattress sutures, then standard skin closure. If the sides of the lateral incision are not equal, a small dog ear may be excised at the temporal portion of the wound edge (Fig. 5D).

The Tenzel rotational flap is quite excellent by itself for smaller full-thickness lower lid defects. As the defects enlarge, there is a tendency for deficiency in the temporal portion of the lower lid since there is no "support structure" for the flap. An attempt to "push the flap too far" will lead to inevitable complications such as lower lid retraction and deficiency of the lid with irritation of the eye. As the size of the defect one wishes to

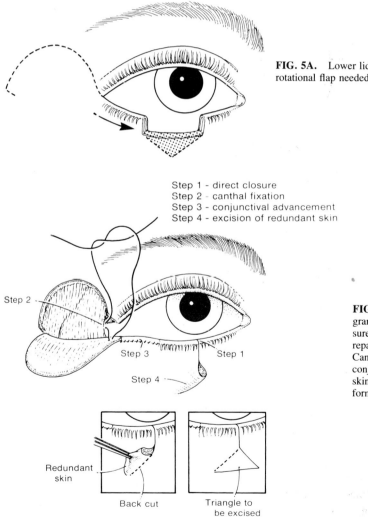

FIG. 5A. Lower lid defect with outline of Tenzel rotational flap needed for closure.

Step 1 - direct closure
Step 2 - canthal fixation
Step 3 - conjunctival advancement
Step 4 - excision of redundant skin

Step 2

Step 3   Step 1

Step 4

Redundant skin

Back cut   Triangle to be excised

FIG. 5B. Composite diagram of Tenzel rotational closure. The medial defect is first repaired using direct closure. Canthal fixation, followed by conjunctival advancement and skin closure, is then performed.

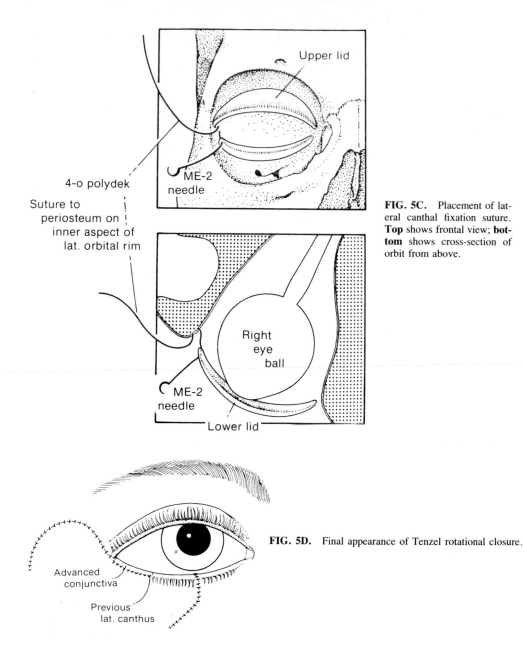

FIG. 5C. Placement of lateral canthal fixation suture. **Top** shows frontal view; **bottom** shows cross-section of orbit from above.

FIG. 5D. Final appearance of Tenzel rotational closure.

repair increases, additional techniques can be used in conjunction with the Tenzel rotational flap to prevent these problems and allow the closure of larger defects in the lower lid.

Tenzel Rotational Flap with Periosteal Flap

The first supplemental procedure that can be performed for the defect slightly larger than standard size is the periosteal strip elevated from the lateral orbital rim that is hinged at the orbital rim. The Tenzel rotational flap is performed in the usual manner, but before closure at the lateral canthal area methylene blue is used to outline the periosteal flap

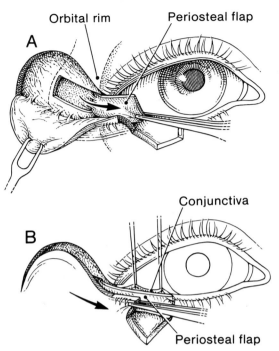

FIG. 6. Tenzel rotational flap with periosteal flap. **A.** A periosteal flap is elevated while remaining hinged at the lateral orbital rim. **B:** The periosteal flap is sutured to the lateral edge of the lower lid tarsus. Conjunctiva is being stretched upward to line the inner surface of the periosteal flap.

based or hinged at the edge of the rim. This rectangular strip of periosteum is elevated from the rim as shown in Fig. 6. Care must be taken to base the flap high enough on the orbital rim to ensure upward pull of the lid. The flap should be placed at least at the midpupillary level. The flap should be slanted so that its base is upward, so that it will pull the lid in the proper direction. As the flap is elevated it is stretched across and anchored as far as possible inside the advanced Tenzel flap. In smaller defects the periosteal flap can be sutured to the edge of the tarsus; however, in some larger defects it is simply tacked to the inner surface of the advanced musculocutaneous flap. Following the periosteal flap addition the Tenzel flap is then closed in the usual manner (Fig. 6).

Tenzel Rotational Flap with Supplemental Ear Cartilage

With larger lower lid defects, in which the lateral edge of the tarsus is pulled further away from the lateral orbital rim as the Tenzel flap is advanced, supplemental procedures of a larger magnitude must be performed to ensure the stability of this lateral portion of the lower lid. In these larger defects even the addition of a periosteal flap may not furnish enough support, and a supplemental ear cartilage graft must be used to "back" the advanced Tenzel flap. The ear cartilage graft is taken as described in Chapter 1 and the graft is "squared off" so that it can be approximated to the edge of the residual tarsal plate in the eyelid. The cartilage should be secured to the edge of the tarsal remnant with two or three 6–0 Vicryl sutures. The edge of the tarsus should also be trimmed to accept the edge of the cartilage. Following this attachment the cartilage is then tensed in a lateral manner toward the lateral orbital tubercle (Fig. 7). After the proper tension is obtained in the lid the cartilage is then trimmed at its lateral edge until it fits in a snug manner with good lid position. It is then sutured to the periosteum with slow-absorbing or permanent

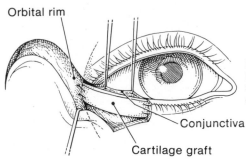

Orbital rim

Conjunctiva

Cartilage graft

FIG. 7.   Tenzel rotational flap with supplemental ear cartilage. The cartilage graft is sutured to the lateral edge of the tarsus, and to the periosteum of the lateral orbital tubercle; this restores firm tension to the lower lid.

sutures. This lateral canthal fixation of the cartilage to the periosteum can be trying because a needle can be successfully passed through the cartilage only one or two times before the cartilage tends to fragment. Wider initial bites must be taken in the cartilage to avoid multiple punctures of the cartilage with the needle. After placement of the cartilage and tensing at the lateral canthal area so that the lower lid has reached the desired position, tension, and contour, the Tenzel flap procedure is then completed in the usual manner. The ear cartilage does not have to be covered with conjunctiva and, indeed, in many cases this is impossible because of the amount of resection. In over 3 to 4 weeks the cartilage will reepithelialize, but it can produce some temporary follicular conjunctivitis, which can be controlled with steroid-antibiotic ointment in the ensuing weeks.

Although not yet used by these authors, it would be possible to combine both the periosteal flap and ear cartilage graft simultaneously in certain lower lid reconstructive procedures.

Modified Hughes Procedure

Larger defects affecting more than 50% (depending on lid laxity) of the lower lid margin ideally are closed with a tarsoconjunctival flap from the upper eyelid (2,3). This technique was originally described by Hughes but has been modified (4). This lid-sharing technique is superior for both cosmesis and lid function, produces a dynamic, moveable lower lid, and is the technique preferred by most ophthalmic plastic surgeons. The disadvantage of the lid-sharing procedure is that it is a two-stage procedure, the first stage requiring that the eye be kept closed for several weeks. After that time, a second procedure is needed to open the lid margins.

The margins of the defect are made perfectly perpendicular from the lid margin to below the tarsus (Fig. 8A). The lower extent of the wound is cut in a rectangular shape. The margins of the defect are gently pulled toward the center until the desired tightness against the globe is achieved. Calipers are then used to measure the horizonal length of the defect in order to determine the correct width of tarsal flap to take from the upper lid. If the lower lid is loose or inelastic, a narrower flap may be used.

The upper eyelid is everted over a Desmarres retractor, and methylene blue is used to mark a superiorly based, three-sided advancement flap on the tarsal conjunctiva (Fig. 8B). The horizontal margin of the flap must be at least 4 mm away from the lid margin. If less than 4 mm of intact upper lid marginal tarsus remains after the procedure, upper lid deformities such as entropion, ectropion, and trichiasis can result. The outlined flap is incised through conjunctiva and tarsus to a plane between tarsus and levator aponeurosis.

Dissection is continued superiorly between Müller's muscle and levator aponeurosis. Care should be taken to avoid damage to Müller's muscle, because this may compromise

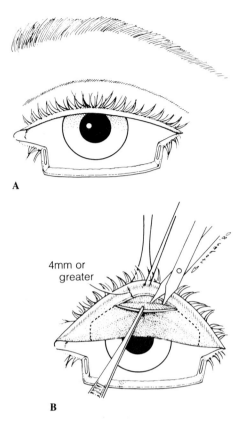

A

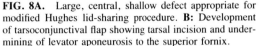

4mm or
greater

B

FIG. 8A. Large, central, shallow defect appropriate for modified Hughes lid-sharing procedure. **B:** Development of tarsoconjunctival flap showing tarsal incision and undermining of levator aponeurosis to the superior fornix.

blood supply to the flap. Blunt dissection with a wet cotton-tipped applicator may facilitate dissection between Müller's muscle and levator aponeurosis. Some surgeons perfer to exclude Müller's muscle from the flap. Although this allows greater ease in separating the lid later, it may compromise the graft vascularity in marginal cases.

When the flap, consisting of tarsus, conjunctiva, and Müller's muscle, is sufficiently mobilized from the upper lid, attention is returned to the lower lid defect. The lateral and medial margins of the tarsal flap are sutured to the cut edges of lower lid tarsus in the manner described under direct eyelid closure (Figs. 1 and 9). The previous upper lid superior tarsal border becomes the lower lid tarsal margin. If no lower lid tarsus at the lateral margin of the defect is available, the tarsal flap from the upper lid can be anchored to the periosteum using lateral canthal fixation in the manner shown in Fig. 5C. If there is an absence of residual tarsus nasally, the flap must be fixed to the posterior reflection of the medial canthal tendon with medial canthal fixation. (Refer to the section on medial canthal defects.) The inferior margin of the flap is sutured to the remaining conjunctiva below with a running 5–0 plain catgut suture. By advancing upper lid tarsus and mucosa on a pedicle flap, the lower lid defect will now have been restored with two of its necessary ingredients. The third ingredient is supplied by a full-thickness skin graft over the composite pedicle flap (Fig. 10). Donor skin may be obtained, in order of preference, from (a) either upper eyelid if sufficient redundancy exists; (b) postauricular skin; or (c) supraclavicular skin. In unusual circumstances, skin may be obtained from the groin or axillary areas. Usually postauricular skin is used.

The skin graft is taken freehand and thoroughly stripped of subcutaneous fat and connective

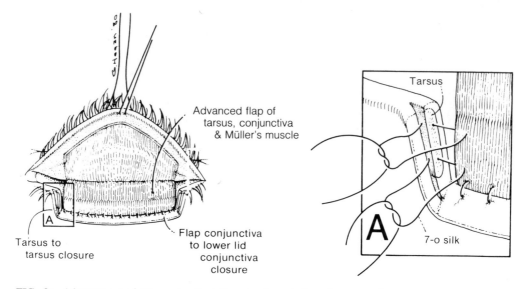

FIG. 9: Advancement of tarsoconjunctival flap showing suturing of tarsus to lower lid conjunctiva. Upper tarsus is sutured to lower tarsus at point A. *Inset:* Close-up view of upper tarsus–to–lower tarsus closure.

tissue with a fine iris scissors. The skin graft is sutured over the composite flap with 7–0 silk. The superior edge of skin is sutured to the conjunctival flap 1 to 2 mm higher than the future lower lid margin. A proper "take" of the graft is obtained by carefully everting the skin edges while the graft is being sutured and covering the graft with Telfa and molded dental wax dressing. This, in turn, is covered by a light pressure dressing consisting of two standard oval eye pads. This light pressure dressing will prevent tenting of the wound edges, which may cause later prominence of the tissue interface. The dressing should be left undisturbed for 5 days until the time of suture removal.

The flap and skin graft are left undisturbed for a period of 6 to 8 weeks. This length of time is crucial not only to allow a new blood supply to develop from the margins of the

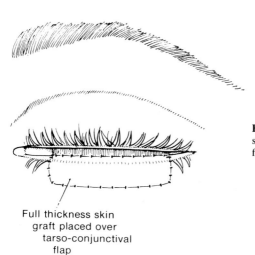

FIG. 10. Final closure of modified Hughes procedure showing full-thickness skin graft covering tarsoconjunctival flap.

graft, but to provide an upward pull during the early phase of wound healing. This counteracts the natural process of wound retraction and sagging caused by gravity.

Separation of the Modified Hughes Flap

The flap is infiltrated with 2% lidocaine (Xylocaine®) with 1 : 100,000 epinephrine added. A grooved director is used to pull the bridge away from the eye to protect the cornea, and the flap is severed as close as possible to its origin under the upper lid with a #15 Bard-Parker blade (Fig. 11A). After everting the released upper lid over a Desmarres retractor, the bed of the previous tarsoconjunctival flap is sharply undermined to the superior fornix. The dissection is carried out in a plane between Müller's muscle fibers and the levator aponeurosis. Müller's muscle will then spontaneously retract to its original level and prevent lid retraction secondary to Müller's advancement (Fig. 11B). Adequate full-thickness incision horizontally must be carried out or upper lid retraction will occur.

After releasing the upper lid, a skin incision is made along the new lower lid margin. Excess grafted skin is removed, but care is taken not to excise the excess mucosa from the released flap. The mucosa is then rolled over the new lid margin and sutured to the anterior mucocutaneous junction with a running 6–0 plain catgut suture tied externally to

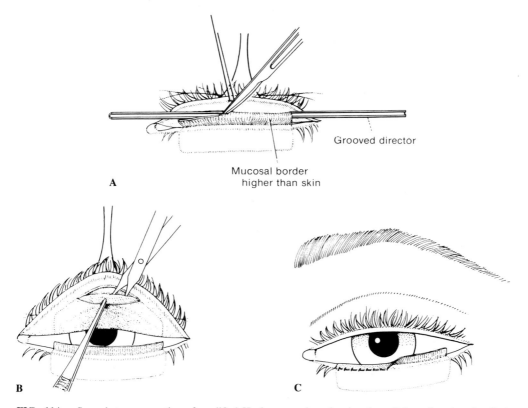

FIG. 11A: Second-stage separation of modified Hughes procedure showing the splitting of conjunctiva flush with the undersurface of upper lid. **B:** After release of tarso conjunctival flap, the advanced Müller's muscle is undermined to the level of the superior fornix. **C:** Final closure of second-stage procedure showing mucosa being draped over margin and sutured to the external cutaneous border.

the lid margin (Fig. 11C). The conjunctiva must completely cover the new lower lid margin or marginal entropion and corneal irritation will occur. The excess conjunctiva on the lid margin will keratinize with time, or with cautery at a later date, and will apear normal.

Hewes' Procedure

A valuable procedure for repair of shallow lower lid defects, particularly those within the temporal half of the lower lid, was described in which a transposition flap of tarsoconjunctiva was placed at the lateral canthal angle, brought into the lower lid defect, and covered with either a full-thickness skin graft or a flap (5). The procedure is somewhat limited in that repair of major defects would be difficult, but is quite excellent for defects not including the entire lower lid margin, particularly those with a major portion of the defect at the lateral canthal area.

The steps of the procedure are shown in Fig. 12. The upper lid is everted and methylene blue is used to outline a flap encompassing the superior tarsal border and the conjunctiva above the superior tarsal border, based at the lateral canthal angle. The flap designed in this manner is a true axial flap in that the peripheral arcade at the superior tarsal edge is included and gives an intact blood supply to the flap. The flap is then dissected into the canthal angle until it moves freely; however, care is taken to spare the arcade as it enters the base of the flap. Stretching of the lower lid to reduce the size of the defect is performed to estimate the true length of flap that is need to produce the proper tension in the lower

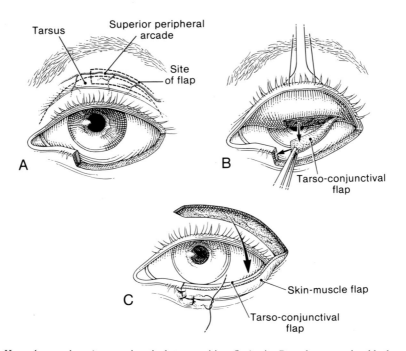

FIG. 12. Hewes' procedure (tarsoconjunctival transposition flap). **A:** *Dotted rectangular block* outlines the flap site. The flap will include the superior border of the upper lid tarsus, the conjunctiva, and part of the superior marginal arcade of vessels. **B:** The upper lid tarsoconjunctival flap has been mobilized and is being transposed into the lower lid defect. **C:** The tarsoconjunctival flap has been secured to the lower lid tarsus. An upper lid musculocutaneous flap, based at the lateral canthal angle, is transposed to the lower lid to cover the tarsoconjunctival flap.

lid. The flap is brought down and is sutured to the tarsus and conjunctiva in the lower lid with the tarsal edge in the downmost position, using absorbable sutures. Care must be taken that too long a flap is not brought down to produce laxity in the lid and possible postoperative ectropion. The transposed tarsoconjunctival flap is then covered with a full-thickness skin graft from a suitable donor site. It is also possible to cover the tarsoconjunctival transposition flap to the lower lid with a musculocutaneous transposition flap from the same upper lid based at the lateral canthal angle. This works particularly well in older individuals with much laxity of the musculocutaneous layer. The advantage is that this is a one-stage procedure and furnishes adequate support and tension to the lower lid at the lateral canthal angle. There is also a cosmetically satisfactory effect, particularly in older individuals.

Mustarde Rotational Cheek Flap

The Mustarde flap is a full-thickness rotational cheek flap that can, when necessary, be relied on to cover virtually any lower lid defect (6). It has the advantage of allowing a complete lower lid reconstruction in one operative procedure. The Mustarde flap is most useful for vertically deep defects, especially those in which the vertical dimension is greater than the horizontal dimension. Nasal defects are better suited to a rotation flap. Objections to this procedure include: (a) the excessively long scar line on the face; (b) the necessity of excising a large triangle of normal tissue, except in rare instances; and (c) the adynamic nature of the reconstructed lower lid.

Atonicity leads to impairment of the lacrimal pump mechanism, and contributes to late occurrence of lateral lower lid sagging and ectropion, which can be complications of the Mustarde technique. Because of these inadequacies, the large rotational cheek flaps are reserved for a few specific indications: (a) a large, vertically deep nasal defect; (b) undesirability of keeping the eye closed for a prolonged period because of ocular disease (such as glaucoma, active corneal disease, or risk of amblyopia in a child); and (c) a patient who is unable to tolerate a second surgical procedure (poor surgical risk).

The rotational cheek flap is begun by infiltrating lidocaine 2% with 1 : 100,000 epinephrine in the cheek and lid area. A large, nasal, superiorly based triangle with the medial edge in the nasolabila fold is outlined (Fig. 13A). A semicircular flap beginning at the lateral canthus and extending to the area immediately adjacent to the auricular tragus is then outlined. The most important requirement of this semicircle is that the superior limit extend at least to the level of the brow or above. Obtaining sufficient height of the flap will help to counteract the inevitable sagging of the lateral lid margin. A corneal protector is placed over the eye, and the medial triangle is exised. The size of the medial triangle may vary with the amount of tissue that needs to be rotated to cover the lid defect. The semicircular flap is then developed and completely undermined beneath the musculocutaneous flap. Two considerations in undermining the flap are to obtain meticulous hemostasis and to avoid branches of the facial nerve. Some surgeons include a winged incision at the end of the flap to prevent tissue puckering during the closure. This can be done more conveniently after the graft has been sutured into position and the exact amount of tissue overlap is known.

Prior to rotation of the undermined tissue, a chondromucosal graft must be obtained. This will provide the supporting and mucosal components of the reconstructed lower lid (Fig. 13B). The nasal septum contains cartilage with its own mucosal backing and has been the usual site for donor material. Autogenous ear cartilage can be used because it

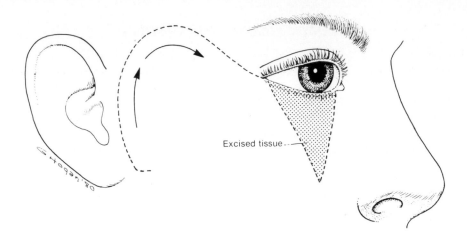

FIG. 13A: Outline of Mustarde rotational cheek flap. *Shaded area* shows excised tissue for one-stage reconstruction of lower lid.

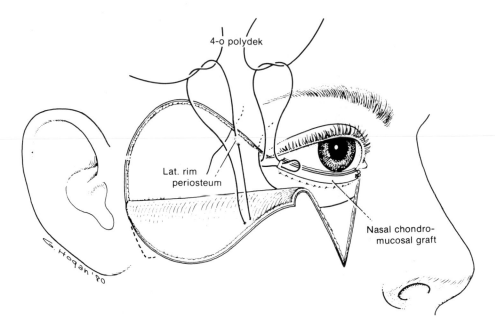

FIG. 13B: Composite drawing of Mustarde reconstruction, showing placement of nasal chondromucosal graft to lateral orbital rim and anchoring of rotated flap to external aspect of lateral orbital rim.

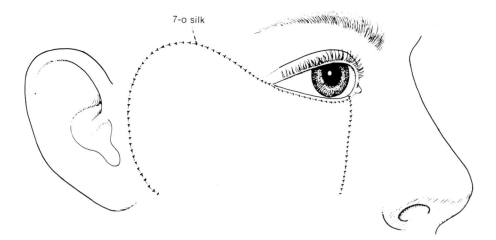

FIG. 13C: Final closure of Mustarde rotational flap.

will epithelialize over a 6-week period. Ocular irritation will be present during this epithelialization period and can be controlled with ointment.

The chondromucosal or ear cartilage graft is then placed with the mucosal surface over the inferior cornea. The inferior margin of the mucosa is sutured to the conjunctival mucosa in the inferior fornix with running 5–0 plain catgut suture. The graft is left temporarily free at the lateral and medial margins.

The rotational cheek flap is then mobilized nasally to fill the nasal triangular defect. The medial canthus is reconstructed by placing a 4–0 Polydek or Mersilene suture through the dermis of the cheek flap and anchoring to the posterior ramus of the medial canthal tendon or to the periosteum of the medial orbital rim. If the lower canaliculus has been reconstructed in the manner described in the section on canalicular defects (see below), the medial canthal suture should be placed posterior to the intubated canaliculus.

After the placement of the medial canthus, the chondromucosal graft is sutured to the posterior margin of the cheek flap at the new lid margin. Running 5–0 plain catgut suture is placed at the mucosal-epithelial border and tied externally to avoid corneal irritation. The lateral canthus is replaced by suturing the dermis of the rotational graft to the superior, inner aspect of the lateral orbital rim with lateral canthal fixation. The placement of the dermal suture should be near the lateral border of the chondral graft. Two to three additional 4–0 nonabsorbable sutures should be placed in the deep tissue of the rotational graft to apply upward traction at the apex of the flap. The skin may now be closed with 5–0 plain catgut subcuticular sutures and 7–0 silk vertical mattress skin sutures (Fig. 14C). The lateral edge of the flap can be closed with a V-to-Y configuration or a triangular excision of redundant skin. Finally, the eyelids are sutured together with a tarsorrhaphy stitch to provide additional upward tension on the flap and to evert the mucosa skin interface during the initial healing period. The tarsorrhaphy and skin sutures may be removed in 5 days.

CANALICULAR RECONSTRUCTION AND CANALICULOSTOMY: MEDIAL CANTHAL FIXATION OF THE LOWER LID

The punctum and a portion of the inferior canaliculus are often a part of the full-thickness defects of the lower lid. Reconstruction of the lower canaliculus in combination with eyelid reconstruction often obviates the need for secondary Jones tube placement for epiphora (7,8).

Rebuilding of the lower canaliculus is possible when as little as one-fourth of the original canaliculus is present (Fig. 14). The distal end of the severed canaliculus is identified. The tissue surrounding the canaliculus is undermined with Westcott scissors to allow stretching of the canaliculus. A Quickert-Dryden intubation of both canaliculi is then carried out as described in Chapter 14.

The medial eyelid margin can now be positioned. If a sliding or rotational lower eyelid flap is being employed, the cut edge of the remaining tarsal plate is sutured to the posterior reflection of the medial canthal tendon (Fig. 15). The direction of the lid margin must be toward the posterior lacrimal sac crest, behind the lacrimal sac. A suture directed toward the anterior reflection of the medial canthal tendon will result in medial ectropion and eyelid malposition.

The medial canthal suture is best carried out with a 4–0 Polydek suture on a ME-2 semicircular needle. The caruncle is first excised to allow greater accuracy in the placement of the medial canthal suture. The lacrimal sac must be retracted anteriorly, and the suture must be placed in the firm tissue posterior to the sac. It is a difficult placement. Some

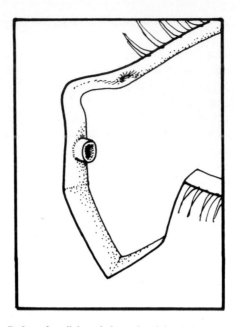

FIG. 14. Defect of medial canthal area involving inferior canaliculus.

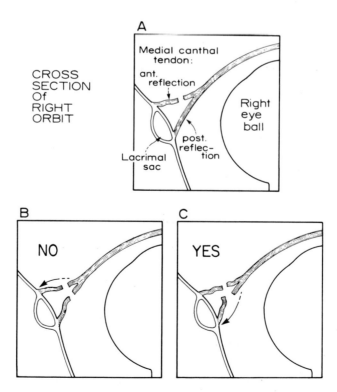

FIG. 15. Correct placement of medial canthal fixation suture. **A:** Location of posterior reflection of the medial canthal tendon behind the lacrimal sac. **B and C:** The posterior direction of the correct fixation point.

extra dissection must expose the posterior tendon, and a small half-circle needle must be used.

Following the reattachment of the medial canthal tendon, a notch on the posterior tarsal plate must be created in order to reattach the new punctum and lower canaliculus (Fig. 16). A small excision of conjunctiva and a triangular portion of tarsus will suffice for this purpose. The residual canaliculus is then stretched along its axis and sutured to the posterior border of the tarsal plate with 8–0 silk suture.

The distal ends of the silicone tubes are recovered through the nasal antrum under the inferior turbinate. The Quickert-Dryden tube ensures the patency of the newly formed punctum and canaliculus and acts as a supporting splint for the lower lid, ensuring proper direction during the healing process (Fig. 17).

After the ends of the Quickert tube in the nasal antrum are tied with a single square knot, the skin incision is closed with a running vertical mattress suture of 7–0 silk. Care

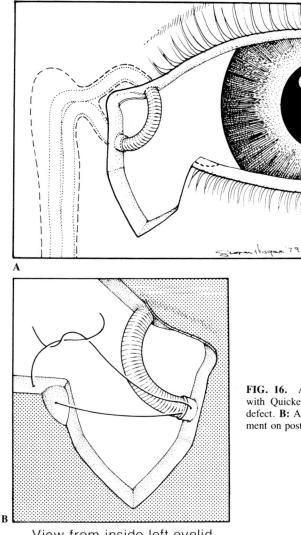

A

B

FIG. 16. A: Intubation of residual inferior canaliculus with Quickert tubing prior to closure of medial canthal defect. **B:** Advancement of inferior canaliculus and placement on posterior notch created on lower lid tarsus.

View from inside left eyelid

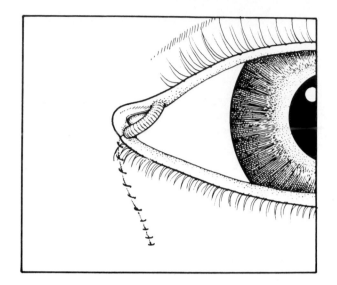

FIG. 17.   Final closure of medial canthal defect after revision of inferior canaliculus.

should be taken to align and evert the skin edges. Additional tension can be taken off the suture line, if necessary, by 4–0 silk horizontal mattress retention sutures.

Sutures are removed in 5 days, but the Quickert tube should be left in position for 3 to 6 weeks.

LATERAL CANTHAL RECONSTRUCTIVE PROCEDURES

Because lateral canthal defects often involve the upper lid as well as the lower lid, reconstruction of this area can be challenging. The order of priorities in planning the reconstruction is to provide: (a) upper lid support, (b) lower lid support, (c) lateral canthal fixation, and (d) skin covering. If possible, it is best to convert the defect into a diamond shape; this allows the greatest ease in closure (Fig. 18A).

Direct Closure of Diamond-Shaped Defect

If at least 70% of both the upper lid and lower lid margins remains, each tarsal plate can be pulled laterally to close the lateral canthal defect. A single 4–0 Polydek suture is placed through the lateral cut edge of both the upper and lower tarsal plates and sutured to the superior, inner aspect of the lateral orbital rim periosteum (see Fig. 5C).

If periosteum is not available for placement of the lateral canthal suture, two drill holes are placed 3 mm posterior to the lateral orbital rim, in the position of the lateral canthal tendon. An arm of the Polydek suture is passed through each drill hole and tied external to the rim and reforms the lateral canthal insertion.

Skin lateral to the canthus is then rotated inwardly by developing two semicircular musculo-cutaneous flaps and advancing one each for the upper lid and lower skin (Figs. 18B and 18C).

Combined Tarsal Flap with Rotational Flap

If as little as 30% of the upper lid tarsal plate is available medially (Fig. 19A), the residual tarsus can be used to provide the supporting framework for the upper lid. The

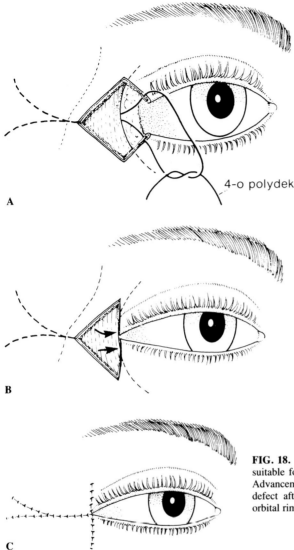

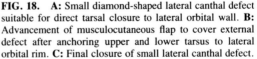

A

B

C

FIG. 18. **A:** Small diamond-shaped lateral canthal defect suitable for direct tarsal closure to lateral orbital wall. **B:** Advancement of musculocutaneous flap to cover external defect after anchoring upper and lower tarsus to lateral orbital rim. **C:** Final closure of small lateral canthal defect.

residual upper lid is everted over a Desmarres retractor or Erhardt clamp. A tarsoconjunctival flap is outlined on the tarsal conjunctiva (Points A and B in Fig. 19B). This flap is similar to the one described in the modified Hughes technique for lower lid reconstruction. It is important to leave intact at least 4 mm of the upper lid tarsal margin to prevent instability of the margin. A careful dissection between the levator aponeurosis and Müller's muscle layer is performed superiorly to the level of the superior fornix. The lateral margin of the tarsal flap is then sutured to the lateral canthus (Point D in Figs. 19C and 19D). If the periosteum of the lateral orbital rim is intact, the flap can be anchored to the periosteum in the manner previously illustrated in Fig. 5C. If the periosteum is absent, two 1-mm burr holes are placed through the lateral canthal wall immediately posterior to point D. The tarsal flap is then anchored to the holes in the orbital wall with nonabsorbable suture. The medial margin of the tarsal flap is then sutured to the lateral cut edge of the original tarsus. Point B in Fig. 19C is sutured to the upper lid margin, and Point C is sutured to

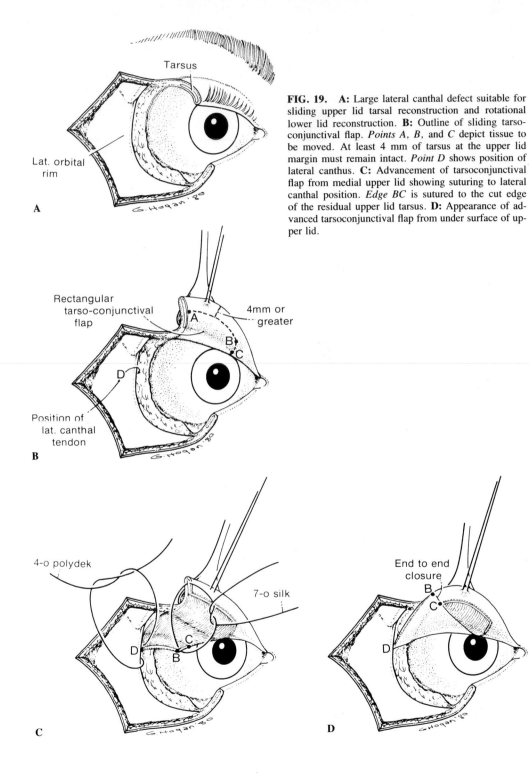

FIG. 19.   A: Large lateral canthal defect suitable for sliding upper lid tarsal reconstruction and rotational lower lid reconstruction. **B:** Outline of sliding tarso-conjunctival flap. *Points A, B,* and *C* depict tissue to be moved. At least 4 mm of tarsus at the upper lid margin must remain intact. *Point D* shows position of lateral canthus. **C:** Advancement of tarsoconjunctival flap from medial upper lid showing suturing to lateral canthal position. *Edge BC* is sutured to the cut edge of the residual upper lid tarsus. **D:** Appearance of advanced tarsoconjunctival flap from under surface of upper lid.

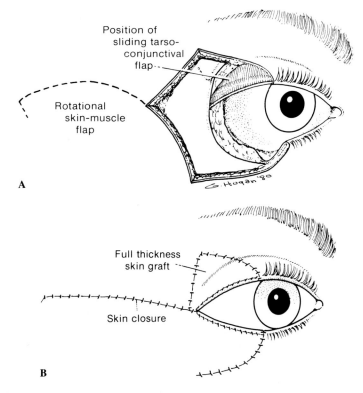

FIG. 20. A: Outline of rotational musculocutaneous flap to close lower lid defect. **B:** Final closure of lateral canthal defect showing skin graft covering upper lid tarsoconjunctival flap. Lower lid conjunctiva has been advanced to margin of lower lid rotated tissue.

the original Point A. This is a technique similar to the "sliding tarsal flap" as described in Chapter 3.

The technique of tarsal closure is the same as that described in Fig. 1. The upper lid conjunctival surface now has the configuration shown in Fig. 19D; the anterior aspect of the upper lid is shown in Fig. 20A. The lower lid and lateral canthus are next reconstructed in the manner described as the lateral rotational flap (see Figs. 5–8). If 50% or more of the original lower lid tarsus is available, additional lid support need not be provided and the rotated cheek tissue can be backed with advanced conjunctiva. If less than 50% of the lower lid tarsus is available and if lid stability is a problem, a nasal chondromucosal graft (see Chapter 1) will provide the necessary support. The skin of the lateral upper lid can also be advanced somewhat, but the residual skin defect of the upper lid can be covered with a full-thickness skin graft from retroauricular tissue (Fig. 20B).

COMPLICATIONS OF LOWER LID RECONSTRUCTION

Eyelid margin positional abnormalities are usually not a serious complication, but they can be annoying to both the patient and the surgeon. They may also require further surgery for correction. The complications of lower eyelid reconstruction include:

1. Marginal ectropion
2. Lateral tissue sag

3. Cicatricial deformity of conjunctiva
4. Upper eyelid instability
5. Corneal injury
6. Orbital hematoma

Lower Lid Ectropion

The three most common reasons for postoperative ectropion are (a) vertical shortage of eyelid skin, complicated by gravitational pull; (b) lower lid laxity with excessive horizontal length; and (c) inadequate canthal fixation.

Vertical shortage of lower lid skin is accentuated by the natural downward pull of gravity and altered lid mobility. The surgeon should not hesitate to use full-thickness skin grafting to the lower lid at the original reconstruction to ensure vertical lower lid skin adequacy. After most lower lid reconstructions, a tarsorrhaphy suture left in place a minimum of 1 week helps to counteract the natural tendency for graft shrinkage. Other authors have performed reconstructive techniques using upward advancement flaps of cheek skin to the lower eyelid defect. Descriptions of these procedures have been omitted deliberately in the chapter, because only rarely can an upward advancement be employed successfully without resulting in contracture and lower lid ectropion.

Ectropion caused by laxity of the lower lid margin may result from the use of sliding tarsoconjunctival flaps of excessive horizontal dimension. Measuring the correct length of horizontal tissue needed to fill a defect should be done with calipers, and with the lower lid stretched to approximate the desired tension on the lower lid margin. The ability of the skin to stretch and cover defects must not be underestimated.

Placement of the lateral canthal fixation suture and medial canthal fixation is an important part of any reconstruction involving the lateral lower lid. Nonabsorbable suture should be used. If the suture does not actually engage the periosteum, incompetence of the lateral canthus will result in lid laxity. Also, because the normal lateral canthal tendon exerts a pull superiorly as well as laterally and posteriorly, placement of the suture should be inside the lateral orbital rim and slightly above the midpupillary line (see Fig. 5C).

Lateral Lid Sag

Sagging of the lateral lower lid in the late postoperative course occurs for many of the same reasons as ectropion. Gravity exerts a constant downward force. When the normal lid mobility has been altered, as it is when large rotational cheek flaps have been used, the effects of gravity are magnified. Although it may be difficult to eliminate totally sagging of the lateral lower lid, several steps may reduce its likelihood. If a rotational flap technique such as the Mustarde or Tenzel miniflap is used, the apex of the semicircle must be sufficiently high to exert an exaggerated upward pull on the lateral lower lid. Nonabsorbable sutures from the repositioned flap to the temporalis fascia can augment this effect. The use of the supplemental periosteal flap and autogenous ear cartilage will augment this support.

Upper Eyelid Abnormalities

Some degree of upper eyelid retraction can occur with the modified Hughes procedure. This can be minimized by careful blunt dissection, using a moist cotton-tipped applicator, of the flap between Müller's muscle and the levator aponeurosis. At the time of separation of the flap, any advanced Müller's muscle must be tenotomized. If significant retraction occurs, it can be corrected easily with a levator recession and a spacer material implant.

Tenting with levator contraction or upper lid instability may occur if the tarsal margin has been violated. A minimum of 4 mm of intact tarsus along the margin of the upper lid is essential for upper lid stability.

Ocular Complications

Areas that appear dry during hypo- or normotensive anesthesia in the operating room may bleed when the blood pressure rises postoperatively, causing an orbital hematoma if the blood dissects retroseptally. The key to avoiding such complications is to cauterize bleeders meticulously and to maintain a respect for the potential hazards of postoperative bleeding. Tight pressure dressings should be avoided over a sighted eye, because vision may be compromised if a hematoma occurs. Patients should always be checked by the surgeon shortly after surgery to detect any problems. Ice compress dressings are safer than compression bandanges and help to prevent eyelid hematoma.

REFERENCES

1. Tenzel, R. R., and Steward, W. B. (1978): Eyelid reconstruction by semi-circular flap technique. *Trans. Am. Soc. Ophthalmol. Otolarygol.,* 85:1164–1169.
2. Hughes, W. H. (1945): Reconstruction of the lids. *Am. J. Ophthalmol.,* 28:1203–1211.
3. Hughes, W. H. (1976): Total lower lid reconstruction: Technical details. *Trans. Am. Ophthalmol. Soc.,* 74:321–329.
4. Cies, W. A., and Bartlett, R. E. (1967): Modification of the Mustarde and Hughes methods of reconstruction of the lower lid. *Ann. Ophthalmol.,* 7:1497–1501.
5. Hewes, E. H., Sullivan, J. H., and Beard, C. (1976): Lower eyelid reconstruction by tarsal transposition. *Am. J. Ophthalmol.,* 81:512–514.
6. Mustarde, J. C. (1971): *Repair and Reconstruction in the Orbital Region,* chpts. 7 and 8. Churchill, Livingston, Edinburgh.
7. Leone, C. R., Jr., and Hand, S. I., Jr. (1979): Reconstruction of the medial eyelid. *Am. J. Ophthalmol.,* 87:797–801.
8. McCord, C. D., Jr. (1980): Canalicular resection and reconstruction by canaliculostomy. *Ophthalmic Surg.,* 11:440–445.

Oculoplastic Surgery, 2nd edition, edited by
Clinton D. McCord, Jr., and Myron Tanenbaum.
Raven Press, New York © 1987.

Chapter 5

System of Repair of Full-Thickness Eyelid Defects

Clinton D. McCord, Jr.

Department of Ophthalmology, Emory University School of Medicine, Atlanta, Georgia 30308

The previous chapters described in detail the specific surgical techniques for repair of full-thickness eyelid defects in different areas. Before applying these techniques to specific defects, certain aspects of the reconstructive procedures previously described must be emphasized because of the key role they play in a successful result, regardless of the type of flap used (1–5).

CANTHAL FIXATION

Medial Canthal Fixation

Special attention was given to the canthal areas emphasizing that, in repair of the inner canthus, fixation of any flap used must be accomplished by directing the flap toward the posterior lacrimal crest, which is located posterior to the lacrimal sac. Inspection of many persons who have prominent medial canthal tendons will show that the anterior reflection of the medial canthal tendon angulates about 30 degrees more anteriorly than the normal direction of the lid contour, which is toward the posterior reflection of the tendon. A common error is to attach the edge of the tarsus of the lower lid to the anterior reflection of the medial canthal tendon, which will cause the lid to be pulled away from the globe.

Lateral Canthal Fixation

With the lateral canthal defects and with lower lid reconstruction, emphasis was also placed on proper fixation of any flap used in this area inside the lateral orbital rim where the normal insertion of the lateral canthal tendon occurs. This lateral canthal fixation is the keystone of most lower lid and lateral canthal reconstructive procedures. Fixation can be performed by suturing to the periosteum or, if the periosteum is absent, by suturing through drill holes placed in the lateral orbital rim at the location of the lateral orbital tubercle. At the lateral canthus the attachment of the eyelid must be inside the lateral orbital rim when using this lateral canthal fixation technique to assure that the lower lid will be flush with the globe in the proper contour and not separated from the globe. This avoids "lower lid sag" and retraction at the lateral canthal area, which has been seen so commonly in the past with many reconstructive techniques.

REPAIR OF LACRIMAL DRAINAGE APPARATUS

If only a small part of the canalicular system is resected in the inner canthal area, residual canaliculus may be intubated with Quickert silicone tubes and a canaliculostomy performed. This technique can be used in conjunction with any of the eyelid reconstructive procedures in that area and may spare the patient the need for a secondary Jones tube placement. If the lacrimal drainage apparatus must be excised completely, then a secondary Jones tube procedure can be performed. This is best done after healing has occurred and the canthal angle has assumed a normal configuration. It is difficult to satisfy the requirement of a normal-shaped canthal angle until healing occurs, but a normal-shaped angle is necessary for the proper placement of the Jones tube. The Jones tube placement is critical, because it must assume the proper attitude in the angle for tear drainage. Usually the Jones tube procedure is performed at a date later than the initial eyelid reconstructive procedure.

LID LAXITY

Eyelid tissue behaves differently in different individuals. Certain individuals, usually those in the older age group, have much more "strechability" of the eyelid and the defect created may be reduced to a smaller size by simple stretching. In other individuals, especially young people, the eyelid is not as lax and the defect cannot be reduced as much in size by stretching. Particularly severe examples of stiff eyelids are those eyelids that have been previously damaged by irradiation, surgery, or burns. Table 1 gives a rule of thumb for classifying defects as small, medium, or large, although each case must be individualized. In general, the rule of thumb would indicate that the defect can be reduced 10% to 15% more in an older person with laxity of tissue than in younger people with tighter lids.

TABLE 1. *Full-thickness defect size according to*
amount of laxity

	Percentage laxity	
Defect size	Young person/ tight lid	Older person/ lax lid
Small	25–35%	35–45%
Moderate	35–45%	45–55%
Large	55–Total	65–Total

FULL-THICKNESS DEFECTS OF UPPER LID

This section discusses a variety of eyelid defects and applies the techniques learned in the previous chapter to these defects.

Central

Small Defects

With small defects in the central portion of the eyelid (Fig. 1), direct closure is accomplished easily since both sides of the defect have normal tarsal tissue of equal width and may be approximated as previously described. Canthotomy and cantholysis of the upper limb of the lateral canthal tendon may be necessary. However, in older patients with more lid laxity, even more than one-third of a full-thickness eyelid defect may be closed in this manner without cantholysis.

Moderate-to-Large Defects

At the lower limits of this defect size, there are obviously some older patients with marked lid laxity whose lids can be repaired with direct closure with cantholysis. In patients with less lid laxity—young patients or patients with rigid eyelids—other techniques must be used, particularly with the larger defects. Central upper lid defects have the advantage of residual tarsal plate being present on either side of the defect. This allows for direct tarsal edge–to–tarsal edge fixation of any flap or graft that may be placed in this position. Some moderate defects of a larger size may be closed in selected cases by advancing tissue at the lateral canthus with an inverted semicircular flap, as described by Tenzel and Stewart (5). However, one should not try to exceed this flap's capability in the upper lid. A special case of central eyelid defects of the upper lid are those of the congenital coloboma, which may or may not be associated with epibulbar dermolipoma. This type of deformity in many cases can be closed directly after the edges of the coloboma have been "freshened." In most cases the repair of the coloboma is successful because the defect is not as great in actuality as it appears, because the tarsus may have "curled up" as opposed to being completely deficient.

With moderate-to-large-to-total defects, the procedure of choice is the Cutler-Beard bridge

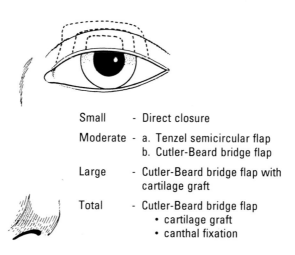

Small   - Direct closure

Moderate - a. Tenzel semicircular flap
                 b. Cutler-Beard bridge flap

Large   - Cutler-Beard bridge flap with
                 cartilage graft

Total   - Cutler-Beard bridge flap
                 • cartilage graft
                 • canthal fixation

FIG. 1.   Methods of repair of full-thickness defects in the central upper lid.

flap technique. This technique has stood the test of time for repairing these defects with an excellent functional and respectable cosmetic result. An "eyelash" graft may be performed before separation of the flap in the desired location with an eyebrow hair–bearing graft. However, the hairs that may be transplanted from the brow or scalp never assume the characteristics of normal cilia. The use of autogenous ear cartilage in conjunction with the Cutler-Beard bridge flap procedure seems to add more stability to the new upper lid in this author's experience.

With aggressive neoplastic disease, total lid defects may be encountered involving the entire upper lid and in many cases a portion of the fornix. In these cases there are no remnants of the tarsal plate left in the eyelid and no residual tissue to be stretched horizontally. The Cutler-Beard bridge flap procedure should be used. Proper medial and lateral canthal fixation of the flaps and the cartilage grafts must be obtained to ensure proper positioning of the new upper lid.

Nasal and Temporal

With smaller defects in these areas (Figs. 2, and 3) direct closure is the procedure of choice combined with the appropriate medial or lateral canthal fixation suture technique. In the moderate-sized nasal and temporal upper lid defects within the lower range of size, a particularly useful technique is the horizontally sliding tarsol-conjunctival flap to the canthus, which is then covered with a full-thickness skin graft (a one-stage procedure). With nasal upper lid defects, the edge of the tarsolconjunctival flap can be attached to the posterior reflection of the medial canthal tendon with a nonabsorbable fixation suture and covered with a full-thickness skin graft. In patients who have extremely loose upper lid skin and muscle, a sliding musculocutaneous flap or skin flap from adjacent upper lid may be stretched and used to cover this tarsolconjunctival flap in some cases as an alternative to a skin graft. The method of repair in larger upper nasal eyelid defects should be the Cutler-Beard bridge flap technique, and it may be the only one that will give an adequate result. Temporal upper lid defects may also be repaired by the sliding tarsolconjunctival flap with a full-thickness skin graft or a musculocutaneous flap, and again the tarsolconjunctival flap must be anchored at the proper point laterally with the lateral canthal fixation suture at the origin of the lateral canthal tendon. Larger defects in the upper lid in this

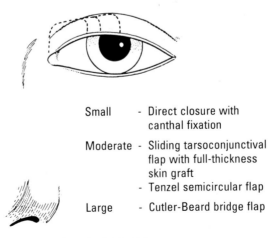

Small   - Direct closure with
            canthal fixation

Moderate - Sliding tarsoconjunctival
            flap with full-thickness
            skin graft
          - Tenzel semicircular flap

Large   - Cutler-Beard bridge flap

FIG. 2.   Methods of repair of full-thickness defects in the nasal upper lid.

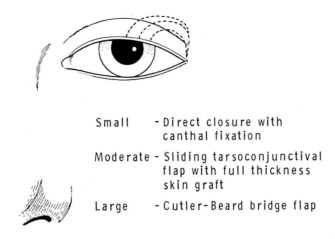

Small — Direct closure with
canthal fixation

Moderate — Sliding tarsoconjunctival
flap with full thickness
skin graft

Large — Cutler-Beard bridge flap

FIG. 3. Methods of repair of full-thickness defects in the temporal upper lid.

area usually require the Cutler-Beard bridge flap technique. Loss of lashes is much more conspicuous in the nasal portion of the upper lid; in some cases it has seemed beneficial to "convert" a nasal upper lid defect to a temporal defect by performing a lateral cantholysis and canthotomy, and sliding the lash-bearing segment of the lid nasally, and then proceeding with the repair of an upper temporal defect.

WIDE SHALLOW DEFECTS

It is not unusual to encounter a lid defect involving mainly the eyelid margin with little vertical involvement of the eyelid (Fig. 4). These shallow defects may occur posttraumatically or in many cases with a "sliding" epithelial neoplastic process. At first glance one may tend to minimize the importance of this defect, but one must recognize that the margin is

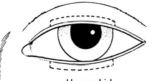

Upper Lid
a) Bridge flap
b) Nasal chondromucosal
graft with musculocutaneous
advancement
c) Pedicle flap from lower lid
d) Composite grafts

Lower Lid
a) Semicircular flap
with inferior relaxing
incision (Reese)
b) Hughes procedure
c) Hewes procedure (for lateral defects)
d) Composite grafts

FIG. 4. Methods of repair of shallow defects or defects confined to the eyelid margin.

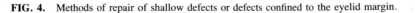

the most important portion of the eyelid with relationship to the preservation of corneal integrity and comfort. The surgeon may be resistent to employing a major reconstructive procedure to repair these shallow defects because in some cases, in order to implement the repair, large amounts of normal tissue may have to be sacrificed or rearranged. If a lesser procedure can be employed to repair the margin, it should be used; however, no shortcuts should be employed that would result in anything less than a completely healthy eyelid margin because of the severe corneal complications that might occur. In most cases one must resort to a full bridge flap from the lower lid to supply the necessary tissue to reconstruct a healthy lid margin in broad, shallow upper lid defects. A possible alternative would be a free nasal chondromucosal graft to this area; however, the graft must be backed by a vertically advanced musculocutaneous flap from the upper lid, which can only be accomplished if there is skin-muscle laxity in the upper lid (in older patients in most cases). Shallow margin defects can be repaired by composite grafts or pedicle margin grafts which will contain lashes.

FULL-THICKNESS DEFECTS OF LOWER LID

Central

Small defects are closed with direct closure (Fig. 5). In the lower lid, some defects at the lower range of moderate size may be repaired by direct closure in patients with extremely lax lids. Central lid defects again have the advantage of residual tarsal plate being present on both sides of the defect, allowing closure to be more precise with normal restoration of the margin. With most moderate-sized defects, the ideal procedure in the lower lid is the semicircular flap, as described by Tenzel and Stewart (5), which can produce excellent results. One must not be tempted to stretch its use too far to the upper range of this size defect. The next procedure of choice with the larger defects would be the modified Hughes procedure. The disadvantage of the Hughes procedure (a two-stage procedure) is in most cases negated by the excellent result, which produces a normal-appearing lid with normal movement.

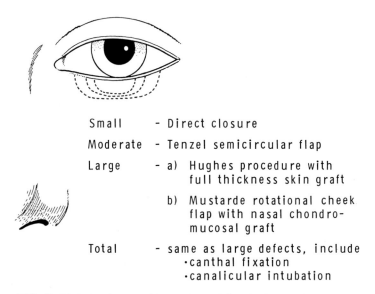

Small   – Direct closure

Moderate   – Tenzel semicircular flap

Large   – a) Hughes procedure with
                    full thickness skin graft

               b) Mustarde rotational cheek
                   flap with nasal chondro-
                   mucosal graft

Total   – same as large defects, include
                    •canthal fixation
                    •canalicular intubation

FIG. 5 Methods of repair of full-thickness defects in the central lower lid.

Some broad, shallow defects in the lower lid margin can be repaired with a horizontally sliding flap that employs the principle of the Tenzel semicircular flap but also includes an inferior relaxing incision as well. This can be used quite successfully if these shallow defects are not too wide (6). In the more extensive broad, shallow defects of the lower lid, one must use a Hughes two-stage procedure to adequately repair this area (see Fig. 7). It does not seem justifiable to excise the extensive amounts of normal lid and cheek tissue that would be necessary to utilize a Mustarde rotational cheek flap for this type of defect (7). The Mustarde rotational cheek flap, however, can be used as an alternative for large lower lid defects in patients who are not willing to tolerate a two-stage procedure or who are poor anesthetic risks.

Repair of total lower lid defects requires canalicular intubation, if possible, together with canthal fixation of the reconstructive flaps.

Nasal

The same reconstructive procedures used for central lower lid defects are available for nasal defects (Fig. 6). However, additional consideration is needed in the medial canthal area for proper fixation of the flaps with use of medial canthal fixation sutures. Canalicular intubation must also be considered in defects in this area.

Lateral

The central theme of repair of lateral canthal defects in the lower lid is the use of the lateral canthal fixation suture regardless of whether the defects are small, moderate, or large. Direct closure, the Tenzel semicircular flap, the Hewes procedure, or the modified Hughes procedure is used for defects of a progressively increasing order of magnitude (Fig. 7).

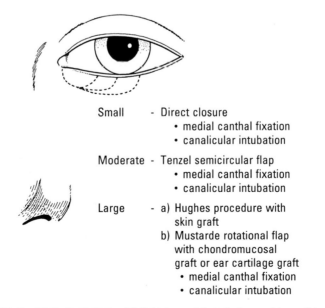

Small   - Direct closure
      • medial canthal fixation
      • canalicular intubation

Moderate - Tenzel semicircular flap
      • medial canthal fixation
      • canalicular intubation

Large   - a) Hughes procedure with
      skin graft
     b) Mustarde rotational flap
     with chondromucosal
     graft or ear cartilage graft
      • medial canthal fixation
      • canalicular intubation

FIG. 6. Methods of repair of full-thickness defects in the nasal lower lid.

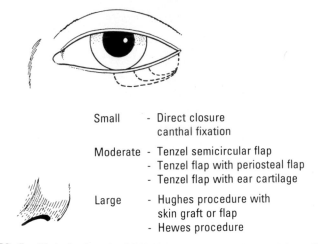

Small	- Direct closure canthal fixation
Moderate	- Tenzel semicircular flap - Tenzel flap with periosteal flap - Tenzel flap with ear cartilage
Large	- Hughes procedure with skin graft or flap - Hewes procedure

FIG. 7. Methods of repair of full-thickness defects in the lateral lower lid.

TOTAL CANTHAL DEFECTS

Total canthal defects in most cases can be considered as a combination of upper and lower lid defects and reconstructed as described in the preceding chapters. In the canthal angles the importance of proper fixation of the flaps to the inner canthal area has been emphasized. In larger resections with removal of bone for neoplastic disease, fixation to the canthal tendon medially or laterally may be impossible because of the absence of bone. In the medial canthal area, in these cases, one may consider the passage of transnasal wires nasally to facilitate fixation of the flap in the proper position. Fixation at the lateral canthus may be obtained with drill holes in the bone or, if the bony wall is absent, may be made to the temporalis muscle.

COMBINED DEFECTS

In many clinical situations a large canthal defect may occur in conjunction with a large defect of the upper and/or lower lid. Combinations of the previously described techniques must be employed to repair these large defects satisfactorily.

Inner Canthus and Upper Lid Defects

In this difficult defect (Fig. 8), the lower lid canthal defect is first closed by advancement of the lower lid with medial canthal fixation. A Cutler-Beard bridge flap procedure is then used as if the lower lid were intact. A flap from the lower lid is brought into the upper lid defect, implanting ear cartilage between the conjunctiva and the musculocutaneous layer of the flap from the lower lid. In this special situation, adequate lower lid margin must be left intact to preserve its integrity because the lid has already been compromised. The lower lid tarsus should not be included in the flap, and this is accomplished by making the horizontal incision across the lower lid at the exact inferior border of the tarsus. The implanted cartilage graft within the flap to the upper lid must be fixed nasally with proper canthal fixation. Any residual canthal skin defect may be covered with a small full-thickness skin graft or a small glabellar flap, or be allowed to granulate.

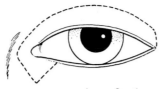

Inner Canthus and Upper Lid

Steps:
1. Advancement of lower lid

2. Bridge flap with autogenous
   ear cartilage graft

3. a) Small glabellar flap
   b) Full skin graft
   c) Granulation

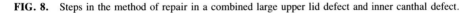

FIG. 8. Steps in the method of repair in a combined large upper lid defect and inner canthal defect.

Outer Canthus and Upper Lid Defects

Again, for upper lid defects (Fig. 9) the Cutler-Beard bridge flap procedure used as if the lower lid were intact is necessary for repair of the upper lid defect, and lateral canthal fixation of the cartilage used is necessary. A Tenzel semicircular flap can then be rotated into the lower lateral canthal defect and attached to the "lower eyelid bridge" portion of the lower eyelid margin. Proper lateral canthal fixation of this semicircular flap repairing the lower lid and canthal defect must be obtained. In smaller defects, the temporal edge of the lower eyelid "bridge" may be attached diectly with lateral canthal fixation.

Inner Canthus and Lower Lid

Large lower lid and inner canthal defects (Fig. 10) can be repaired well with the modified Hughes procedure in which the tarsoconjunctival flap is brought into the lower lid defect and then stretched nasally and attached to the inner canthal area with medial canthal fixation. A full-thickness skin graft can then be used to cover the flap to the lower lid and also to

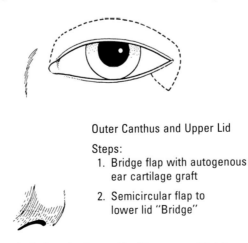

Outer Canthus and Upper Lid

Steps:
1. Bridge flap with autogenous
   ear cartilage graft

2. Semicircular flap to
   lower lid "Bridge"

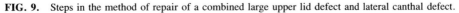

FIG. 9. Steps in the method of repair of a combined large upper lid defect and lateral canthal defect.

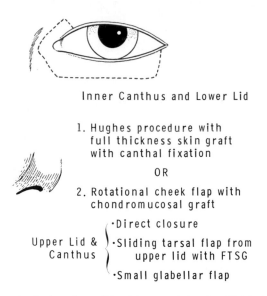

Inner Canthus and Lower Lid

1. Hughes procedure with
   full thickness skin graft
   with canthal fixation

OR

2. Rotational cheek flap with
   chondromucosal graft

Upper Lid & ·Direct closure
Canthus   ·Sliding tarsal flap from
                upper lid with FTSG
            ·Small glabellar flap

FIG. 10.   Methods of repair of a large lower lid and inner canthal defect. FTSG, full-thickness skin graft.

cover defects in the inner canthal area. A very acceptable alternative for large lower lid defects involving particularly the inner canthal area is the Mustarde rotational cheek flap with the chondromucosal graft. The situation in which the Mustarde rotational cheek flap seems to be best used is when the lower lid defects are confined mainly to or in combination with inner canthal defects. The vertical suture line that extends on the facial area following this type of rotational flap falls in a more normal orientation when the defects are located in this area and produces the least amount of scarring. The portion of the defect that extends into the upper lid may be repaired by a direct advancement of the upper lid or, in larger defects, a sliding tarsolconjunctival flap with a full-thickness skin graft may be used. In some cases a small glabellar flap could be rotated into the upper canthal defect area or simple granulation may provide filling of the defect over a period of time.

Outer Canthus and Lower Lid Defects

For large defects in the lower lid including the outer canthus, this author has had the best results with the modified Hughes tarsolconjunctival flap that is brought into the lower lid defect and then brought laterally and fixed inside the lateral orbital rim (Fig. 11). A full-thickness skin graft is then applied over the flap and the defect at the lateral canthus and lower lid. A small Tenzel-type semicircular flap at the lateral canthus may be used to supplement closure in that area.

PROBLEM CASES

From time to time the ophthalmic surgeon will encounter a total eyelid defect with an inability to share the opposing eyelid tissue because it has been previously reconstructed or damaged in some way by trauma or by irradiation and is unsuitable to use in a lid-sharing procedure. In some rare injuries or defects, both eyelids may be unuseable. Another problem, in addition to the absence of the opposing eyelid, is the absence of adjacent

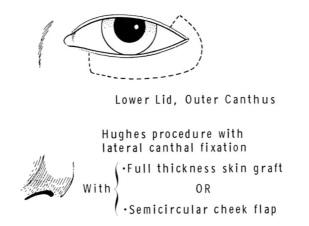

Lower Lid, Outer Canthus

Hughes procedure with
lateral canthal fixation

With { •Full thickness skin graft

OR

•Semicircular cheek flap

FIG. 11. Methods of repair of a large lower lid and outer canthal defect.

tissue in the cheek area that may be rotated; this is a particular problem in the lower lid. In these problem cases, one's priority must be to protect the eye and secondarily to introduce appropriate tissue into the area to prepare the foundation for formation of a new eyelid. Any tissue that will cover the surface of the globe must be lined with mucous membrane whose epithelial layer faces the cornea. This mucous membrane must be covered in most cases with a flap of thicker skin or muscle that can be brought in from a peripheral area. The most readily available vascularized skin flap is the median forehead flap or temporal forehead flap, as described in Chapter 3. If upper and lower forniceal conjunctiva is present, it can be dissected free from either the upper or lower or both forniceal areas to form the lining for the flap. If conjunctival remnants are not present, then one must utilize a free graft of buccal mucous membrane or nasal chondromucosal mucous membrane to line the inner surface of the flap, and one must accept the tenuous nature of a free graft lining the inner surface of a primary flap. In a similar situation in the lower lid a flap from the nasolabial area based nasally may be rotated upward to the lower lid. Full-thickness skin grafts may be needed to cover the donor site. The general surgeon may rarely encounter the need for this type of procedure; however, knowledge of the technique may be useful in extreme situations.

REFERENCES

1. Leone, C. R., Jr., and Hand, S. I., Jr. (1979): Reconstruction of the medial eyelid. *Am. J. Ophthalmol.*, 87:797–801.
2. Hewes, E. H., Sullivan, J. H., and Beard, C. (1976): Lower eyelid reconstruction by transposition. *Am. J. Ophthalmol.*, 81:512–514.
3. Hecht, S. D. (1970): An upside down Cutler Beard bridge flap. *Arch. Ophthalmol.*, 84:760–764.
4. Cies, A. W., and Bartlett, R. E. (1975): Modification of the Mustarde and Hughes methods of reconstruction of the lower lid. *Ann. Ophthalmol.*, 7:1497–1501.
5. Tenzel, R. R., and Steward, W. B. (1978): Eyelid reconstruction by semi-circular flap technique. *Trans. Am. Ophthalmol. Soc.*, 85:1164–1169.
6. Reese, A. B. (1976): Epithelial tumors of the lid, conjunctiva, cornea, and lacrimal sac. In: *Tumors of the Eye*, 3rd ed. p. 50. Harper & Row, New York.
7. Mustarde, J. C. (1979): *Repair and Reconstruction in the Orbital Region*, Chpts. 7–9. Churchill/Livingston, Edinburgh.

Oculoplastic Surgery, 2nd edition, edited by
Clinton D. McCord, Jr., and Myron Tanenbaum.
Raven Press, New York © 1987.

Chapter 6

Acute Orbital Trauma: Diagnosis and Management

*Arthur S. Grove, Jr. and **Clinton, D. McCord, Jr.

*Department of Ophthalmology, Harvard Medical School, and Massachusetts Eye and Ear Infirmary,
Boston, Massachusetts 02114; and **Department of Ophthalmology, Emory University School of
Medicine, Atlanta, Georgia 30308*

Orbital trauma can damage soft tissues, embed foreign bodies, and cause fractures. Soft tissue injuries may involve the eye as well as any other structures within the orbit. Foreign bodies may be extremely difficult to detect and localize, particularly if they are not radiopaque. Fractures of the orbit may be extensive and may involve the midfacial skeleton and the skull. Orbital injuries may be associated with damage to the brain, the paranasal sinuses, or the nasolacrimal pathways. Carotid cavernous sinus (CCS) fistulas and cerebrospinal fluid (CSF) leaks may be associated with orbital trauma and with fractures that involve the base of the skull (1).

An orderly sequence of diagnostic steps, including a careful history and physical examination, should be used to evaluate a patient who has sustained orbital trauma. Most of the basic principles of orbital examination and the diagnostic techniques available to study patients who suffer orbital trauma are described in Chapter 10.

GENERAL PRINCIPLES OF ORBITAL TRAUMA DIAGNOSIS

History and Physical Examination

In most cases ocular or orbital abnormalities occur shortly after the trauma that caused them. However, some traumatic abnormalities first appear long after the injury has occurred and been forgotten. Therefore, even in the absence of recent trauma, a patient with an orbital disorder should be questioned about past injuries that may have produced chronic abnormalities such as CCS fistulas or blood cysts. Foreign bodies may lie dormant for years before they cause an abscess or bony erosion. Fractures may produce enophthalmos, which mimics contralateral exophthalmos (pseudoexophthalmos).

A detailed ocular examination should include measurement of visual acuities and intraocular pressures. Anterior segment and fundus details should be evaluated. Neurological and orbital examinations should be performed to determine eye movements, pupil reactions, sensory abnormalities, and positions of the eyes. Photographs and sketches are useful to document clinical features for future reference.

Diagnostic Studies

The most valuable diagnostic studies for the evaluation of patients who have sustained orbital trauma are plain and tomographic X-rays and computed tomographic (CT) scans, Ultrasonography is useful for the evaluation of intraocular injuries, especially when direct visualization of the fundus is prevented by hemorrhage or lens opacity. However, ultrasonography is not as useful as radiographic studies or CT scans for the evaluation of extraocular trauma (1–4). On occasion, other diagnostic studies such as metrizamide CT scans or arteriograms may provide useful information about the presence of CCS fistulas or the location of CSF leaks (1,5).

MANAGEMENT OF ORBITAL TRAUMA

Soft Tissue Injuries

Hemorrhage into the orbital soft tissues may cause exophthalmos and limited movements of the eye and eyelids. In adults the posterior surface of the globe is usually less than 20 mm from the optic foramen, whereas the orbital segment of the optic nerve is approximately 25 mm long. Therefore, exophthalmos may occur without damaging the optic nerve by stretching. Drainage or aspiration of an orbital hemorrhage is seldom necessary, unless visual function is compromised by compression of the optic nerve or the globe. Extravasated blood usually resorbs, although a chronic blood cyst may sometimes form and require surgical removal.

Optic neuropathy may sometimes result from direct injury (contusion of the nerve), from secondary vascular ischemia, or from damage caused by foreign bodies or bone fragments. Generally speaking, if the loss is very abrupt and simultaneous with the accident itself, there is irreversible nerve damage because of contusion or avulsion of the nerve, and chances for recovery of vision are slim (6,7). The patients who initially have fairly good vision but whose vision diminishes over intervening time are those with salvageable vision. The nerve is usually compromised by intraorbital or nerve sheath edema and a medical treatment of this edema in many cases suffices. A ''medical decompression'' with high-dose intravenous steroids (10 mg Decadron i.v. q. 6 hr) many times can dramatically reverse this situation. In all of these cases CT scans (axial and coronal views) should be obtained to visualize the anatomy of the orbit and rule out an optic nerve sheath hematoma, which may require a surgical sheath decompression. In some cases if the vision deteriorates even in the presence of high-dose steroids and significant edema is present, some decompressive procedure, including unroofing the bony optic canal (8,9), can be tried; this has given restoration of vision in some patients.

Limited movement of the extraocular muscles (Fig. 1) or levator can be caused by either soft tissue injury to nerves or muscles alone, or by mechanical restriction associated with orbital fractures. It is important to distinguish between neuromuscular injury, which often improves spontaneously, and mechanical restriction associated with fractures, which may require surgical exploration. Fortunately, many orbital fractures do not mechanically restrict eye movements or cause significant cosmetic facial deformity and therefore do not require surgical intervention.

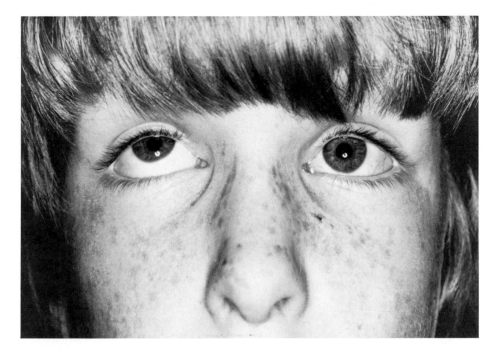

FIG. 1. Blowout fracture of left orbital floor, with limited elevation of left eye in upgaze.

Many patients whose eye movements are limited in both horizontal and vertical gaze will have spontaneous improvement to at least some movement. Limitation of eye movements chiefly in upgaze and downgaze is more likely to be the result of mechanical restriction of movement of the inferior rectus muscle and possibly of the inferior oblique muscle. The forced traction test is useful to determine if eye movements are mechanically restricted. It must be remembered that mechanical restriction with a positive forced traction test can occur with a hematoma of the extraocular muscle sheath, or marked orbital edema, in addition to frank entrapment·of orbital tissues. Four percent cocaine on a cotton pledget may be applied to the inferior surface of the globe and allowed to remain in place for several minutes. The insertion of the inferior rectus muscle is then firmly grasped and the globe is moved up and down by the examiner. Restriction of such passive movements suggests that the muscle is mechanically bound by direct entrapment within a fracture, by connective tissue septa between a muscle and the fracture, or by secondary adhesions.

Decreased sensation in the distribution of the infraorbital nerve is common in patients who suffer fractures of the orbital floor. This numbness may involve the lower eyelid, the cheek, the palate, and the upper lip, but usually improves spontaneously.

Nasolacrimal obstructions may result from fractures of the medial orbit or nose. Lacrimal sac mucoceles, dacryocystitis, and epiphora can result from such obstructions and may require dacryocystorhinostomy to reestablish tear drainage into the nose. Medial orbital trauma may also disrupt attachments of the medial canthal tedon and cause displacement of the medial canthus and eyelids. Orbital emphysema and epistaxis are frequent sequelae of medial orbital fractures because of injury to the ethmoid sinus.

Frontal sinus mucoceles may result from fractures that involve the frontal bones, the orbital walls, and the nose. The frontal sinuses normally drain into the nasal cavities by the nasofrontal duct. If this duct is lacerated or obstructed so that it cannot be repaired, it may be necessary to obliterate the sinus with adipose tissue. Such an obliteration may be performed by an osteoplastic approach as recommended for the treatment of frontal sinus mucoceles (10,11).

CCS fistulas sometimes result from tears in the wall of the segment of the internal carotid artery that lies within the cavernous sinus. These injuries are usually associated with basal skull fractures. A bruit is usually heard when such a fistula is present. Dilated, tortuous vessels are usually seen on the surface of the eye (Fig. 2). CT scans with contrast enhancement and carotid arteriograms (Fig. 3) may visualize these vascular communications with minimal risk to the patient. Fine anatomic details of these vessels can be seen by using positive contrast arteriography with selective injections and radiographic subtraction.

CSF leaks into the nose (rhinorrhea) sometimes occur after severe midfacial trauma. Such leaks should be suspected if the patient notes the drainage of clear fluid from the nose or frequently swallows when recumbent. Fluorescein dye may be injected by lumbar puncture to determine if CSF is leaking into the nose. Metrizamide has also been injected by lumbar puncture so that radioactivity can be detected by nasal pledgets or followed by CT scanning.

Orbital Foreign Bodies

The detection, localization, and removal of foreign bodies from the orbit is often extremely difficult. Although bone details are usually adequately seen with conventional X-rays, these are of little value in the detailed study of soft tissues and low-density foreign bodies such as plastic, glass, or wood. Even radiopaque foreign bodies are sometimes difficult to accurately

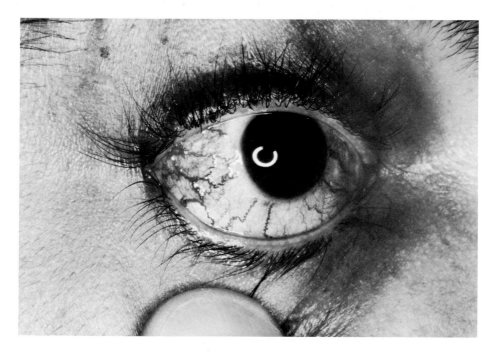

FIG. 2. Carotid cavernous sinus (CCS) fistula causes dilated, tortous episcleral vessels.

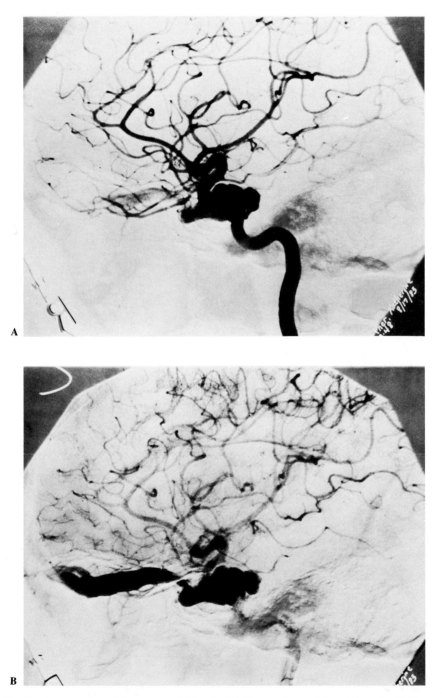

FIG. 3. Arteriogram of carotid cavernous fistula: **A:** Arteriogram demonstrates contrast dye in the cavernous sinus following injection of dye through the internal carotid artery. **B:** Later phase in arteriogram shows filling of cavernous sinus and a markedly enlarged superior ophthalmic vein. (Courtesy of Robert H. Spector, M.D.)

localize with X-rays unless mathematical computations or devices such as contact lenses are used (1). By using X-rays alone it may be impossible to determine the position of foreign bodies in reference to the globe, the optic nerve, or the extraocular muscles.

CT scans visualize most soft tissue, bone details, and foreign bodies regardless of their density. Accurate foreign body localization as well as fracture evaluation by CT scanning can be most effectively achieved by using narrow density windows and three-dimensional tomography with both axial (CAT) and coronal (CCT) sancs (Fig. 4). To rule out the

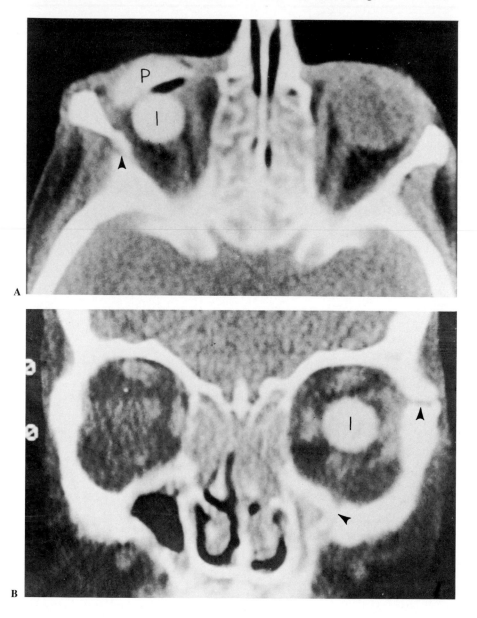

FIG. 4. Plastic foreign bodies and fractures localized by three-dimensional CT scanning. **A:** Axial (CAT) scan shows enucleation implant (I), prosthesis (P), and fracture (*arrow*) of lateral orbital wall. **B:** Coronal (CCT) scan shows enucleation implant (I) surrounded by rectus muscles. Fractures (*arrows*) are present in floor and lateral wall of left orbit.

possibility of an intraorbital wooden foreign body one must specifically request that the CT scanner view the orbit in the ''measure mode'' or ''narrow window,'' which will show up densities of material between that of soft tissue and bone. Many wooden foreign bodies have been missed because of failure to employ this scanning technique (see Fig. 5). The capabilities of magnetic resonance imaging (MRI) in the detection of intraorbital foreign bodies has yet to be determined.

Clinically, it is very important to maintain a high index of suspicion that a foreign body may be embedded within the orbit after a penetrating wound has occurred. Wooden

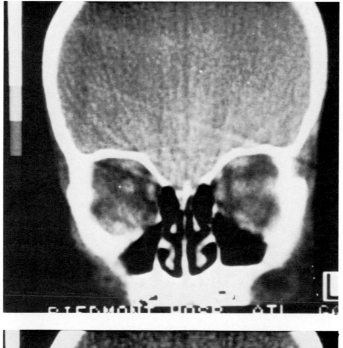

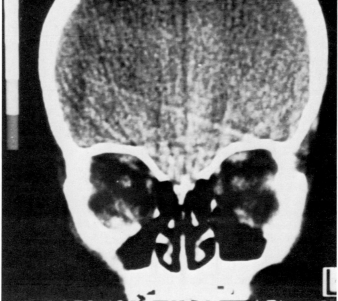

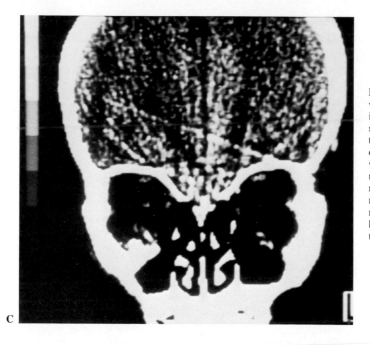

FIG. 5. CT scans of intraorbital wooden foreign body demonstrating the sensitivity of narrow-density windows. **A:** Standard sensitivity coronal CT scan of orbits cannot clearly identify intraorbital wooden foreign body. **B:** A more narrow-density window CT scan reveals the foreign body in the right inferior orbit. **C:** Very narrow-density windows strikingly highlight the presence of the intraorbital wooden foreign body.

objects may lacerate the eyelid or the conjunctiva and appear to be completely withdrawn from the point of entry. However, portions of these objects may remain buried within the orbit and may be initially asymptomatic. Vegetable matter foreign bodies, such as wood fragments, may cause chronic abscesses that drain to the skin surface through a fistula. By surgically following such a fistula tract, these fragments may sometimes be reached and removed even from remote areas of the orbit. The most likely position of an embedded foreign body may sometimes be predicted by reconstructing the direction of entry into the orbit and then approaching the orbital wall that lies opposite to the original wound.

When a foreign body has entered the orbit, general principles of management include culturing the wound or culturing the foreign body if it is removed and administering systemic antibiotics. Foreign objects should usually be removed if they are composed of vegetable matter, if they are anterior in the orbit, or if they have sharp edges. Objects may sometimes be safely left in place if they are inert, if they are in the posterior orbit, or if they have relatively smooth surfaces.

Orbital Fractures

Most fractures of the middle segment of the face involve at least a portion of the orbit (12). These midfacial fractures may be classified into the following categories: (a) Le Fort fractures, (b) zygomatic fractures, (c) orbital apex fractures, (d) orbital roof fractures, (e) medial orbital fractures, and (f) orbital floor fractures. Some of the soft tissue injuries that may be associated with these fractures have already been discussed.

Le Fort Fractures

Le Fort fractures involve the maxilla and can be divided into three categories. Le Fort I (Guérin) fractures are low transverse maxillary fractures that do not involve the orbit.

Le Fort II fractures are pyramidal fractures that involve the maxilla, the nasal bones, and the medial orbital floors (Fig. 6). Le Fort III fractures are complex fractures that extensively involve both orbits to produce separation of the maxilla from the skull (craniofacial dysfunction or free-floating maxilla). These fractures are often complex and asymmetric, with more damage to one side of the face than the other. Treatment of these maxillary fractures may require reduction of displaced bone fragments with fixation and dental stabilization. Severe Le Fort fractures are frequently associated with skull fractures and intracranial injuries that require neurosurgical treatment (13).

Zygomatic Fractures

The zygoma (cheekbone or malar bone) forms a significant portion of the floor and the lateral wall of the orbit. The zygoma is composed of an arch, which extends laterally over the temporalis muscle to articulate with the temporal bone, and a body, which produces the prominence of the cheek. Zygomatic fractures may involve the arch alone, without extension into the orbit. If a zygomatic fracture involves the body, it is sometimes termed a tripod fracture since breaks almost always occur in three locations: the zygomatic arch, the lateral orbital rim, and the inferior orbital rim. If the bones are not significantly depressed or rotated, no reduction or fixation may be required. Simple fractures that produce a cosmetic deformity or limit jaw motion may sometimes be treated by reduction without fixation. Some fractures require both reduction and open fixation by wires, suspension, or packing (13,14). In some cases it may be appropriate to repair the orbital floor if the bones are severely comminuted. It is uncommon for extraocular muscle entrapment to occur with zygomatic fractures.

Orbital Apex Fractures

Fractures of the orbital apex usually occur in association with other fractures of the face, orbit, or skull. Le Fort fractures may extend posteriorly to the orbital apex, and complex zygomatic fractures may extend medially through the sphenoid wings. Orbital apex fractures may encroach upon the optic canal and the base of the skull with damage to the optic nerves or production of CCS fistulas or CSF leaks. When visual acuity is decreased in patients with orbital fractures and with no significant intraocular injury, involvement of the orbital apex and optic canal should be suspected.

Orbital Roof Fractures

An orbital roof fracture is a potentially life-threatening condition (15). Priority is directed toward evaluation for intracranial injury, specifically brain injury, an intracranial foreign body, intracranial air (pneumocephalus), or a dural tear with CSF leakage (16). Neurosurgical consultation is required in those emergency situations where intracranial complications result from orbital roof fractures. Beyond the primary injury, the development of meningitis or brain abscesses is the major risk in many of these cases. The neurosurgical management of these complicated cases is beyond the scope of this text, but the interested reader may refer to the reference list (17–20). It should be noted that CSF leakage following closed head trauma has a very high rate of spontaneous cessation.

Beyond the intracranial complications, the oculoplastic surgeon must be ready to deal with numerous other problems. Orbital roof fractures can involve the frontal sinus or nasofron-

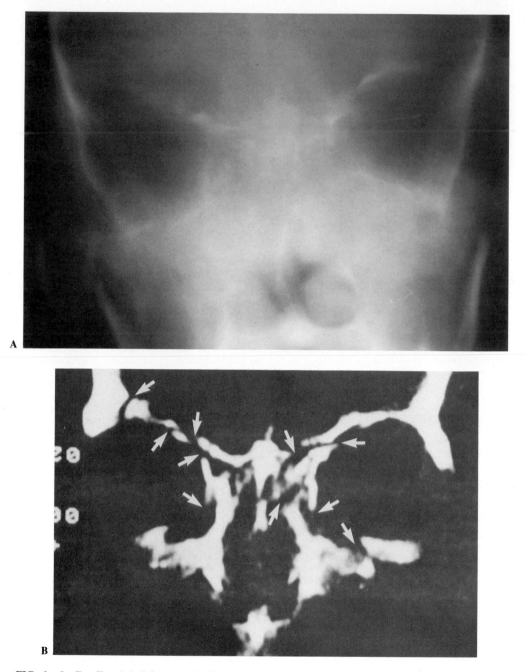

FIG. 6.   Le Fort II and skull fractures. **A:** Hypocycloidal tomographic X-ray (Polytome) demonstrates obscured bone features as a result of multiple fractures of both orbits and skull. **B:** CAT scan with narrow-density window demonstrates multiple fractures (*arrows*) more clearly than X-rays.

tal duct. Sinus obliteration may be considered at the time of initial surgical repair in order to avoid the delayed-onset complication of frontal sinus mucoceles (10,11). Rarely repair of large orbital roof defects may be necessary in the presence of significant exophthalmos secondary to orbital herniation of the anterior cerebrum.

These large orbital roof defects are frequently contiguous with a frontal sinus fracture. With an exposed sinus the risk of infection is increased; therefore, thin autogenous bone grafts should be used to repair the defect rather than alloplastic materials.

It may be necessary to reduce displaced bone fragments that mechanically restrict the superior rectus muscle or impinge on the levator muscle. With blunt trauma, it should be remembered that there are other, more common causes of extraocular muscle imbalance and ptosis. In the absence of significant displaced bony fragments, extraocular muscle surgery and ptosis repair are generally delayed for 6 months following trauma.

Medial Orbital Fractures

Medial orbital fractures are usually the result of direct trauma to the nose or to the medial orbital rim. Such direct fractures may involve the frontal process of the maxilla, the ethmoid labyrinth (including the lamina papyracea, or paper plate), and the lacrimal bone (21). Medial orbital direct fractures may damage the lacrimal sac or nasolacrimal duct to cause epiphora or a lacrimal sac mucocele. Cosmetic deformity may be produced by damage to the nose or displacement of the medial canthus and eyelids (22).

Indirect, or blowout fractures are those in which the orbital rims are intact and only the bony wall is fractured. The mechanism of most blowout fractures is believed to be the hydraulic transmission of forces produced by a blow to the globe or eyelids (23). Since the lamina papyracea is one of the thinnest surfaces of the orbit, this portion of the medial wall is frequently fractured by such injuries. In many patients, medial orbital blowout fractures produce few consequences and may be overlooked. Epistaxis and orbital emphysema may occur but are usually self-limited and do not require treatment except to avoid blowing the nose. Occasionally, movement of the medial rectus muscle may be mechanically restricted by a medial orbital fracture and may require surgical exploration. Prolapse of orbital fat and other tissues into the ethmoid sinus may play a role in the production of enophthalmos in some patients (Fig. 7).

Orbital Floor Fractures

Orbital floor fractures may also be either direct or indirect, depending upon whether or not the orbital rims are fractured. Direct fractures of the floor are those that involve the inferior orbital rim. Since much of the inferior orbital rim is a part of the zygoma, these injuries are usually classified as zygomatic fractures. Although the floor may have to be repaired in some severe zygomatic fractures, it is unusual for true entrapment of the extraocular muscles to occur with such injuries.

Indirect, or blowout, fractures, as previously explained, are those in which the inferior orbital rim is intact and the bony injury usually results from hydraulically transmitted forces (23). In most instances the injury is due to a sudden increase in intraorbital pressure applied by a nonpenetrating object such as a fist or a ball (13,24).

Orbital X-rays often demonstrate defects in the orbital bones and soft tissues (Fig. 8). Tomographic X-rays usually provide increased details of bone distortion (see Fig. 9). Computed tomographic scans, particularly CCT scans, are valuable because they demonstrate

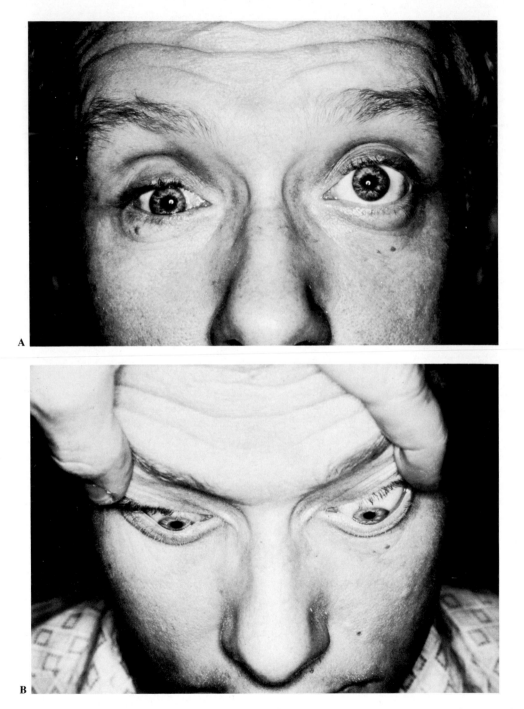

FIG. 7. Blowout fractures of medial wall and floor of right orbit. **A:** Ptosis of right eye (drop of eye toward maxillary sinus). **B:** Enophthalmos of right eye.

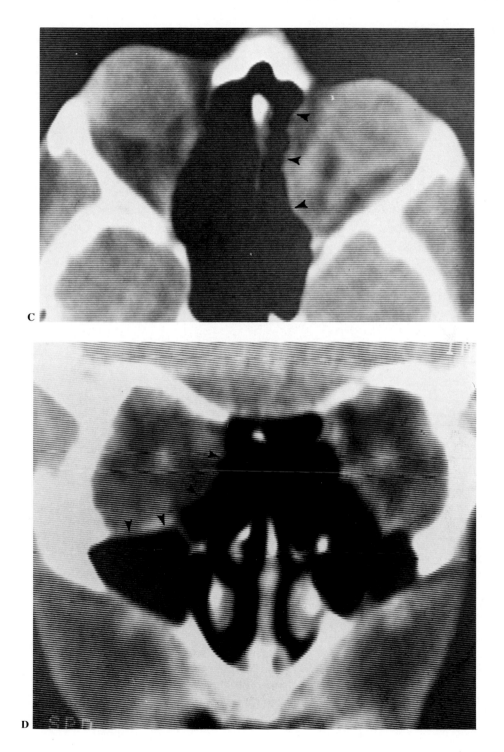

FIG. 7. (*cont.*)   **C:** CAT scan shows displacement of medial wall (*arrows*) of right orbit with enophthalmos.
D: CCT scan shows displacement of medial wall and floor (*arrows*) of right orbit.

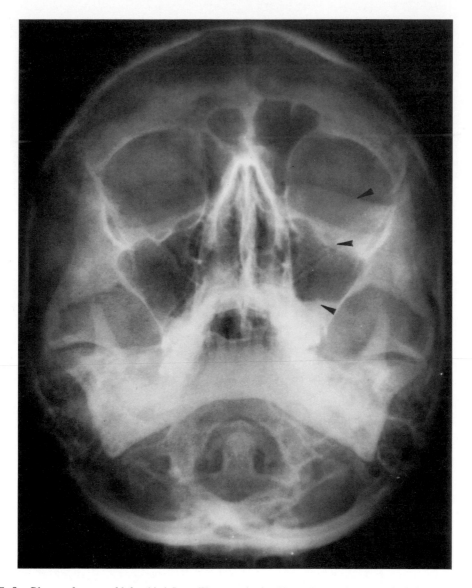

FIG. 8. Blowout fracture of left orbital floor. Waters projection X-ray shows edematous cheek (*upper arrow*), depressed orbital floor (*middle arrow*), and air-fluid level (*lower arrow*) in maxillary sinus.

both orbital bones and soft tissues, including the extraocular muscles (Fig. 10) (2,3,4,25).

Decreased sensation in the distribution of the infraorbital nerve is common in patients with blowout fractures of the orbital floor, since the bones covering the infraorbital canal are very thin and are subject to fragmentation. Orbital floor fractures may lead to displacement of the eye or to mechanical restriction of eye movement. These two features are the most common indications for surgical repair of blowout fractures of the orbital floor (Fig. 11) (26).

Displacement of the eye may take the form of enophthalmos (decreased prominence) or ptosis of the globe (drop of the eye toward the maxillary sinus). The mere presence of

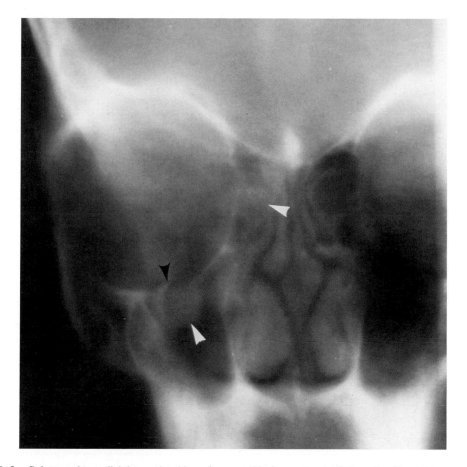

FIG. 9. Polytome shows slightly angulated bone fragment (*black arrow*) and soft tissue densities (*white arrows*) in maxillary and ethmoid sinuses.

measurable enophthalmos is not always an indication for surgical repair. Significant enophthalmos or ptosis of the globe usually occurs only in patients with relatively large bony defects. It is common for blowout fractures to involve both the floor and the medial wall of the orbit. The medial wall defect may be the cause of persistent enophthalmos even after the floor defect has been repaired. In some cases the presence of enophthalmos may be responsible for abnormal eye movements because of a shift of the plane of action through which the vertical rectus muscles move. Although it may be possible to arrest the progress of enophthalmos by covering the fracture defect wih a plate such as a plastic prosthesis, it is often difficult to correct enophthalmos that has already occurred (13). Surgical repair of an orbital floor fracture may be indicated when a significant cosmetic defect seems to evolve because of progessive enophthalmos or ptosis of the globe.

Restriction of eye movements in patients with orbital floor fractures may be due to generalized orbital edema or hemorrhage, to neuromuscular injury, or to mechanical restriction of the vertical rectus muscles. In most cases any surgical repair should be delayed until significant orbital edema and hemorrhage have been resolved. If eye movements are chiefly restricted in vertical fields of gaze, a forced traction test may confirm that the eye

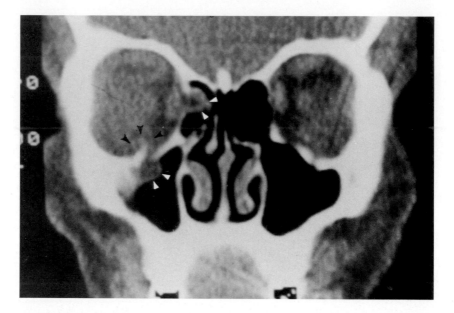

FIG. 10. CCT scan visualizes orbital component of entrapped inferior rectus muscle (*black arrows*)and prolapsed soft tissues (*white arrows*) in maxillary and ethmoid sinuses.

either is or is not mechanically restricted. Surgical repair may be indicated when the forced traction test is positive (when passive movements are restricted), when double vision is present in a functionally important position of gaze (usually in primary gaze or down-gaze), and when the diplopia fails to abate after several days of observation.

In general, the best time for surgical exploration of an orbital floor fracture is within the first 2 weeks after injury. However, if the eye or the optic nerve has been damaged, a longer delay is usually appropriate. If eye movements are restricted but seem to be improving, then surgery may be delayed for weeks or months. Except when a linear fracture is actually compressing the inferior rectus muscle and causing fibrosis, a delay of several weeks probably has little effect on the ultimate results of surgical repair. In many patients with mechanical limitation of eye movement, the restriction may be due to connective tissue septa extending between the fracture and the extraocular muscles (27,28). However, in some patients the muscles themselves may actually be entrapped within the fracture, necessi-tating surgical release.

The surgical approach to blowout fractures that we prefer is the inferior fornix approach via the swinging lower lid flap (see Fig. 12) (29,30). Lidocaine 2% with epinephrine 1:100,000 and hyaluronidase (Wydase) is infiltrated into the inferior fornix, along the floor of the orbit, and over the lateral canthal region. The exposure of the inferior fornix begins with a lateral canthotomy incision horizontally through the skin and the lateral canthal tendon to the periosteum of the lateral orbital rim (Fig. 12A). The lid is placed on gentle inferior traction with a retractor or lid sutures and the inferior limb of the lateral canthal tendon is detached from the lateral orbital rim (Fig. 12B). This procedure fully exposes the inferior fornix, which is then incised with a sharp scissors. The subconjunctival tissue can be severed with an incision directly to the periosteum of the inferior orbital rim (Fig. 12d). It is important to retract the skin to avoid buttonholes. A malleable retractor pressed against the rim can guide the incision and protects the globe and the orbital contents.

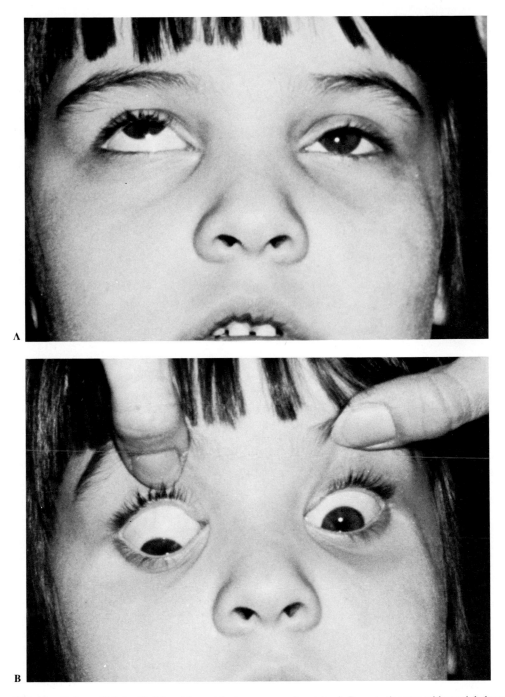

FIG. 11. Patient with left orbital floor blowout fracture: preoperative state. **A:** Preoperative state with enophthalmos of left eye and markedly limited upgaze. **B:** Preoperative limitation in downgaze with blowout fracture of left orbit.

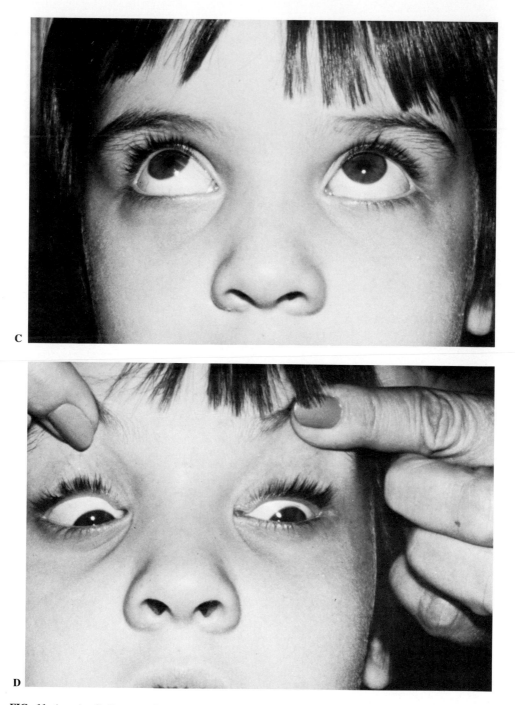

FIG. 11. (*cont.*) **C:** Postoperative state showing excellent return of upgaze function in left eye. **D:** Excellent return of downgaze following reduction and repair of left orbital floor blowout fracture.

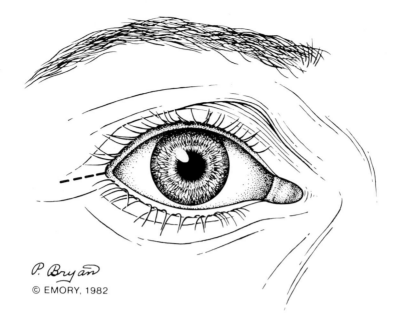

FIG. 12. Exposure of the orbital floor through an inferior fornix incision with cantholysis: the "swinging lower lid flap." **A:** Methylene blue skin marking before performing initial incision.

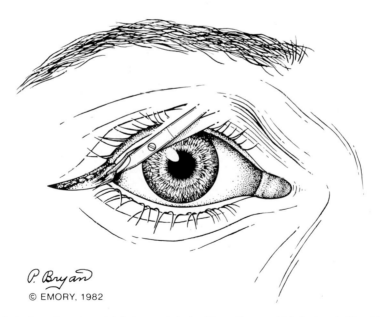

FIG. 12B. Lateral canthotomy and inferior cantholysis. (From Shore and McCord, ref. 30, with permission. © 1984, American Academy of Ophthalmology.)

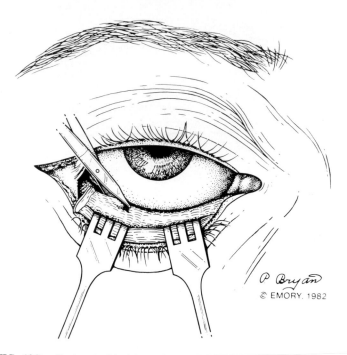

FIG. 12C.   Conjunctival incision at junction of bulbar and palpebral conjunctiva.

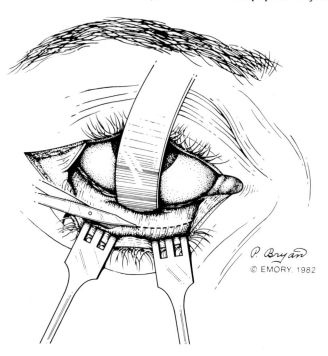

FIG. 12D.   After the conjunctival incision, the capsulopalpebral fascia is held under tension and incised directly over the inferior orbital rim. (From Shore and McCord, ref. 30, with permission. © 1984, American Academy of Ophthalmology.)

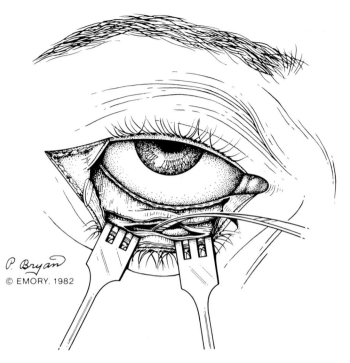

FIG. 12E. The periosteum of the inferior orbital rim is incised and the periorbita of the orbital floor is elevated.

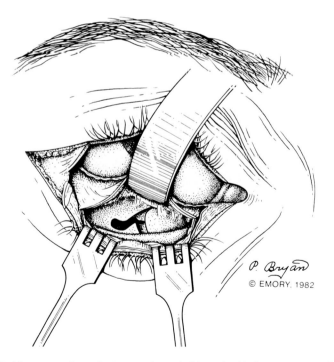

FIG. 12F. A malleable retractor is used to retract the periorbita and orbital contents upward to give excellent exposure of the fracture site in the orbital floor. (From Shore and McCord, ref. 30, with permission. © 1984, American Academy of Ophthalmology.)

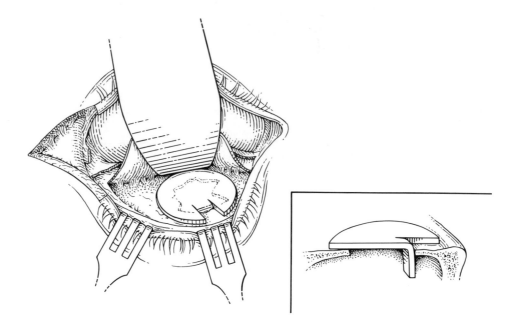

FIG. 12G. An alloplastic plate covers the fracture defect; the tab in the anterior aspect of the plate reduces the chance of implant migration (see inset).

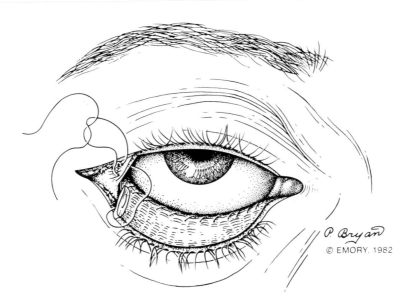

FIG. 12H. Following implant placement, the conjunctiva is closed with a running 6–0 plain suture and the canthal tendon is refixated. (From Shore and McCord, ref. 30, with permission. © 1984, American Academy of Ophthalmology.)

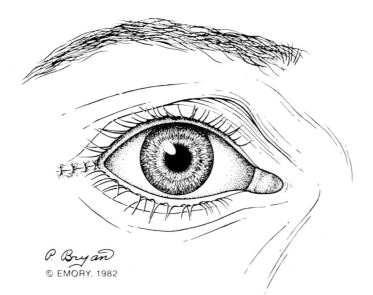

© EMORY, 1982

FIG. 12I. Final closure. (From Shore and McCord, ref. 30, with permission. © 1984, American Academy of Ophthalmology.)

An incision is made in the periosteum. The floor of the orbit can then be exposed by elevating the periosteum with a Tenzel periosteal elevator (Storz #E-4595) and by placing a large malleable retractor, which elevates the orbital contents superiorly (Fig. 12F). The floor of the orbit may be viewed easily using this technique.

The floor of the orbit is explored to visualize the fracture (Fig. 12F). Further elevation of the periosteum allows for visualization of the medial and lateral orbital walls if necessary. Entrapped orbital tissues are removed from the fracture site. If surgery is performed within the first 7 to 10 days following the trauma, blunt dissection may be used to separate the orbital contents from sinus tissues. By 10 to 14 days following trauma, firm adhesions will bind together the orbital and maxillary sinus tissues. To reduce these fractures after the first 2 weeks following trauma, sharp dissection is necessary to disentrap the orbital tissues. We commonly use the needle Bovie unit or Westcott scissors for this maneuver. It is very important to have a traction suture placed under the inferior rectus muscle insertion. This allows the surgeon to identify the muscle during surgery and avoid traumatizing or cutting it. Loose bone chips can be grasped with a forceps and removed. The bony defect is generally covered with an alloplastic plate (Fig. 12G). The plate must not tether the orbital contents, so forced duction testing of globe rotations is repeated before final closure. Excessively large plates should not be used because they may compress the optic nerve posteriorly, as well as having a higher incidence of extrusion.

Closure of the inferior fornix orbitotomy with lateral canthotomy and inferior cantholysis is accomplished by closing the conjunctiva with a running absorbable suture, but the periosteum is not closed. The inferior lid retractors are reapproximated with the conjunctival closure; 6–0 Vicryl sutures have been used for this purpose. The reattachment of the inferior limb of the lateral canthal tendon is accomplished by approximating severed tendon to the periosteum of the lateral orbital rim utilizing 4–0 Prolene sutures with a semicircular needle (Fig. 12H). A firm grasp on the lateral tarsal elements is essential for the placement of the suture. The suture into the periosteum is slightly above the horizontal line and

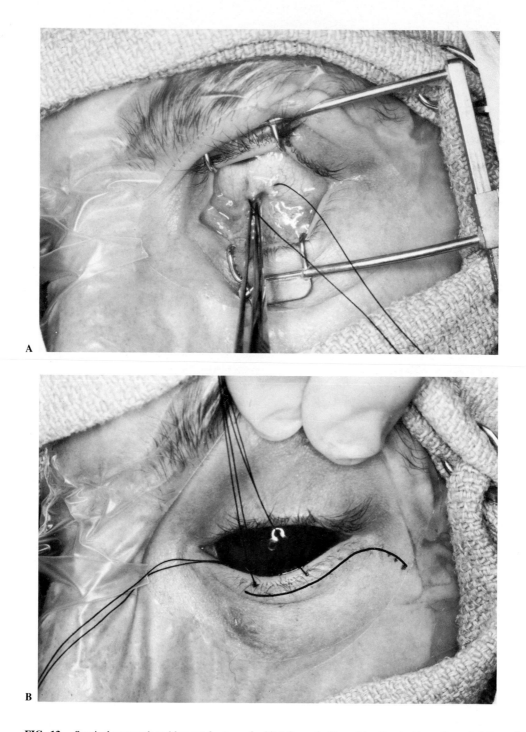

FIG. 13. Surgical approach to blowout fracture of orbital floor. **A:** Forced traction test is performed at time of surgery to determine whether movement of globe is mechanically restricted. Suture is passed beneath insertion of inferior rectus to aid in muscle identification. **B:** Skin incision (*curved line*) is placed several millimeters beneath lashes of lower lid.

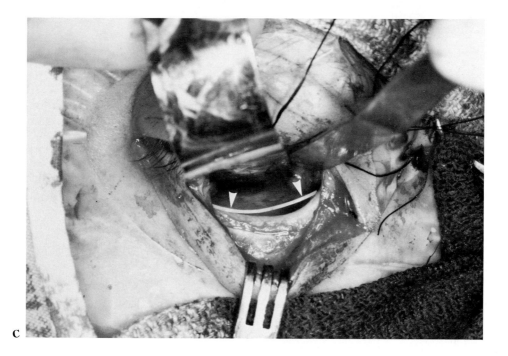

C

FIG. 13 (*cont.*)   **C:** After periosteum has been elevated from orbital floor and prolapsed tissues (if any) are removed from fracture, defect is covered by plastic prosthesis (*arrows*).

internal to the lateral orbital rim. When the knot is tied, appropriate tension is placed on the suture, adjusting the contour to match the opposite lower eyelid margin. The skin of the lateral canthus is then closed with a series of running or interrupted nonabsorbable sutures (Fig. 12I). Post operatively only ice compresses are used to combat swelling.

Another common surgical approach to blowout fractures of the orbital floor is a skin incision (blepharoplasty incision) placed several millimeters beneath the lashes of the lower lid (Fig. 13). A suture is usually passed under the insertion of the inferior rectus muscle so that it may be identified during surgery. The forced traction test should be performed once again to determine if movement of the globe is mechanically restricted. A skin and muscle flap is dissected free from the underlying orbital septum until the inferior orbital rim is reached. The periosteum is elevated from the orbital floor until the area of the fracture is located. Entrapped or prolapsed tissues are removed from the defect and the continuity of the orbital floor is restored, if necessary. The bony defect is usually covered by a plastic prosthesis such as a Silastic or Supramid implant. It is important to avoid using an unnecessarily large prosthesis so that the risk of optic nerve damage and implant extrusion is minimized. Sometimes no implant is needed, especially when the fracture is small. Small defects may be covered with Gelfilm, which is rapidly absorbed but which may prevent secondary adhesions from forming during the postoperative period. Some surgeons prefer to cover the defect with autogenous cartilage or bone.

Complications of blowout fracture surgery include diplopia, lower eyelid retraction, infraorbital nerve damage, implant extrusion, and blindness (24,31). Loss of vision has sometimes occurred several days after orbital fractures, even when surgery was not performed.

REFERENCES

1. Grove, A. S., Jr. (1977): New diagnostic techniques for the evaluation of orbital trauma. *Trans. Am. Acad. Ophthalmol. Otolaryngol.*, 83:626–640.
2. Grove, A. S., Jr., Tadmore, R., New, P. F., and Momose, J. K. (1978): Orbital fracture evaluation by coronal computed tomography. *Am. J. Ophthalmol.*, 85:679–685.
3. Grove, A. S., Jr. (1982): Computed tomography in the management of orbital trauma. *Ophthalmology*, 89:433–440.
4. Grove, A. S., Jr. (1980): Orbital trauma and computed tomography. *Ophthalmology*, 87:403–411.
5. Grove, A. S., Jr. (1975): Evaluation of exophthalmos. *N. Engl. J. Med.*, 292:1005–1013.
6. Walsh, F. B. (1976): Pathological clinical correlations. I. Indirect trauma to the optic nerves and chiasm. II. Certain cerebral involvements associated with defective blood supply. *Invest. Ophthalmol.*, 5:433–449.
7. Anderson, R. L., Panje, W. R., and Gross, C. E. (1982): Optic nerve blindness following blunt head trauma. *Ophthalmology*, 89:445–455.
8. Niho, S., Yasuda, K., Sato, T., et al. (1961): Decompression of the optic canal by the transethmoidal route. *Am. J. Ophthalmol.*, 51:659–665.
9. Fukado, Y. (1975): Results in 400 cases of surgical decompression of the optic nerve. *Mod. Probl. Ophthalmol.*, 14:474–481.
10. Gross, C. W., Teague, P. F., and Nakmura, T. (1972): Reconstruction following severe nasofrontal injuries, *Otolaryngol. Clin. North Am.*, 5(3):653–665.
11. Montgomery, W. W. (1971): Surgery of the frontal sinuses. *Otolaryngol. Clin. North Am.*, 4(1):97–126.
12. Neuman, P. R., Zilkha, A. (1982): Use of the CAT scan for diagnosis in the complicated facial fracture patient. *J. Plast. Reconstr. Surg.*, 70:683–693.
13. Converse, J. M. (1974): Fractures of the zygoma. In: *Surgical Treatment of Facial Injuries*, Vol. 1, 3rd ed., pp. 287–306. Williams & Wilkins, Baltimore.
14. Nunery, W. R. (1985): Lateral canthal approach to repair of trimalar fractures of the zygoma. *Ophthalmic Plast. Reconstr. Surg.*, 1:175–183.
15. McLachlan, D. L., Flanagan, J. C., and Shannon, G. M. (1982): Complications of orbital roof fractures. *Ophthalmology*, 89:1274–1278.
16. Waring, G. O., and Flanagan, J. C. (1975): Pneumocephalus: A sign of intracranial involvement in orbital fracture. *Arch. Ophthalmol.*, 93:847–850.
17. Leech, P. J., and Paterson, A. (1973): Conservative and operative management for cerebrospinal fluid rhinorrhea after closed head trauma. *Lancet*, 1:1013–1015.
18. Jamieson, K. C., and Yelland, J. D. N. (1973): Surgical repair of the anterior fossa because of rhinorrhea, aerocele or meningitis. *J. Neurosurg.*, 39:328–331.
19. Maxwell, J. A., and Goldware, S. I. (1973): Use of tissue adhesive in the surgical treatment of cerebrospinal fluid leaks. Experiences with isobutyl 2-cyanoacrylate in 12 cases. *J. Neurosurg.*, 39:332–336.
20. McCabe, B. F. (1976): The osteo-mucoperiosteal flap in repair of cerebrospinal fluid rhinorrhea. *Laryngoscope*, 86:537–539.
21. Converse, J. M., and Smith, B. (1963): Naso orbital fractures. *Trans. Am. Acad. Ophthalmol. Otolaryngol.*, 67:622–634.
22. Beyer, C. K., Fabian, R. L., and Smith, B. (1982): Naso orbital fractures: Complications and treatment. *Ophthalmology*, 89:456–463.
23. Smith, B., and Regan, W. F. (1957): Blow out fracture of the orbit. Mechanism and correction of internal orbital fracture. *Am. J. Ophthalmol.*, 44:733–739.
24. Converse, J. M., and Smith, B. (1978): On the treatment of blow out fractures of the orbit. *Plast. Reconstr. Surg.*, 62:100–104.
25. Grove, A. S., Jr. (1978): Coronal computed tomography (CCT) of the orbit. In: *Ocular and Adnexal Tumors*, edited by F. A. Jakobiec, pp. 271–280. Aesculapius, Birmingham Alabama.
26. Wilkins, R. B., and Havins, W. E. (1982): Current treatment of blow out fractures. *Ophthalmology*, 89:464–466.
27. Koornneff, L. (1979): Orbital septa: Anatomy and function. *Ophthalmology*, 86:876–880.
28. Koornneff, L. (1977): *Spatial aspects of Orbital Musculo-Fibrous Tissue in Man.* Suets and Zeitlinger, Amsterdam.
29. McCord, C. D., and Moses, J. L. (1979): Exposure of the inferior orbit with fornix incision and lateral canthotomy. *Ophthalmic Surg.*, 10(6):53–63.
30. Shore, J. W., and McCord, C. D., Jr. (1984): Delayed repair of orbital and adnexal deformities following trauma. In: *Ophthalmic Plastic and Reconstructive Surgery*, edited by W. B. Stewart, pp. 400–412. American Academy of Ophthalmology, San Francisco.
31. Nicholson, D. H., and Guzak, S. V. (1971): Visual loss complicating repair of orbital fractures. *Arch. Ophthalmol.*, 86:369–375.

Oculoplastic Surgery, 2nd edition, edited by
Clinton D. McCord, Jr., and Myron Tanenbaum.
Raven Press, New York © 1987.

Chapter 7

Orbital Fractures and Late Reconstruction

*Clinton D. McCord, Jr., **John W. Shore, and †James L. Moses

*Department of Ophthalmology, Emory University School of Medicine, Atlanta, Georgia 30308;
**Department of Ophthalmology, Wilford Hall U.S.A.F. Medical Center, Lakeland, Texas 78236
and †Department of Ophthalmology, Ohio State University, Columbus, Ohio 43210*

Extensive acute orbital trauma may cause displacement of orbital bones together with soft tissue injuries that may go untreated because of other life-threatening problems. Also, in many cases, despite acute repair of facial fractures, residual posttraumatic deformities may require secondary repair and reconstruction. This chapter will emphasize the evaluation of the late complications of orbital fractures and procedures for their reconstruction, with particular emphasis placed on the problems of globe malposition, diplopia, and posttraumatic telecanthus.

GLOBE MALPOSITION

Enophthalmos, or posterior displacement of a normal-sized eye, may occur from a number of mechanisms. It may occur secondary to traumatic enlargement of the orbit with loss of orbital support, to loss of orbital contents through a fracture site, or to cicatricial changes causing orbital fibrosis drawing the globe posteriorly with possible absorption of orbital tissues. In some cases enophthalmos may occur as a combination of all three of the above (1).

Hypoophthalmos refers to the inferior displacement of the globe that occurs when there is a marked disruption of the supporting elements of the globe, including the orbital floor and Lockwood's ligament. It may be seen unilaterally with extensive orbital rim or orbital floor fractures as well as bilaterally with facial fractures in which the maxilla is detached and "free floating." Hypoophthalmos may occur in combination with enophthalmos.

Evaluation and quantitation of the amount of enophthalmos or hypoophthalmos may be aided by the use of full-face and lateral photographs. Exophthalmometry may determine the amount of enophthalmos when the lateral orbital rims are intact and in normal position. In some cases radiologic evaluation may be needed to determine the integrity of the orbital bones in order to plan surgical correction. In patients with globe malposition, work-up must always include documentation of the visual acuity, ocular rotations, and pattern of

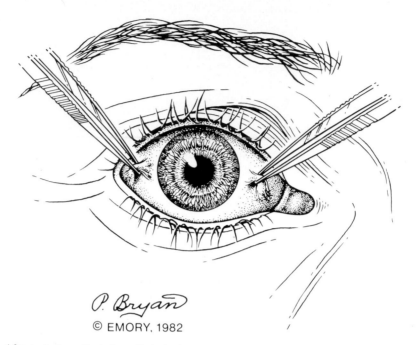

P. Bryan
© EMORY, 1982

FIG. 1. After topical anesthesia is applied, the forward traction test is performed by grasping the insertions of the medial and lateral rectus muscles. The globe is prolapsed anteriorly. Increased resistance is encountered in proportion to the amount of orbital fibrosis.

associated diplopia, in addition to a routine ocular exam, because this information will be required for medical-legal-insurance purposes. Before planning surgical correction of enophthalmos, a forward traction test should be performed (Fig. 1) (1). This test is essental to rule out the diagnosis of significant orbital fibrosis that may be tethering the eye posteriorly. This condition is commonly seen in those patients with generalized restriction of ocular motility. After applying topical proparacaine hydrochloride (Ophthaine®) and subconjunctival lidocaine (Xylocaine®), forward traction of the globe is performed by grasping the tendons of the medial and lateral rectus muscles with Bishop-Harmon forceps and pulling forward. If the globe is tightly fibrosed into the orbit, anterior "reducibility" or prolapse will be limited. Orbital volume replacement with subperiosteal implantation, which will be described in this chapter, should not be used in patients with significant orbital fibrosis, because the volume implant pushes the globe superiorly rather than forward in most cases.

General Principles in the Treatment of Orbital Deformities[1]

Before extraocular muscle surgery is performed, the patient who has displacement of the eye with diplopia must have the globe restored to its normal position. Some surgeons feel that late restoration of the bony orbital skeleton is best carried out by osteotomies and open reduction of bone malunion. Other surgeons recognize this approach can be fraught with complications and recommend the safer use of volume implants and the application of alloplastic or autogenous materials over the bone to restore the configuration of the orbit and to reposition the globe. Repositioning the eye to its normal position in the orbit yields an excellent cosmetic result; nevertheless, diplopia normally persists, particularly in patients with angulating displacement

---

[1] Extracted portions of this chapter are modified from ref. 2 with permission of the American Academy of Ophthalmology. ©1984.

of the globe. Fortunately, diplopia can fequently be eliminated with appropriate eye muscle surgery. The adjustable suture technique is ideally suited for these cases. (2)

Implantation Materials

Autogenous bone (3,4), including cancellous bone from the iliac crest, rib bone, and calvarium bone grafts, has been used for orbital volume augmentation, as have fascia lata and ear or rib cartilage. With autogenous materials infection and migration are unlikely, and rejection does not occur. Absorption of the implanted autogenous material remains a significant drawback. Surgery to repeat the orbital volume augmentation is not uncommon when autogenous implants are used primarily.

Synthetic materials such as bone cement (methyl methacrylate) (5), silicone (6), and proplast (7), have been used to supplement orbital volume. In our experience, bone cement (Surgical Simplex P®, Howmedica) has been the easiest and most predictable material to use for orbital volume augmentation. Its use avoids the additional surgery needed to obtain bone, and it will not reabsorb with time. Infection is a concern when using bone cement in the presence of an exposed sinus or chronic sinusitis. In those patients with an exposed sinus or with very large defects in the orbital floor, our approach of choice is to initially implant an autogenous bone graft and secondarily, if needed, augment the orbital volume with bone cement implanted on top of the previously placed subperiorbital bone graft. This secondary implantation of the bone cement is frequently necessary because the bone graft may reabsorb with time. With this staged surgical approach, the bone cement implant is well tolerated.

Surgical Correction of Globe Malposition

In the absence of significant orbital fibrosis, enophthalmos associated with increased orbital volume and/or loss of orbital support may be corrected by restoring the position of the bony orbital floor and repositioning the globe by supplementing the orbital volume with a subperiosteal volume implant. Exposure of the orbital floor can be obtained through a standard subciliary eyelid incision; however, we prefer a transconjunctival fornix approach to the orbital floor (8) because it provides wide exposure of the inferior orbit and orbital floor, yet avoids a cutaneous scar in the eyelid, which can interfere with lower eyelid movement and, in some patients, lead to a cicatricial ectropion.

The surgical technique is the same regardless of the material to be implanted. Chapter 6 describes in detail the inferior fornix incision and lateral cnathotomy technique for exposure of the orbital floor.

When using bone cement, exposure of the orbital floor should be accomplished prior to preparing the augmentation material. The powder and solution contained in the Howmedica bone cement kit is then mixed in an open plastic dish or an Evacutainer that is connected to a suction system and stirred vigorously to dissipate the monomer produced. The toxic fumes from the mixing process are not liberated into the room environment if an Evacutainer is utilized. After several minutes, the bone cement has assumed a doughy consistency and placement in the orbit is then possible (Fig. 2). At this time, the material is placed in the space between the periosteum and the bone and, in the case of enophthalmos, is forced posteriorly. This is done using moistened Q-tips to push the "doughy" substance into the space. Posterior orbital placement for enophthalmos may be facilitated by applying anterior tranction on the globe utilizing 4–0 silk bridle sutures, which have been previously placed

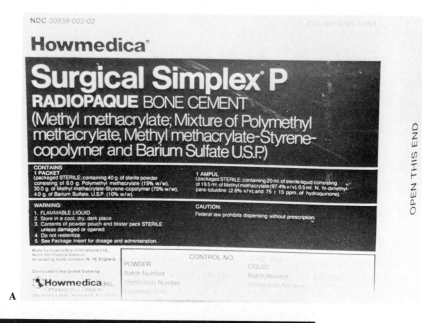

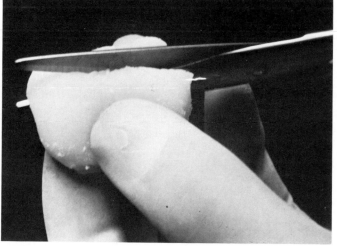

FIG. 2. Bone cement. **A:** Howmedica bone cement kit. **B:** The bone cement has assumed a doughy consistency and is trimmed to the correct size with scissors.

around the rectus muscles (Fig. 3). The amount of material needed can only be estimated after experience with the procedure is gained. In general, bone cement is added to create a slight overcorrection. One should be conservative when placing the material. If too much material is placed, some tethering of the globe is possible if the inferior muscles are very fibrotic, and in these cases, some secondary muscle surgery may be necessary.

Correction of hypoophthalmos is accomplished by placing the bone cement material more anteriorly in the floor of the orbit, elevating the globe. Care should be taken to apply only the amount of bone cement that appears to be appropriate.

When volume augmentation is performed in the presence of a seeing eye, indirect ophthalmoscopy should be performed intraoperatively to evaluate the optic nerve and central retinal artery for signs of vascular compromise.

Visualization of the external position of both eyes during the procedure is essential to aid in estimating the correction that has been produced. Excessive implantation material

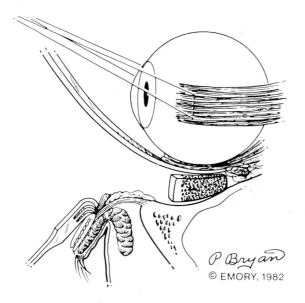

FIG. 3. Cross-sectional view of orbit showing subperiorbital placement of implant material. Traction sutures on the recti muscles and elevation of the globe with a malleable retractor facilitate placement of the implant material posteriorly in the subperiorbital space.

© EMORY, 1982

may extend beyond the anterior orbital rim, producing an irregular orbital margin, and should be removed while soft.

While the bone cement material is hardening, the globe may be rotated using the rectus muscle bridle sutures. This maneuver may prevent possible restriction in extraocular muscle movement, particularly if there are fibrotic inferior muscles or fibrotic adhesions. Again, in the cases of muscle fibrosis, subsequent muscle surgery may still be necessary and the patient must be so informed.

Following volume implantation, conjunctival closure and lateral canthal fixation are performed as described in Chapter 6.

With most patients, particularly those without fibrotic muscles, the results of orbital augmentation are gratifying, but this surgical procedure for correction of hypoophthalmos and enophthalmos may be associated with various complications. Poor hemostasis may produce increased orbital pressure with edema and chemosis. Postoperative systemic steroids used routinely will reduce this tendency. Excessive bone cement material may cause exophthalmos. Upward displacement of the globe occurs if orbital fibrosis is present. Diplopia with restriction of upgaze can occur in the presence of inferior rectus fibrosis. Subsequent inferior muscle recession alleviates this problem in many cases.

If residual enophthalmos is present after orbital augmentation has been conducted, a minimal ptosis procedure may help to mask it. In some cases of hypoophthalmos, the globe may be restored to a normal position but the upper eyelid may not follow. A ptosis procedure may also be required to complete the restoration, elevating the upper lid to correct the secondary ptosis.

DIPLOPIA

Diplopia following orbital trauma may result from neuromuscular paralysis or cicatricial restriction. In cases of vertical displacement of the eye, the malposition may or may not be associated with significant double vision. The presence or absence of double vision

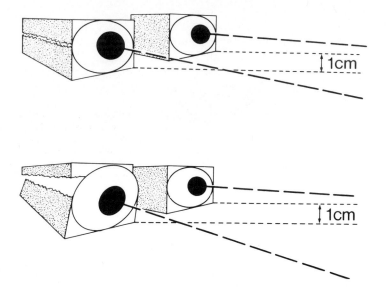

FIG. 4. Schematic demonstration of two types of vertical displacement of the globe. **Top:** Translatory displacement with a minimal induced vertical phoria. The optical axes are parallel but the globes are at different levels. **Bottom:** Angulating displacement frequently induces a manifest hypertropia with subjective diplopia.

may be explained by the type of displacement (Fig. 4) (9). If the globe is displaced without angulation, the eye may be moved vertically (as much as 1 cm) with little effect, i.e., 1 prism diopter at 1 m on binocular single vision. With angulation of the globe, despite relatively small actual vertical displacement, a large amount of hypertropia may result, producing diplopia. This may be seen when there is a displacement in the globe in association with restrictive or paralytic extraocular muscle changes. Vertical muscle imbalance must be documented by prism-cover testing or diplopia fields. Cover-uncover testing may be utilized. Extraocular muscle surgery is almost always necessary following repositioning of the globe. The most common type of posttraumatic strabismus is a vertical muscle imbalance secondary to restriction of the inferior rectus muscle, which may be corrected in many cases by inferior rectus muscle recession with an adjustable suture.

For the surgical correction of diplopia in posttraumatic cases, it is often necessary to recess a fibrotic muscle. The amount of suitable recession can be difficult to predict. Recession of the involved muscle with an adjustable suture may greatly improve the patient's field of single binocular vision.

The surgical technique of adjustable sutures for extraocular muscle surgery is described briefly here (see Chapter 8 for a detailed description of the adjustable suture technique). Jampolsky has popularized several techniques using absorbable and nonabsorbable adjustable strabismus procedures (10). These techniques provide for intraoperative and postoperative adjustment of the recessed extraocular muscle. After the conjunctiva at the limbus has been incised and a radially oriented relaxing incision has been made, the muscle is secured with a double-armed dyed synthetic 6–0 Vicryl suture. The muscle is detached from the globe and the intrascleral passage of the suture is in the anterior direction at the muscle insertion. The 6–0 Vicryl suture is tied temporarily with the muscle in a position of slightly exaggerated recession. The conjunctiva is recessed from the limbus and closed with 6–0 plain sutures.

Postoperative adjustment is done under topical conjunctival anesthesia. The patient should be as alert as possible. Systemic analgesics and relaxants should be avoided because of their effect on extraocular muscle function. The muscle is adjusted depending on the amount of residual deviation, determined by cover-uncover testing, and in part on the subjective response of the patient. The suture endings can then be secured permanently on the conjunctival surface.

TELECANTHUS

Midfacial fractures may be associated with an increase in the distance between the medial canthal angles, which is known as telecanthus, and may be secondary to underlying skeletal changes from splaying out of nasal bone, soft tissue injury, or a combination of hard and soft tissue disruption causing a rounded appearance in the area of the medial canthal tendon (11). The horizontal displacement may be bilateral or may be predominantly unilateral. Repositioning of the medial canthal angles with transnasal wires may correct the deformity of posttraumatic telecanthus (12,13,14). Palpation of the area can readily identify the presence of bony abnormalities. Anterior tomography of the orbital bones and medial aspects of both orbits identify the extent of underlying bony abnormalities. This information is necessary to determine if enough bone is present to support the posterior placement of the transnasal wires. Also, the possible complication of herniation of central nervous system tissue via the area of bony defect may be determined utilizing anterior tomography.

Disruption of the lacrimal drainage apparatus occurs frequently in these patients either because of disruption of the soft tissues in the medial canthus, or, more commonly, from associated fractures in the lacrimal sac fossa or nasolacrimal canal. Generally speaking, lacrimal drainage should be reestablished prior to correcting telecanthus to prevent late, post-traumatic dacryocystitis. If this requires insertion of a Jones' tube, however, the telecanthus will have to be corrected first, since one major requirement for a functional Jones' tube is to have a normally-shaped medial canthal angle. (2)

Surgical Technique of Transnasal Wiring

The transnasal wiring technique is the procedure of choice for the correction of posttraumatic and congenital telecanthus (2). The surgical techniques used to correct unilateral and bilateral deformities are different and are described in the following sections.

Unilateral Transnasal Wiring (Fig. 5)

The superior aspect of each nasal cavity is packed with Webril moistened with a mixture of oxymetazoline hydrochloride (Afrin®) 0.05% and phenylephrine hydrochloride (Neo-Synephrine) 0.25%. The medial canthal angle is infiltrated with lidocaine 2% with epinephrine 1:100,000 and hyaluronidase (Wydase®). The local anesthetic mixture is injected into the ethmoid air cells by passing the needle through the medial orbital wall. This, in conjuction with the nasal packing, will greatly aid hemostasis during surgery.

The skin and subcutaneous tissue just anterior to the medial canthus on the unaffected or normal side is likewise injected. A crescent-shaped skin incision is made 2 mm anterior to the canthal angle on the affected side with the apex centered over the canthal angle pointing towards the dorsum of the nose. The incision is carried down to include the periosteum. Any abnormal subcutaneous tissue is excised before reflecting the periosteum temporally. Hypertrophic scar tissue is usually found following trauma to this area and must be trimmed to get a good result.

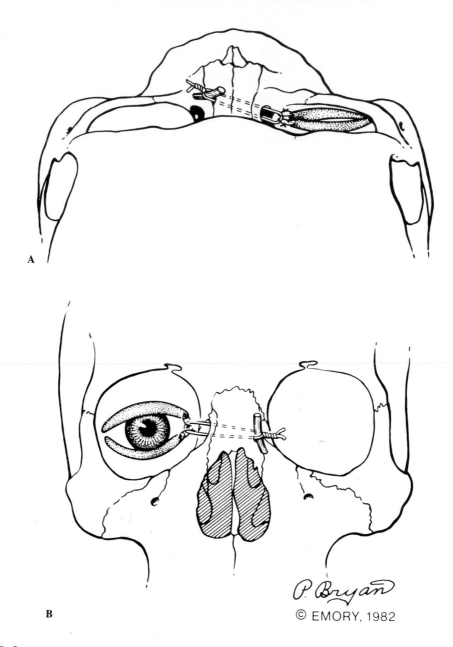

FIG. 5. Unilateral transnasal wiring. **A:** Posterior fixation of the transnasal wire is performed only on the side with horizontal displacement of the medial canthal angle. **B** A pin is fashioned from the stylet of a 16-gauge angiocath to hold the transnasal wire on the side opposite from the medial canthal fixation loop.

Damage to the lacrimal canaliculi and sac must be avoided during the dissection which is continued until the anterior and posterior lacrimal crests and the superior portion of the lacrimal sac fossa are exposed. The periosteum may be quite adherent to bone in this area following naso-orbital fractures making the dissection difficult; however, the periosteum and adherent scar tissue must be dissected off the bone before proceeding.

When the proper exposure has been obtained, a medium sized dental burr on a rotary osteotome or air-pneumatic drill is introduced into the area and the splayed-out bone in the region of the posterior lacrimal crest is thinned down completely to the level of the ethmoidal air cells. This hyperostotic bone is formed during the healing of nasoethmoidal fractures and may extend inferiorly into the lacrimal sac fossa and nasolacrimal canal. Adequate bone removal must be accomplished by thinning to restore the bony canthal configuration prior to transnasal wiring. In order to reform the canthal angle properly, the direction of pull on the eyelids must be toward the posterior lacrimal crest, and that must be the level of passage of the transnasal wires. There must be intact bone present anterior to this level to prevent the wires from migrating to a more forward position. The bone anterior to the posterior lacrimal crest can be thinned a great deal to restore contour; however, it must not be completely removed as that might allow forward migration of the wires, although occasionally an intact nasal septum will stabilize the wires posteriorly. Anterior migration can result in poor eyelid apposition to the globe postoperatively, an undersirable result that can be avoided by proper fixation of the wire.

The nasal packing is now removed . . . and a small hole is drilled in each lateral nasal wall where the wires will subsequently be passed. A [14] gauge trochar is passed transnasally from the normal to the abnormal side through the holes previously created in the side of the nose [Fig. 6]. (2)

In most cases the trochar must be tapped through the bone and septum with the help of a small mallet. It is important to protect both globes during the passage of the trochar, and an assistant must watch for the appearance of the tip of the trochar. Protective scleral contact lenses should be placed on the globe and a malleable retractor should be positioned to prevent possible penetration of the globe by the point of the trochar.

When the trochar has been passed, the stylet is removed and a [32] gauge stainless steel wire is bent on itself and the loop of the wire passed through the lumen of the trochar transnasally so that the loop of the wire rests on the side to be wired. The trochar is then removed leaving the loop of wire in place. The wire has usually been pinched at the apex of the loop during passage through the trochar creating a weak spot in the wire. The ends of the wire should be adjusted to bring this kink back through the nose to the normal side where it is cut off leaving a smooth loop of wire for later fixation to the eyelids.

The tissue in the area of the medial canthal tendon is sutured to the wire on the looped side with 4-0 non-absorbable suture [e.g., Prolene]. The wire itself should not be passed through the canthal tendon as it may "cheese wire," leading to recurrence of the telecanthus. The wire is now ready for tightening. To fixate the wire, a metal bolster pin is fashioned by cutting an 8 mm length from the central portion of the stylet of a 19 gauge angiocath. The pin is bent slightly in the middle and held against the lateral nasal bone with a vertical orientation resting between the ends of the wire which are now twisted over the pin, anchoring the pin against the bone and giving excellent purchase for further tighening to the wire. The wire loop is tightened by simultaneously pulling on the ends of the wires and twisting them over the pin until the telecanthus is slightly overcorrected. The twisted wire is cut and bent into the hole in the lateral nasal bone. The skin is meticulously closed with 6-0 nylon sutures.

Nose pads are usually not required in unilateral cases; however, if necessary they can be

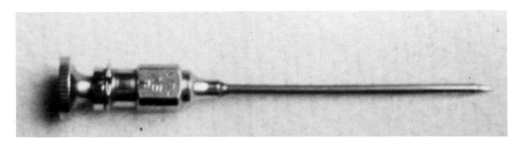

FIG. 6. A 16-gauge trochar with stylet used for passage of 32-gauge transnasal wires.

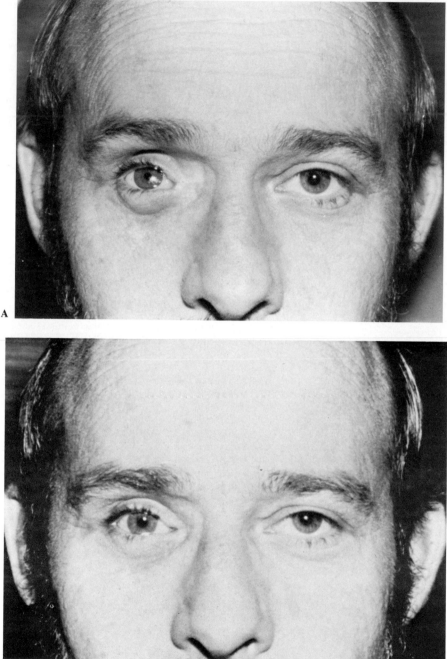

FIG. 7. Preoperative and postoperative results in a patient with unilateral telecanthus. **A:** Patient with posttraumatic anophthalmic socket (prosthesis in place) and unilateral telecanthus shows a rounded appearance of the right medial canthal angle. **B:** Postoperative result with restoration of normal contour and placement to right medial canthal angle.

applied. A decision to use them will have to be made before the trochar is removed. If they are to be used, a second loop of [32] gauge wire is passed through the trochar and tagged. After the transnasal wiring has been completed, but before [final skin closure], the tags are removed and the loop of wire is cut leaving two [external wires] exiting each skin incision. The skin is closed around these wires. The end of each wire is then passed through one of two silicone nose pads fashioned from cut-down silicone ocular conformers. The wires on each side are then twisted together over dental rolls to compress the skin in the canthal region, thus flattening out epicanthal folds and restoring consistency to the soft tissue in the canthal area. The nose-pads and skin sutures are left in place for 7 to 10 days, at which time the skin wires are clipped and the nose pads [are] removed. The deep, looped transnasal wire remains in place permanently.

The 6-0 nylon skin sutures are removed approximately 7 days after removal of the nose pads (Fig. 7).

Bilateral Transnasal Wiring (Fig. 8)

The surgical technique for bilateral transnasal wiring differs only slightly from that described for unilateral cases. The crescent-shaped skin incision is made bilaterally just anterior to the canthal angles. If an epicanthal fold exists, a small amount of skin may be excised; however, if no epicanthal fold is present, the skin excision is omitted [Fig. 8A]. The subsequent dissection and removal of excess subcutaneous tissue and the thinning of hyperostotic bone is completed bilaterally just as described for unilateral cases. (2)

Again, penetration of the bone must be at the level of the posterior lacrimal crest bilaterally, and intact bone should be left anterior to that position if possible to avoid forward migration of the wires postoperatively.

Once the trochar has been passed and the stylet removed, two looped 32-gauge stainless steel wires are threaded intraluminally through the trochar, which is then removed, leaving the loops of wire in place (Fig. 8B). One loop, along with its two ends on the opposite side, is tagged with hemostats and becomes the external fixation wires. The other loop and its ends fix the canthal tendons bilaterally. The tissue in the medial canthal area is now sutured to the wire on the looped side with a 4-0 nonabsorbable suture such as Prolene. In the bilateral cases,

the two ends of the wire opposite the loop are twisted on themselves forming a second loop which is sutured to the medial canthal tendon on that side with 4-0 non-absorbable suture. By tightening the looped wires, each canthal angle will be pulled toward the base of the nose reforming the canthal angles bilaterally. The [external wires] will protrude through the skin and be tied over nose pads to restore concavity to the soft tissues in the canthal angles. The tightening of the looped wire which repositions the tendons in the canthal angles of the base of the nose is performed by three manipulations taking place simultaneously. As the twisted wires are tightened, countertraction pulls the loop on the opposite side tight, and at the same time the non-absorbable sutures on the twisted side are pushed inward toward the base of the nose with forceps. The sutures will slide very easily down the wire toward the base of the nose as the twisting takes place. After proper tightening of the tendons corrects the telecanthus, the twisted wire is cut short and the ends inverted in the deep tissue. The skin is closed with 6-0 nylon. The tags are removed from the [external wires and] the loop cut, leaving two free wires which are used to fixate the silicone nose pads and dental rolls, exactly as described for unilateral cases [Fig. 9]. The [external wires and nose pads] are removed in 7 to 10 days. The deep transnasal wire is left in place permanently. (2)

Skin sutures are removed 7 days following removal of the nose pads.

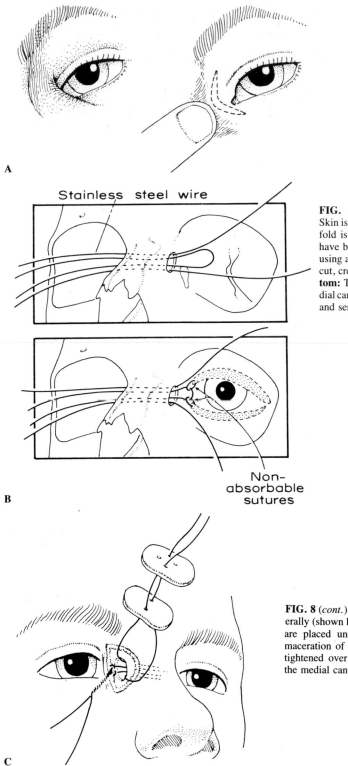

A

Stainless steel wire

Non-absorbable sutures

B

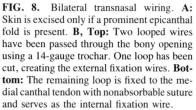

FIG. 8. Bilateral transnasal wiring. **A:** Skin is excised only if a prominent epicanthal fold is present. **B, Top:** Two looped wires have been passed through the bony opening using a 14-gauge trochar. One loop has been cut, creating the external fixation wires. **Bottom:** The remaining loop is fixed to the medial canthal tendon with nonabsorbable suture and serves as the internal fixation wire.

FIG. 8 (*cont.*)   **C:** The nose pads are applied bilaterally (shown here prior to skin closure). Telfa pads are placed under silicone conformers to prevent maceration of the skin. The external wires will be tightened over dental rolls to provide pressure on the medial canthal tissue.

C

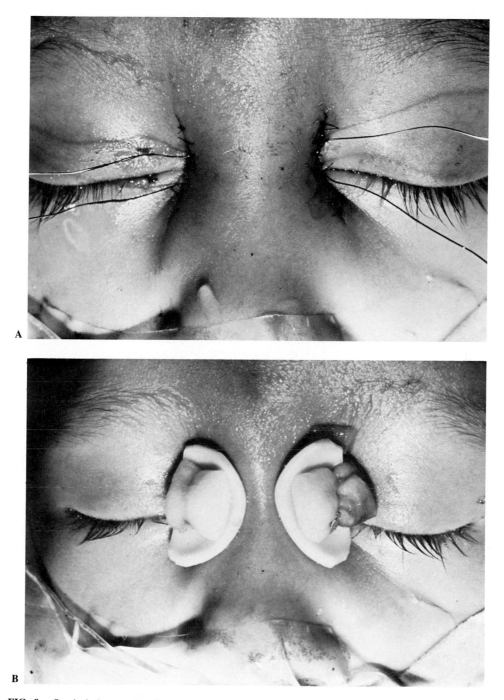

FIG. 9. Surgical photographs of nose pad placement in bilateral transnasal wiring. **A:** The skin incisions have been closed with 6–0 nylon sutures and the two external wires are exposed on each side. **B:** The external fixation wires have been threaded through Telfa pads and silicone conformers, and tightened over dental rolls.

ASSOCIATED INJURIES

Extensive midfacial and orbital trauma is commonly associated with injuries to the lacrimal drainage system and eyelids. The lacrimal drainage system may be disrupted by injury to the bone that forms the lacrimal fossa. These bones are often fractured and displaced, impinging on the lacrimal sac or nasolacrimal duct, and such damage is associated with chronic recurrent dacryocystitis and epiphora. Correction of these problems may be accomplished by standard dacryocystorhinostomy procedure or by the placement of a Jones Pyrex tube. These procedures can be performed after restoration of the canthal angles has been made. Correction of posttraumatic ptosis may be obtained by utilizing various procedures, depending on the amount of levator function and the amount of associated restriction and scarring. Correction of lid malposition in part may be accomplished by reforming severed components of the medial and lateral canthal tendons. Procedures to correct lacrimal system dysfunction may be performed in conjunction with or after correction of globe malposition, diplopia, and telecanthus. In general, Jones tube procedures and correction of eyelid malposition are best done after globe position is restored and a canthal angle as normal as possible has been formed.

REFERENCES

1. Converse, J. M., Smith, B., Obear, M. F., and Wood-Smith, D. (1967): Orbital blowout fractures: A ten year survey. *Plast. Reconstr. Surg.,* 39:20–36.
2   Shore, J. W., and McCord, C. D., Jr. (1984): Delayed repair of orbital and adnexal deformities following trauma. In: *Ophthalmic Plastic and Reconstructive Surgery,* edited by W. B. Stewart pp. 407–410. American Academy of Ophthalmology, San Francisco.
3. Kaye, B. L. (1966): Orbital floor repair with antral wall bone grafts. *Plast. Reconstr. Surg.,* 37:62–65.
4. Pike, R. L., and Boyne, P. J. (1973): Composite autogenous marrow and surface-decalcified implants in mandibular defects. *J. Oral Surg.,* 31:905–912.
5. McCord, C. D., Jr. (1977): Orbital fractures. In: *Ophthalmic Plastic Surgery,* edited by B. Silver, 3rd ed., pp. 285–286. American Academy of Ophthalmology and Otolaryngology, San Francisco.
6. Soll, D. B. (1971): Correction of the superior lid sulcus with subperiosteal implants. *Arch. Ophthalmol.,* 85:188–190.
7. Epstein, L. I. (1979): Clinical experiences with proplast as an implant. *Plast. Reconstr. Surg.,* 63(2):219–223.
8. McCord, C. D., Jr., and Moses, J. L. (1979): Exposure of the inferior orbit with fornix incision and lateral canthotomy. *Ophthalmic Surg.,* 10(6):53–63.
9. McCord, C. D., Jr. (1977): Orbital fractures. In: *Ophthalmic Plastic Surgery,* edited by B. Silver, 3rd ed., pp. 282–283. American Academy of Ophthalmology and Otolaryngology, San Francisco.
10. Jampolsky, A. (1978): Adjustable strabismus surgical procedures. In: *Transactions of the New Orleans Academy of Ophthalmology* (*Symposium on Strabismus*), pp. 321–349. Mosby, St. Louis.
11. Beyer, C. K., Fabian, R. L., and Smith, B. (1982): Naso-orbital fractures, complications, and treatment. *Ophthalmology,* 89:456–463.
12. Converse, J. M., and Smith, B. (1963): Naso-orbital fractures. *Trans. Am. Acad. Ophthalmol. Otolaryngol.,* 67:622–634.
13. Smith, B., and Beyer, C. K. (1969): Medial canthoplasty. *Arch. Ophthalmol.,* 82:344–348.
14. McCord, C. D., Jr. (1980): The correction of telecanthus and epicanthal fold. *Ophthalmic Surg.,* 11:446–454.

Oculoplastic Surgery, 2nd edition, edited by
Clinton D. McCord, Jr., and Myron Tanenbaum.
Raven Press, New York © 1987.

Chapter 8

Graves' Ophthalmopathy

*Myron Tanenbaum and **Clinton D. McCord, Jr.

*Bascom Palmer Eye Institute, Department of Ophthalmology, University of Miami School of Medicine,
Miami, Florida 33101; and **Department of Ophthalmology, Emory University School of Medicine,
Atlanta, Georgia 30308*

The term Graves' opththalmopathy is applied to an inflammatory orbital disorder usually associated with thyroid disease (1,2). There is confusion as to the underlying mechanism and there are clinical subsets of the disorder. Regardless of etiology, it appears that this inflammatory disorder primarily affects the ocular muscles and lacrimal gland, with all ocular and eyelid signs and symptoms occurring secondarily. Patients with Graves' ophthalmopathy may be hyperthyroid, euthyroid, or hypothyroid.

PATHOGENESIS

There is clinical, humoral, and cellular evidence that Graves' ophthalmopathy is an immunologic disorder (2,3). Clinically, patients with Graves' ophthalmopathy have increased incidence of other autoimmune diseases, including myasthenia gravis, Addison's disease, vitiligo, and pernicious anemia. In certain patients with Graves' ophthalmopathy, systemic corticosteroid (prednisone) therapy will effect a rapid improvement in the orbital signs and symptoms (4). Humoral evidence at present revolves around the presence of thyroid-stimulating immunoglobulin (TSI), a G class immunoglobulin that is present in over 90% of thyrotoxic patients with Graves' ophthalmopathy. While TSI levels may coincide with exacerbations of thyrotoxicosis, there is no demonstrable correlation between TSI levels and clinical Graves' ophthalmopathy. On a cellular level the histopathology of this disorder demonstrates lymphocyte, plasma cell, and macrophage infiltration of the extraocular muscles and other tissues. In addition, patients with Graves' ophthalmopathy appear to have a suppression of T lymphocyte subpopulations as measured by erythrocyte rosette formation (5,6).

Presently much evidence implicates the extraocular muscle as a target organ in Graves' ophthalmopathy. Kriss and co-workers studied the binding of thyroglobulin and thyroglobulin-antithyroglobulin immune complexes to human and bovine extraocular muscle membranes (7). Although it is not anatomically demonstrated, Kriss has proposed the existence of a direct thyroid-orbit lymphatic pathway whereby thyroglobulin and thyroglobulin-antithyro-globulin immune complexes could reach the orbit via retrograde flow. (8).

Jakobiec believes that a breakdown in T lymphocyte function is central to the immune derangement of Graves' ophthalmopathy (1). This is evidenced by diminished numbers of rosette-forming T lymphocytes in patients with severe orbitopathy. However, much remains either unexplained or unknown. Among the key unanswered questions are:

What is the true relationship between thyroid dysfunction and orbitopathy?

Which patients with thyroid dysfunction will develop orbitopathy typical of Graves'?

Following treatment of thyroid dysfunction, why does the Graves' ophthalmopathy improve in some patients and worsen in others?

What parameters could predict the clinical course of a given patient with Graves' ophthalmopathy?

What immunologic differences underlie corticosteroid-responsive patients verses Graves' patients nonresponsive to steroids?

What mechanisms explain the apparent different subsets of patients with Graves' ophthalmopathy, for example, the young female patient with minimal extraocular muscle enlargement and maximal proptosis, versus the older patient with maximal extraocular muscle enlargement with restrictive motility patterns and compressive optic neuropathy yet minimal proptosis?

In reference to surgical intervention in patients with Graves' ophthalmopathy, what parameters best determine if the patient's clinical course is stable?

PATHOPHYSIOLOGY

A primary autoimmune reaction against the extraocular muscles can cause all of the characteristic features of Graves' ophthalmopathy. According to Jakobiec, the earliest inflammation occurs within the endomysium or connective tissue spaces of the extraocular muscles (1). Endomysial fibroblasts are stimulated to produce both mucopolysaccharides and collagen. Mucopolysaccharide deposition predominates in the early phases of acute disease, and in the later stages of chronic disease it is collagen deposition that predominates. The extraocular muscles enlarge and undergo degeneration and fibrosis. It is extraocular muscle fibrosis that accounts for motility restriction, and increased volume of orbital soft tissue. Proptosis of the eye can only partially relieve an increasing orbital pressure. The inflammatory process that is occurring facilitates pathologic fluid transudation and resultant orbital tissue edema. Orbital edema is further exacerbated by increased orbital pressure and venous congestion due to apical venous compression, with resultant stasis of interstitial fluid due to diminished outflow of interstitial fluids from the orbit. Increased orbital pressure and interstitial fluids account for lacrimal gland enlargement, eyelid edema with fat prolapse, and conjunctival chemosis. Inflammatory cells accompany the orbital interstitial fluid as it moves anteriorly into the eyelids. This explains the ''spot welding'' effect between eyelid tissue planes, that is so characteristic of Graves' ophthalmopathy (9). Fibroblast proliferation and fibrosis of the levator muscle account for the upper eyelid retraction and actual restriction of the upper eyelid when one attempts forcibly to pull the lid down. The extraocular muscle fibrosis and enlargement is great in the middle and posterior third of the muscle belly. It is posteriorly, at the annulus zinnii, that enlarged extraocular muscles cause compressive optic neuropathy and visual loss.

The above-stated pathophysiologic mechanism is the present theory based on clinical and immunopathologic observations.

DIAGNOSIS

There are different modes of presentation of Graves' disease. The signs and symptoms may be unassociated with a known thyroid disorder. They also may be separated in time from known thyroid treatment. Simple complaints of a "wide-eyed look" or "bulging eye" (exophthalmos and lid retraction) are common. Nonspecific irritation, continual tearing (hypersecretion), and foreign body sensation are common symptoms in patients with excessive proptosis, eyelid retraction, and possibly limited Bell's phenomenon due to inferior rectus muscle restriction. It is common for patients to experience diplopia in certain fields of gaze, and this may be a presenting sign. The patient may present with a nonspecific ocular inflammatory disease, complaining of red eyes and eyelid swelling. Visual loss due to compressive neuropathy is often overlooked by the patient until a very advanced state is reached, particularly if only mild exophthalmos is present.

Attempts to classify the signs and symptoms have been made in the past. The Werner "NO SPECS" classification of stages in orbital Graves' disease may be helpful as a mnemonic device but is of little practical value in terms of staging clinical disease for patient assessment (10). Upper eyelid retraction may be the most common early sign of Graves' ophthalmopathy. The normal anatomic position of the upper eyelid is approximately 1 mm below the superior limbus. In more elderly patients with Graves' disease dermatochalasis and involutional eyelid changes may mask upper eyelid retraction. Lower eyelid retraction is also very common in patients with Graves' ophthalmopathy; the lower eyelid normal anatomic position should be right at the inferior limbus. Stare or infrequent blinking is a common sign. The likely mechanism is that edema and inflammation lead to secondary fibrosis and contracture of the eyelid retractors, that is, the levator muscle in the upper lids and the capsulopalpebral fascia in the lower lids. This mechanical stiffness of the eyelid is evidenced by lid lag (the upper eyelids lag behind the eyeball when the eyeball moves in pursuant motion from upgaze downward), difficulty in everting the stiff retracted upper eyelid, and a positive forced duction of the upper eyelid when attempting to pull it downward. Orbital tumors as a rule do not cause lid retraction. If one is faced with a patient with lid retraction and possibly proptosis and the computed tomography (CT) scan shows an "orbital tumor," one must carefully evaluate the coronal and axial CT views because the "tumor" will most likely be an enlarged extraocular muscle.

Proptosis, either unilateral or bilateral, is a hallmark sign of Graves' ophthalmopathy. Hertel exophthalmometric measurements will vary within a normal range depending on age, sex, and race of the patient (11). As a general rule, the upper limits of normal in white adult patients is approximately 21 mm and in black adult patients is approximately 24 mm. An asymmetry between the patient's two eyes of more than 2 mm is usually pathologic. Patients with proptosis may simply complain of cosmetic disfigurement, or show evidence of punctate epithelial errosions due to corneal drying and exposure. Untreated severe proptosis can lead to corneal ulcerations and perforation. Lagophthalmos is invariably present in these patients. Generalized redness and dilation of the conjunctival and episcleral blood vessels is commonly seen in patients with advanced proptosis. Intense conjunctival injection over the rectus muscle insertion is a frequent finding.

Certainly the most common cause of limitation of upgaze in adults is Graves' ophthalmopathy affecting the inferior rectus muscle. There is an unexplained predilection for enlargement and fibrosis of the inferior rectus, and the medial rectus is the next most frequently involved extraocular muscle. The abnormal motility patterns in these patients with restrictive myopathy show positive forced duction testing. In patients with unilateral or highly asymmetric proptosis. CT scan or standardized echography will usually demonstrate extraocular muscle enlargements in both orbits, a significant differentiating feature with other conditions that cause enlarged extraocular muscles. The differential diagnosis of enlarged extraocular muscles includes: Graves' ophthalmopathy, inflammatory myositis, carotid cavernous fistula, and neoplastic disease (12).

Compressive optic neuropathy is among the most worrisome sequelae of Graves' orbitopathy. In its early stages, compressive optic neuropathy is frequently unrecognized or misdiagnosed (13), and visual loss may be severe and permanent. It addition to visual acuity testing, it is essential to test the patient with color plates. Evidence of dischromatopsia cannot be explained by corneal epithelial erosions but rather indicates optic nerve dysfunction. Other signs of Graves' ophthalmopathy are indicative of the generalized orbital inflammatory process and associated edema. Eyelid edema and boggy conjunctiva are common during acute flare-ups of the condition. Patients may complain of nonspecific irritation and frequent tearing that may appear to be nothing more than staphylococcal blepharoconjunctivitis. Associated findings such as eyelid retraction, proptosis, and motility restriction will lead to a correct diagnosis of Graves' ophthalmopathy. Amid other acute findings of typical Graves' orbitopathy, an enlarged lacrimal gland should not cause undue concern.

Probably no other ocular condition has as many eponyms as Graves' ophthalmopathy. The more common include von Graefe's lid lag sign, Dalrymple's signs of eyelid retraction and stare, and Stellwag's sign of infrequent blinking.

Laboratory Tests

When clinical features suggestive of Graves' ophthalmopathy are present, a few basic laboratory tests should be performed to assess thyroid function. There are no tests, however, that can predict the clinical course of a patient with Graves' ophthalmopathy, nor is there a test to determine if a patient's ocular and orbital condition is stable.

The most useful battery of initial tests to measure thyroid function are: throxin (T_4) level, triiodothyronine (T_3) level, and T_3 resin uptake. If the above tests indicate a euthyroid state in the face of clinical evidence of Graves' ophthalmopathy, a thyrotropin-releasing hormone (TRH) test is indicated. This easy-to-perform, highly sensitive test has generally replaced the Werner suppression test and is even used by some authorities as an initial screening test in the evaluation of a patient's thyroid function. In performing the TRH test, one must first obtain a baseline measurement of thyrotropin (TSH). The patient is given an intravenous injection of TRH. A normal response is a three- to fivefold increase in the serum TSH levels when measured in 20 to 30 min. With great sensitivity, this test detects an abnormal or autonomous pituitary-thyroid axis. The measurement of isolated TSH levels may be a sensitive indicator for the presence of hyperthyroidism, although TSH levels are of greater value as part of the TRH test in a measurement of TSH responsiveness. In some laboratories, radioimmunoassay methods of measuring thyroxin-binding globulin (TBG) are being used. This direct measurement of TBG may replace the T_3 resin uptake eventually.

CT scans are of great value in the diagnosis and evaluation of patients with Graves' ophthalmopathy (14). The classic findings are enlargement of the muscle bellies with relative sparing of the anterior tendon insertions. The lacrimal glands may be enlarged, although the fat is generally uninvolved and is radiolucent. Inferior orbital ''tumors'' seen on axial CT scan projections are revealed to be enlargement of the inferior rectus muscle when studied with coronal CT scan projections. CT scan evaluation of patients with unilateral proptosis due to Graves' ophthalmopathy will often reveal bilateral rectus muscle enlargement. Standardized echography (A-mode and B-mode ultrasound) can also be helpful in evaluating patients with Graves' ophthalmopathy (15). Standardized A-mode echography will show high internal reflectivity in affected extraocular muscles and can be useful in measuring actual thickness of the extraocular muscles. It is anticipated that magnetic resonance imaging (MRI) with surface coil adaptation for orbital study will be of great value in the future in studying patients with Graves' ophthalmopathy.

TREATMENT

There are two situations in which the surgeon will have to manage Graves' patients after the initial diagnosis has been made: the active inflammatory phase, which may be progressive, and the inactive fibrotic phase, in which the anatomic changes in the lids and orbit must be surgically corrected. In patients with Graves' orbitopathy during the active inflammatory phase, the underlying autoimmune process causes progressive orbital and eyelid changes that vary in severity and may continue for as long as 6 months to a year (Fig. 1). During this period nonsurgical management of symptoms and possible antiinflammatory therapy are used. The only situation in which surgical intervention may become necessary in this phase is in patients with visual loss with compressive neuropathy who do not respond to medical treatment. All other corrective surgical procedures are performed when the patient reaches the healed fibrotic state.

Medical Treatment

From the standpoint of the hyperthyroid state, endocrinologic care is of primary concern in the management of the Graves' ophthalmopathy patient. It should be remembered that the treatment of the orbitopathy and dysthyroid state seem to be independent of one another; therefore, systemic treatment of the dysthyroidism may have no effect on the state of the orbitopathy. Mild forms of Graves' ophthalmopathy produce patients with symptoms mostly related to corneal drying. The frequent use of artificial teardrop preparations and lubricating ointments at bedtime can be very helpful in alleviating symptoms. Occasional patients with exopthalmos and nightime lagophthalmos may require eyelid taping. Moisture-chamber glasses can be of great help to some patients, especially during wintertime in the cooler climates. Head elevation during sleep reduces edema. Fresnell "paste on" prisms are

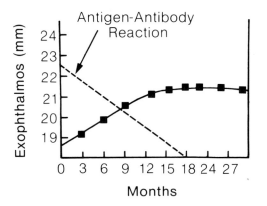

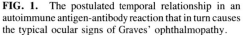

FIG. 1. The postulated temporal relationship in an autoimmune antigen-antibody reaction that in turn causes the typical ocular signs of Graves' ophthalmopathy.

useful in treating mild diplopia, are less expensive than permanent prisms ground into prescription glasses, and can be easily interchanged as a given patient's treatment course mandates. For advancing degrees of horizontal and vertical strabismus, treatment options become a choice between botulinum toxin (Oculinum®) injections or extraocular muscle surgery (16). The preliminary experience with botulinum toxin injections indicates favorable results when treatment is given for "early" phases of extraocular muscle imbalance, but much less effective results for "late" phases of the disease when advanced extraocular muscle fibrosis results in a severe, restrictive myopathy. This generalization regarding botulinum toxin injection usage probably also applies to the injection of the upper eyelid levator muscle for the treatment of eyelid retraction. Botulinum toxin injection therapy is usually effective for a period of 60 to 90 days. Surgical procedures, other than in emergency situations, should generally be deferred until the clinical findings are stable for 6 months, although the exact time to reach stability is not known and may vary.

Corticosteroid therapy and supervoltage radiation therapy are two major antiinflammatory treatment modalities in the physician's armementarium. Corticosteroid therapy maintains an important role in the treatment of compressive optic neuropathy and in patients with progressive inflammatory disease. Patients with the acute, congestive signs of Graves' ophthalmopathy are most likely to respond to corticosteroid therapy. Sergott and co-workers have studied the T lymphocyte populations in patients with Graves' ophthalmopathy (4). It appears that patients with depressed T lymphocyte counts show the most favorable therapeutic response to corticosteroids. Patients who have reached the fibrotic stage are generally refractory to treatment with corticosteroids. Initial treatment is usually oral prednisone 100 mg or more daily. In cases of compressive optic neuropathy, evidence of clinical improvement should occur within 2 weeks of starting high-dose prednisone therapy (17). A survey of the responsiveness of patients with compressive neuropathy in 1983 showed that approximately one-fourth of patients will respond to steroids alone (see Fig. 2) (18). Visual loss from compressive optic neuropathy may be irreversible; therefore, the physician must be prepared to implement other modalities of treatment in those patients refractory to high-dose corticosteroid therapy. To date, periocular or intraorbital steroid injections have not been shown to be effective.

Supervoltage radiation therapy has been used successfully for the treatment of compressive neuropathy and other acute changes (19,20). It yields the best results when used to treat

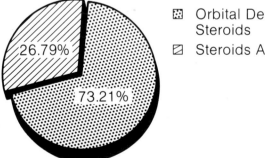

FIG. 2.   Among the patients (293 cases) who underwent a trial of high-dose steroids for compressive neuropathy, greater than 73% subsequently required orbital decompression in order to achieve "best final vision." (From McCord, ref. 18, with permission of Lippincott/Harper & Row.)

the same group of patients that best respond to corticosteroid therapy, i.e., radiation is most effective in patients with recent-onset symptoms and the acute, congestive signs of Graves' ophthalmopathy, and least effective in the treatment of the fibrotic stage of the disease. Nonetheless, it must be remembered that patients refractory to one treatment modality may show a good response to a different one. Most patients treated with radiation receive 1,500 to 2,000 rads of supervoltage divided over 10 daily fractions. Radiation treatment is aimed at the orbital apices via a lateral port. In experienced hands, there should be minimal or no morbidity to the globe or intraocular contents.

Plasmapheresis, thymus gland extirpation, and systemic immunosuppression remain experimental modalities of treatment and play an uncertain role at present in the medical management of patients with Graves' ophthalmopathy.

Surgical Treatment

After the inflammatory orbital and eyelid changes become quiescent, surgical correction of exophthalmos, restrictive myopathy, and eyelid malposition may be undertaken. The single biggest decision facing the oculoplastic surgeon before undertaking surgery is deciding when the disease is stable. There is no laboratory test to answer this question, and good history taking is critical in this regard. The patient should report stability of proptosis and eyelid retraction for a period of at east 6 months before surgery in order to reduce the chances of undergoing further changes in globe or eyelid position. In some patients, unusual progressive changes have been noted to occur over a period of years. Orbital decompression alters eyelid position and muscle balance, and eye muscle surgery influences eyelid position. If the patient with more severe changes is considered to require surgical correction in all of the above areas, the correct sequence of staged surgery would be orbital decompression first, eye muscle surgery second, and eyelid surgery third. This section will address these topics separately.

Orbital Decompression

Over the years every orbital wall, separately or in combination, has been resected in an attempt to decompress the orbit in patients with Graves' ophthalmopathy. This section will describe the two-wall antral-ethmoidal decompression by both the lower lid fornix approach and the Caldwell-Luc transantral approach, and the three-wall decompression. The interested reader may refer to references regarding transfrontal decompression of the orbital roof (21), the four-wall decompression of Kenerdell-Maroon (22), and the Leforte III osteotomy orbital expansion (23). The two indications are orbital decompression in patients with Graves' ophthalmopathy are compressive optic neuropathy with visual loss and proptosis with corneal exposure and facial disfigurement (Fig. 3).

Antral-ethmoidal decompression via inferior fornix approach
The inferior fornix incision with lateral cantholysis provides excellent exposure for the two-wall or three-wall decompression (24). This technique can usually achieve 4 to 6 mm of retroplacement of the globe (18,25,26). It is used for noncompressive neuropathy patients for correction of exophthalmos. It is a more anterior decompression and is not as effective for correction of compressive neuropathy as the transantral decompression, which is more posterior (18). It has much less adverse effect on motility than the transantral approach

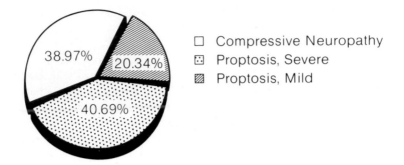

FIG. 3.   Three-year total cases (531), showing the indications for decompression used by the surgeons participating in the compressive neuropathy survey. (From McCord, ref. 18, with permission of Lippincott/Harper & Row.)

and gives excellent retroplacement of the globe. Preoperative orbital CT scans are evaluated for sinus disease and anatomic variants.

Surgical technique.   The night before surgery oral steroids and decongestants are given to reduce mucosal inflammation and edema. Attention to any clotting abnormalities, including medicines that affect blood clotting, is crucial. In the operating room, the patient is positioned in a slight head-up position and all arm boards are omitted from the operating table to allow the surgeon better positioning. Lidocaine 2% with 1:100,000 epinephrine is infiltrated over the lateral canthal tendon, transconjunctivally into the inferior fornix along the floor of the orbit, and injected into the ethmoid sinus. A nasal speculum and bayonet forceps are used to pack the nose along the inferior turbinate with cottonoid sponges soaked in 0.25% phenylephrine hydrochloride (Neo-Synephrine®) and oxymetazoline hydrochloride (Afrin®). Moistened Gelfoam pads are useful in protecting the cornea during surgery since protective scleral shells often do not remain in place in patients with severe exophthalmos.

Methelyne blue is used to mark the skin laterally and a #15 blade is used to perform the lateral canthotomy incision (Fig. 4). The needle Bovie is used to perform the cantholysis of the inferior crus of the lower lid. Blair retractors are used to evert the lower lid and expose the inferior fornix. The Bovie is used to incise the conjunctiva and dissect through lower lid retractors down to the inferior orbital rim. A periosteal elevator is used to reflect the periosteum and periorbita up off the floor of the orbit. It is important to identify the intraorbital neurovascular complex (infraorbital nerve and artery) so as to avoid damaging it. An osteotome and mallet are used to crack the orbital floor medial to the infraorbital neurovascular complex. Pituitary forceps are used to fracture and remove the floor of the orbit in a piecemeal manner. A Durden suction cautery is helpful to cauterize the sinus mucosa as removal progresses. It is important to remove the junction between the floor of the orbit and the medial wall. The orbital floor is removed back to the posterior aspect of the maxillary sinus. The surgeon usually unroofs the infraorbital neurovascular complex. Removal of the orbital floor lateral to the infraorbital neurovascular complex will increase the amount of retroplacement achieved; however, it will also increase the tendency of postoperative globe ptosis. The advantages and disadvantages of removing this lateral portion of the orbital floor must be judged individually in each case.

With the orbital floor resected, attention is turned to the medial orbital wall. Pituitary forceps are useful in removing the medial orbital wall and ethmoid air cells. Suction cautery is invaluable in maintaining visualization and achieving hemostasis. A fiberoptic head lamp worn by the surgeon is necessary for good illumination of this area. The subtotal ethmoidectomy is accomplished close to the level of the frontoethmoidal suture. Dissection beyond this important landmark can result in injury to either the anterior or posterior ethmoidal artery or penetration through the cribriform plate with a subsequent cerebrospinal fluid leak. Hemostasis is achieved, and a hemostatic surgical sponge (Surgicel) is applied to the ethmoidal area. The surgeon then proceeds to the opposite side for the bony decompression, leaving the Surgicel in place and the periorbita intact.

Following the bony decompression on the other side, the surgeon then returns to the first side to open the periorbita. Up to this point in the operation it is important not to have incised the periorbita because prolapsing deep orbital fat would obscure visualization. To open the periorbita, a Westcott scissors is used. An incision is made across the width

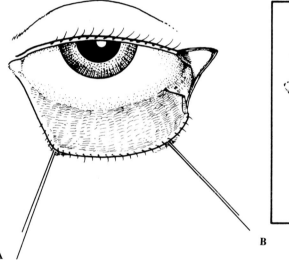

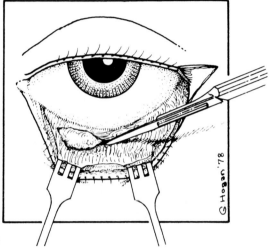

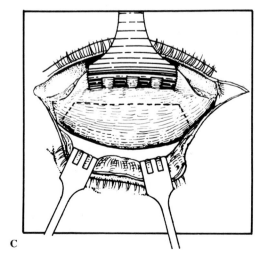

FIG. 4. Antral-ethmoidal decompression via inferior fornix approach. **A:** Eversion and outward swinging of the lower lid after lateral canthotomy and cantholysis has been performed; this exposes the lower formix for the incision to the inferior orbital rim. **B:** Incision through capsulopalpebral fascia and orbital fat to the orbital rim after the cut conjunctival edge has been retracted. In this step a ribbon retractor is placed in front of the globe and is pressed against the inferior orbital rim to guide the incision and protect the globe. **C:** Exposure of the inferior periosteum of the orbit after it has been elevated from the floor and nasal wall with a periosteal elevator. Dotted line shows site of future incision to open orbital contents.

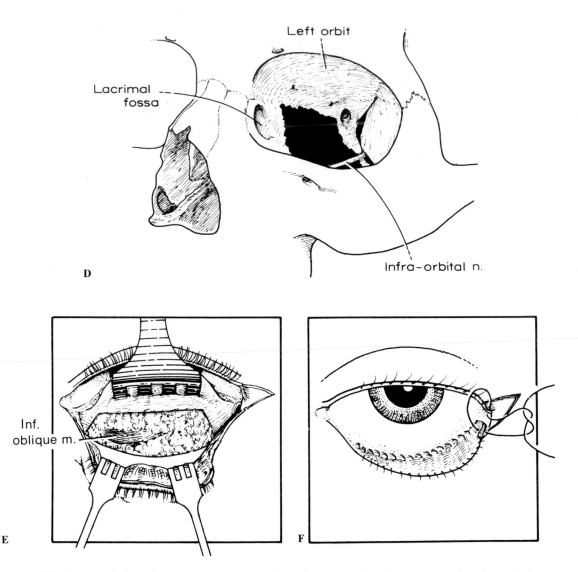

FIG. 4 (*cont.*)   **D:** Area of bone removed with antral-ethmoidal decompression showing preservation of infraorbital neurovascular bundle. The bony orbital floor and inferior ethmoids are removed completely along with the sinus mucosa. **E:** Diagram showing opening of the periosteum of the inferior orbit with a horizontal anterior incision and two posterior relaxing incisions. The anterior leading edge of the periosteum is pushed and peeled backwards and excised. The inferior oblique muscle is practically always encountered and is quite enlarged. **F:** Diagram showing closure of the inferior fornix incision with a running absorbable suture and reattachment of the lateral canthal tendon to the lateral orbital tubercle.

of the orbit while also making axial relaxing incisions. A malleable retractor can be slid under the periorbita to protect the orbit. A hemostat is then used to grasp the periorbita and tear out a large strip of periorbita from the inferior and medial orbit. Gentle pressure on the globe and teasing maneuvers will allow orbital fat to prolapse into the sinus openings that have been created. The retrodisplacement of the globe should be quite apparent at the time of this maneuver. In some cases of Graves' ophthalmopathy with fibrosis and scarring, much less retrodisplacement of the globe will be achieved from the orbital decompression because of the stiffness of the tissue.

The conjunctiva of the inferior fornix is closed with a loose, running, 6-0 plain suture. Lateral canthal fixation is achieved with 4-0 Polydek. The lateral canthotomy incision is closed with interrupted 6-0 nylon suture. The nasal packing is removed so that a nasoantral window can be fashioned. The anterior tip of the inferior turbinate is excised with a cutting cautery. A sharp Wener rasp is used to punch an opening into the maxillary antrum. The antrostomy is enlarged with a curved rongeur. Care is taken to avoid injury to the nasolacrimal duct (Fig. 5). A #12 red rubber catheter is inserted up into the maxillary sinus and cut flush with the external nare. A drip bandage is applied to the patient's nose. The nasal antrostomy is important to allow drainage of fluid and any blood from the maxillary sinus postoperatively, thus avoiding any pressure buildup in the orbit. Postoperative care includes

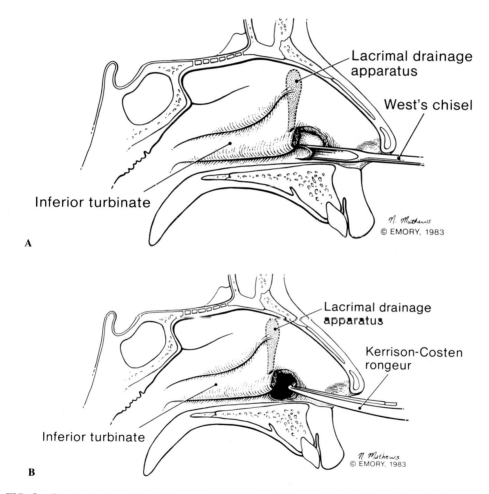

FIG. 5. Steps in the formation of the nasoantral window. **A:** The anterior tip of the turbinate has been excised with a cutting cautery and the mucosa in the lateral wall is being elevated away from the proposed site of placement with a chisel. Note the proximity to the nasolacrimal duct. (From McCord, ref. 18, with permission of Lippincott/Harper & Row.) **B:** Enlargement of the nasoantral window after puncture into the antrum has been performed using a rongeur, hemostat, or Weiner rasp. (From McCord, ref. 18, with permission of Lippincott/Harper & Row.)

light ice compresses (pressure dressings are avoided); oral prednisone, tapered over a 1-week period; and prophylactic antibiotics and oral decongestants.

Three-wall decompression

Three-wall decompression combines resection of the medial wall and orbital floor (2-wall) with resection of the lateral orbital wall (Fig. 6A). This technique may enhance the reduction of exophthalmos achieved by the two-wall decompression technique. (27).

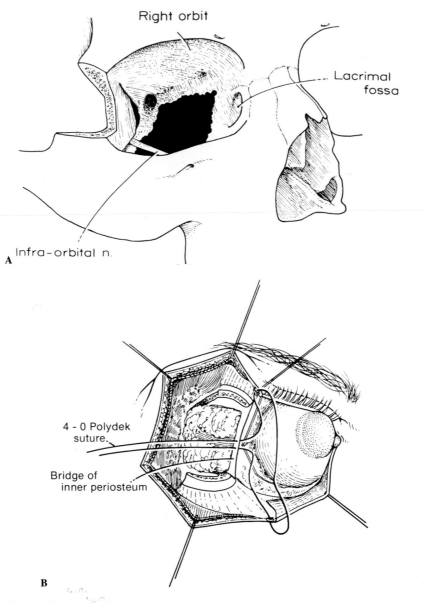

FIG. 6. Three-wall decompression via inferior fornix approach. **A:** Bony removal with three-wall orbital decompression showing excision of the lateral wall and removal of the floor of the orbit and inferior ethmoids, sparing the infraorbital neurovascular bundle. **B:** The fornix incision has been closed with a running plain suture. The upper and lower limb of the canthal tendons are reattached to the anterior edge of a periosteal bridge tag to reform the lateral canthus before closure of the lateral incision.

The lateral orbital wall may be removed through a canthal incision using standard lateral orbitotomy techniques as described in Chapter 11. This is followed by a fornix incision for inferior and medial orbital exposure and completion of the antral-ethmoidal decompression as previously described. The lateral periorbita, bone flap, and temporalis muscle in the area are excised and removed completely. Closure of the lateral canthus requires a piece of periorbita for reformation of the lateral canthal attachment (Fig. 6B).

Antral-ethmoidal decompression via transantral approach

In the authors' opinion the transantral exposure for the antral-ethmoidal decompression is the best procedure for relief of compressive neuropathy (18,28–30). This technique allows removal of more of the posterior ethmoids and more decompression of the orbital apex than does the inferior fornix approach. In patients with visual loss from compressive optic neuropathy, the transantral approach yields better visual recovery than does the inferior fornix approach (18). However, one-third of patients will develop new diplopia following transantral orbital decompression. Patients with preoperative strabismus have a significant risk of worsened motility imbalance following transantral decompression; therefore, we do not use it in noncompressive neuropathy patients (31,32). Figure 7 compares the effect on motility of the transantral and the translid (transfornix) two-wall decompression (18).

Surgical technique. To obtain the standard Caldwell-Luc exposure, the patient is positioned in a semi-sitting position with the head at a 45° angle without arm boards and with the endotracheal tube midline. Lidocaine 2% with epinephrine and hyaluronidase are used

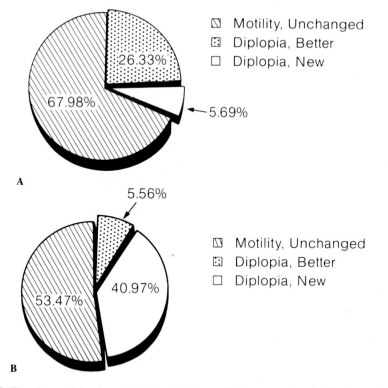

FIG. 7. Motility changes following antral-ethmoidal (two-wall) decompression. **A:** The change in motility in those patients undergoing antral-ethmoidal decompression through the transfornix (translid) approach. **B:** The number of patients undergoing changes in motility following antral-ethmoidal decompression via the transantral approach. (From McCord, ref. 18, with permission of Lippincott/Harper & Row.)

to infiltrate the ethmoid air cells, the floor of the orbit, and the buccogingival mucosa. Army-Navy retractors are used to retract the upper lip. A buccogingival sulcus incision is made with a #15 blade, leaving a cuff of gingiva above the toothline. Mucoperiosteum is then reflected up off the anterior wall of the maxillary antrum with a peanut dissection. The infraorbital nerve should be identified and preserved. A standard Caldwell-Luc antrostomy through the canine fossa and anterior wall is made with an osteotome. A rongeur is used to enlarge the antrostomy as wide as possible laterally and nasally. Laterally, care should be taken to avoid injury to Stenson's duct. The mucosa of the superior nasal aspect of the maxillary antrum is removed with a currette.

The ethmoidectomy is performed first. A Frazier suction or Durden cauterizing suction is used to scratch back and forth in the superior nasal aspect of the antrum, which is the inferior ethmoidal sinus (Fig. 8). The nasolacrimal canal may be prominent, obstructing direct access to the ethmoidal air cells. In these cases it may be inwardly fractured without causing lacrimal obstruction. Patient rubbing and fracturing of the air cells with the suction tip followed by removal with pituitary forceps allows a complete ethmoidectomy to be performed in the posterior area. When air cell removal is completed, the white frontal bone is seen in the superior aspect of the ethmoidal cavity. The surgeon should not veer nasally to avoid penetrating the cribriform plate, or laterally where the orbit would be encountered. The medial orbital wall is removed only after the ethmoidectomy is complete.

Attention is next turned to the orbital floor, where the infraorbital groove containing the infraorbital neurovascular complex is identified. It appears as a dark line running along the floor of the orbit in a posterolateral–to–anteromedial direction. The floor of the orbit (roof of the maxillary antrum) is removed from the orbital rim to the apex of the sinus. A hinged incision is made in the periorbita. A hemostat is used to grasp the hinge and tear away a strip of periorbita from the medial orbit and orbital floor. Gentle pressure on the globe should cause orbital contents to prolapse down into the sinus opening. A nasal antral window is then performed as previously described.

When good hemostasis has been achieved and a satisfactory decompression accomplished, the buccogingival incision is closed with interrupted 4-0 Vicryl sutures through the mucosa. A red rubber catheter is inserted in this antrostomy to maintain patency and allow drainage over the first few postoperative days. Ice compresses, oral prednisone, antibiotics, and decongestants are used. Pressure dressings are avoided.

In the learning stages of orbital decompression surgery it is very instructive to the surgeon to compare preoperative and postoperative CT scans (axial and coronal views). This allows the surgeon to compare the bone removal seen intraoperatively with radiologic anatomy and improves intraoperative surgical judgment (Fig. 9).

Surgery on Extraocular Muscles

The restrictive myopathy of Graves' ophthalmopathy may cause patients to suffer from diplopia. When chronic fibrosis of the extraocular muscle is severe, botulinum toxin injections are generally ineffective and surgery on the extraocular muscles becomes the procedure of choice. The most commonly affected extraocular muscles are the inferior rectus and medial rectus muscles, making limitation of upgaze and decreased abduction the most common deficits. Demonstrated stability over a minimum 6-month period should be a prerequisite to surgery on the extraocular muscles.

Surgical technique

We typically perform motility surgery under general anesthesia, although local anesthesia is certainly satisfactory. Topical phenylephrine hydrochloride eye drops or subconjunctival lidocaine 2% with epinephrine and hyaluronidase can be used to aid hemostasis. Forced duction testing is performed at the start of the procedure (33). This technique is performed with a toothed forceps and the surgeon may either grasp the conjunctiva–Tenon's capsule layer near the limbus or actually grasp the rectus muscle insertion. A firm grasp is necesary so as to rotate the globe and not merely stretch the conjunctiva. The most common extraocular muscle surgery in Graves' ophthalmopathy will be recession of the inferior rectus. To expose the inferior rectus, the conjunctiva is opened at the limbus and a fornix-based flap

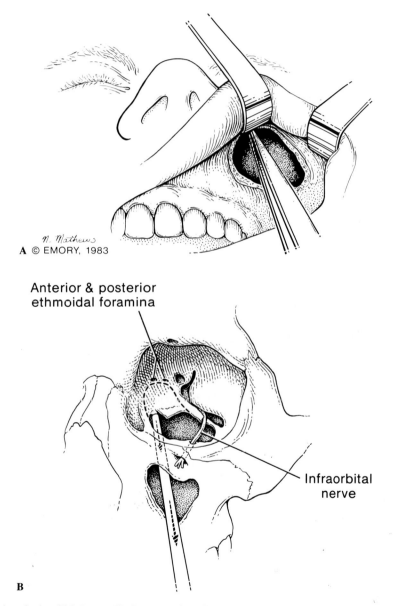

FIG. 8. Antral-ethmoidal (two-wall) decompression via transantral (Ogura) approach. **A:** Surgical exposure required in the Ogura procedure for removal of ethmoid air cells and orbital floor. (From McCord, ref. 18, with permission of Lippincott/Harper & Row. **B:** Typical bone removal via the transantral antral-ethmoidal decompression. In this diagram the Frazier suction tip is positioned to remove the ethmoid air cells.

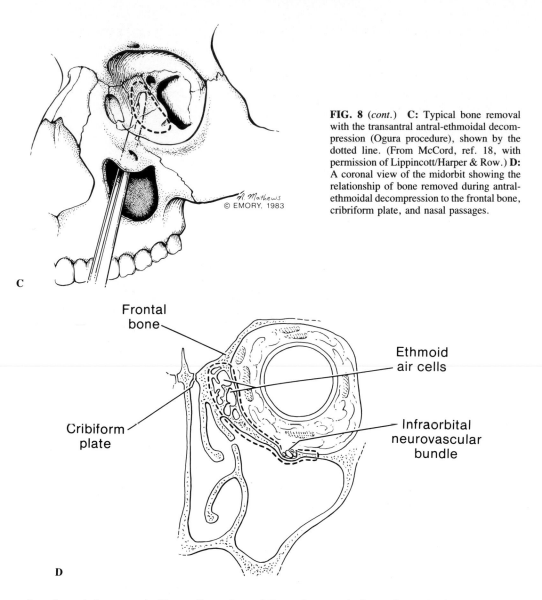

FIG. 8 (*cont.*)   **C:** Typical bone removal with the transantral antral-ethmoidal decompression (Ogura procedure), shown by the dotted line. (From McCord, ref. 18, with permission of Lippincott/Harper & Row.) **D:** A coronal view of the midorbit showing the relationship of bone removed during antral-ethmoidal decompression to the frontal bone, cribriform plate, and nasal passages.

is reflected downward. Sharp dissection of Tenon's capsule is performed with a Westcott scissors. Dissection of the check ligaments and the intermuscular septae, as well as any adhesions, is important is obtaining a good motility result as well as minimizing postoperative lower eyelid retraction. A double-armed 6-0 Vicryl suture is sewn through the muscle and securely locked at each border. A Westcott scissors is used to disinsert the rectus muscle from the globe, and the double-armed Vicryl suture is then sewn directly through the stump of the tendon insertion.

Our strong preference is to use an adjustable suture technique whenever possible. The adjustable suture technique allows for a postoperative alteration of the "best estimate" surgical repositioning of the muscle (34). This if of great importance in the Graves' ophthalmopathy patient, in whom abnormal muscle length and elasticity cause unpredictability of conventional strabismus surgery. The scleral-muscle suture tract is enlarged by a to-and-fro sawing motion of the 6-0 Vicryl suture. This maneuver will facilitate the final postoperative adjustment. When planning a recession, e.g., a fibrosed inferior rectus muscle, it is best to overrecess the muscle, because postoperatively it is easiest to pull up on the muscle rather than cause it to recess back farther. The conjunctiva is closed with 6-0 plain suture. The conjunctival flap is recessed to the level of the tendon insertion so as not to encumber te 6-0 Vicryl suture during postoperative adjustment. A 6-0 Prolene suture is sewn into

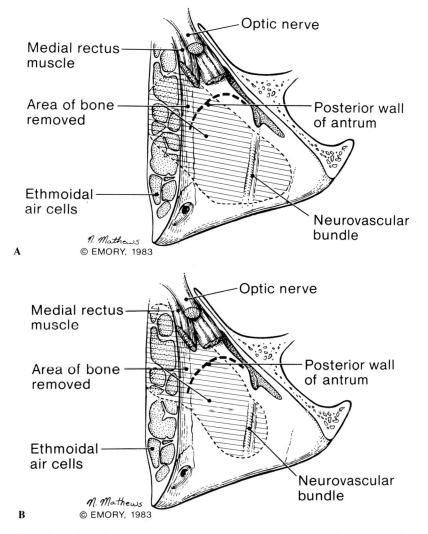

FIG. 9. Comparison of transfornix and transantral two-wall decompression techniques. Area of bone removed under direct visualization. **A:** Usual bony defect in the floor and ethmoids obtained through the transfornix (translid) approach to antral-ethmoidal decompression. The *shaded area* represents bone that is most often excised by the surgeon with reasonably good visualization. Additional bone can be removed through this approach without good visualization, but visualized bone is the most likely to be removed in any decompression procedure. (From McCord, ref. 18, with permission of Lippincott/Harper & Row.) **B:** The usual bony defect obtained in antral-ethmoidal decompression via the transantral approach. It is to be emphasized that the *shaded area* is the bone most often removed by the surgeon with adequate visualization. Obviously, different configurations could be removed, but would in general be undertaken without visualization. (From McCord, ref. 18, with permission of Lippincott/Harper & Row.)

the sclera in the event that traction is required on the globe during adjustment. The double armed 6-0 Vicryl suture and the Prolene suture are draped over the eyelid and the eye covered lightly with a patch. Ophthalmic ointment is not instilled because this may hamper postoperative adjustment.

We generally complete the adjustment on the first postoperative day. Postoperative suture adjustments may be performed a few hours following surgery if the patient is awake and alert and all local anesthetic has worn off. For adjustment, topical anesthetic drops are instilled in the conjunctival cul-de-sac. Motility balance is examined by cover-uncover testing at distance and near in important fields of gaze. Cover-uncover testing may be repeated several times during suture adjustment. Two empty needle holders are used to grasp the 6-0 Vicryl suture arm and easily pull up an overrecessed muscle. To further recess a muscle, the 6-0 Prolene traction suture is held to fixate the globe, while the patient looks in the direction of the muscle being adjusted. This will generate contraction of that muscle and thus further recess it as needed. When satisfactory adjustments have been made in muscle balance and ocular rotations, the 6-0 Vicryl suture is tied permanently and cut and the 6-0 Prolene is removed. Topical antibiotics and steroid preparations are used during the first postoperative week. Forced duction testing must be performed preoperatively, intraoperatively, and postoperatively in these patients because a tightly fibrosed inferior rectus muscle may cause both limitation of elevation and limitation of abduction, and this can only be determined once the tight inferior rectus muscle is disinserted from the globe.

Surgery for Eyelid Retraction

Corneal and conjunctival exposure and cosmetic disfigurement are the most common indications for surgical correction of eyelid retraction. As with other surgeries for patients with Graves' ophthalmopathy, stability is of paramount importance in the treatment of eyelid retraction. As stated previously, the appropriate order of staged surgical procedures is orbital decompression first, followed by extraocular muscle surgery, and finally eyelid surgery.

There are a variety of contributing factors to upper lid retraction in Graves' disease. In the hyperthyroid state, sympathetic stimulation may cause contraction of Müller's muscle with resulting eyelid retraction, which resolves in many patients with a euthyroid state or treatment with propranolol hydrochloride (Inderal®) or guanethidine eye drops. In euthyroid cases the underlying cause of eyelid retraction is fibrosis and shortening of the eyelid retractor muscles (levator and Müller's) in the upper and lower lid. The many inflammatory adhesions that are present between the levator, orbital septum, and orbital fat may also cause retraction and lagophthalmos. Tethering of the inferior rectus muscle can cause upper lid retraction with the effort involved in upgaze.

When seen in the office, many patients will minimize their eyelid retraction with involuntary squinting. It is important to gain complete relaxation of the eyelids to the resting state in order to measure the true amount of needed correction. Topical anesthetic drops may be used to accomplish this.

Patients wtih asymmetric lid retraction can present problems in two areas. Unequal recession of the levator can produce an unequal eyelid crease. Also, these patients can mask lid retraction in the lesser involved eye that can and will become manifest after unilateral or asymmetric surgery, necessitating secondary surgery. The importance of the possible need for revisional surgery in these patients should be emphasized, particularly with regard to the lid crease. In the upper eyelid, it is our opinion that recession of the fibrosed and shortened levator-Müller's muscle complex without spacer material can be performed and gravity will help counteract further tendencies toward upper eyelid retraction. This is in contradistinction to the situation in the lower eyelid, where release or resection of the capsulopalpebral fascia and inferior sympathetic muscle in some cases is insufficient. In the lower lid, spacer material and supraplacement of the lateral canthal tendon are needed to counteract gravitational effects. An upper lid recession technique with and without spacer material will be described here. We acknowledge the work of Grove (9,35), Doxanas and Dryden (36), Putterman (37), Harvey and Anderson (38), Waller (39), and Baylis et al. (40). Again, the importance of the stabilization of Graves' ophthalmopathy before surgery cannot be overemphasized.

Surgical correction of upper eyelid retraction

The upper eyelid is infiltrated with lidocaine 2% with 1:100,000 epinephrine and hyaluronidase. Because these patients bleed more than normal, the surgeon should allow at least 10 min for the epinephrine effect before beginning the operation. The lid crease is marked in methylene blue in a manner identical to the standard upper lid blepharoplasty approach (Fig. 10). A 4-0 silk traction suture is placed through the upper eyelid margin. Downward traction greatly facilitates dissection of the eyelid tissues and the invariably present tissue adhesions. A #15 blade is used to make a skin excision following the lid crease marking. Redundant skin is usually excised as in blepharoplasty. The needle Bovie is used to dissect through the orbicularis muscle and thus expose the levator aponeurosis. The orbital septum is usually opened and the preaponeurotic fat removed.

Using a 0.3 forceps to lift up on the levator, the Bovie is used to incise the levator

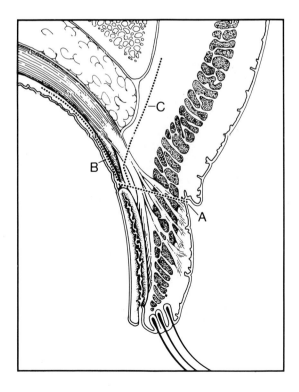

FIG. 10. Cross-sectional diagram of the upper eyelid. **Line A:** The skin incision and dissection at the level of the lid crease. **Line B:** Dissection of the levator-Müller's muscle complex up off the conjunctiva. **Line C:** Dissection of preaponeurotic adhesions, which are typical of Graves' ophthalmopathy.

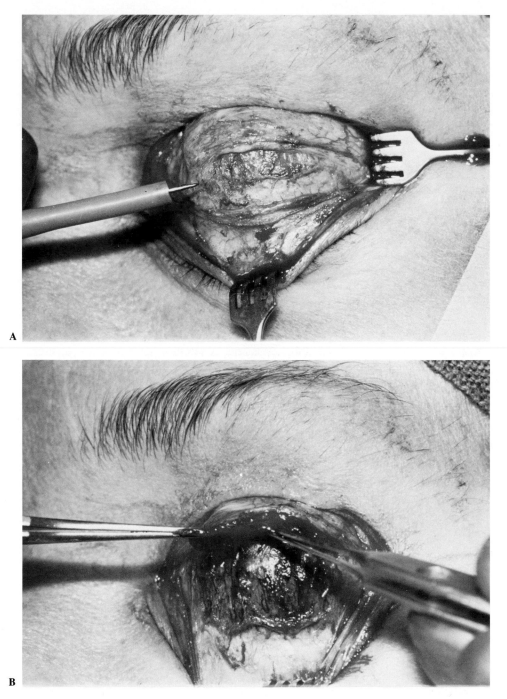

FIG. 11. Surgical steps of levator recession. **A:** With the upper lid held under tension, the levator aponeurosis is incised with the needle Bovie unit. **B:** With the eyelid and conjunctiva retracted downward under tension, Müller's muscle is dissected up off the conjunctiva.

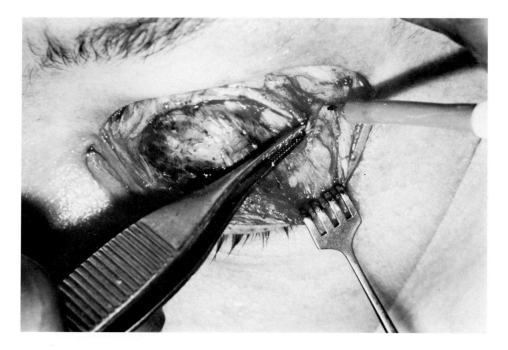

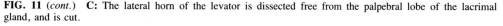

FIG. 11 (*cont.*) **C:** The lateral horn of the levator is dissected free from the palpebral lobe of the lacrimal gland, and is cut.

across its entire horizontal width (Fig. 11A). This incision exposes Müller's muscle and the superior marginal arcade of vessels that is just above the tarsal border. Above the level of the superior arcade, Müller's muscle is dissected free from the conjunctiva (Fig. 11B). A large block resection of Müller's muscle is then performed. Again, it is essential to have firm, downward retraction on the eyelid and conjunctiva to perform this dissection of Müller's muscle from the conjunctiva. A meticulous dissection is necessary to avoid creating buttonholes in the conjunctiva, although some may be unavoidable. At this point, the surgeon should observe the lid and allow the levator to retract upward. It is common to require further dissection of the levator muscle so that it may be freed from the tissue adhesions. More extensive dissection is required at the lateral horn, which as a rule should be completely cut (Fig. 11C). The lateral horn of the levator aponeurosis must first be dissected free of the palpebral lobe of the lacrimal gland before it is cut. This step of the operation is tedious but is necessary to avoid residual upper eyelid retraction laterally.

When adequate dissection of the levator is accomplished, the edge of the recessed levator is sutured in mattress fashion to the upper third of tarsus with a double-armed 6-0 silk suture (Fig. 12A). This 6-0 silk mattress suture acts as a suspender of the upper eyelid, attaching the recessed levator to the tarsus. As a guideline to the amount of levator recession, the surgeon can use a lid-gapping method (Fig. 12B). The surgeon should reduce the intraoperative measured eyelid gapping under general anesthesia or sedation by an equivalent number of millimeters to the preoperative eyelid retraction. As an example, a patient with 4 mm of upper eyelid retraction preoperatively may demonstrate 8 mm of eyelid gapping intraoperatively. The levator muscle should then be recessed to decrease the lid gapping by 4 mm. This rule of thumb is meant to serve as a starting point for the individual

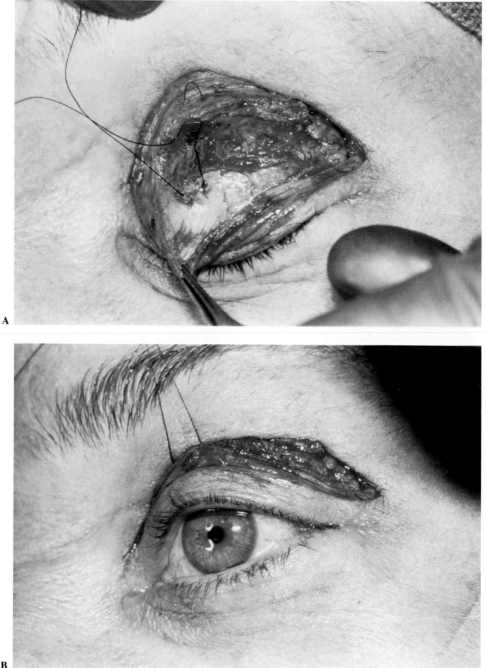

A

B

FIG. 12. Upper lid levator recession with a suspender suture. **A:** A 6–0 silk mattress suture is used as a suspender between the recessed levator aponeurosis and the upper lid tarsus. **B:** With the suspender suture tied temporarily, the eyelid height and contour are examined and adjusted as necessary.

surgeon's own technique. Certainly in the awake patient having surgery under local anesthesia one can observe the contour and height of the eyelid with the patient holding his or her eyes open. However, local anesthesia, and sedation, may have a variable effect.

Closure is achieved with interrupted 6-0 nylon sutures and the skin-muscle edges are sutured to the superior border of the tarsus to form a lid crease, which avoids upward migration and irregularity of the lid crease. As mentioned, this lid crease incision approach to eyelid retraction is readily combined with upper lid blepharoplasty in patients with redundant skin and protuberant fatty pads.

As an alternative to the suspender suture (nonspacer) technique of upper lid recession, traditional spacer material can be used, and is described here for completeness. Following the dissection of the levator aponeurosis with severance of the lateral horn and the excision of Müller's muscle, spacer material (e.g., fascia lata) may be inserted instead of placement of the suspender suture. With adequate dissection, the vertical width of the spacer material at the midpupillary level need be only the amount of recession that one wishes to obtain. The temporal width is wider to compensate for proptosis and the tendency for undercorrection in that area (Figs. 13 and 14). In our experience the results are superior with the suspender suture, but it may be necessary to use spacer material in some reoperated cases or in those patients with increased fibrosis.

Surgical correction of lower eyelid retraction

A significant component of the corneal and conjunctival exposure in Graves' ophthalmopathy may be due to lower eyelid retraction. The three principles of correcting lower lid retraction are: supraplacement of the lateral canthal tendon, release of the lower eyelid retractors, and insertion of spacer material in the eyelid.

Lidocaine 2% with 1:100,000 epinephrine and hyaluronidase are infiltrated across the width of the lower lid on both the cutaneous and conjunctival surfaces. Additional local anesthetic is infiltrated over the lateral canthal tendon. Ample time is alloted for the epinephrine hemostatic effect. A 4-0 silk traction suture is placed through the lower lid margin. Methylene blue is used to mark the skin over the lateral canthal tendon. A #15 blade is used to incise the skin and perform a lateral canthotomy. Cantholysis of the inferior limb of the lateral canthal tendon is then performed with the needle Bovie. A 4-0 double-armed Prolene suture with a semicircular needle is sewn through the tarsus laterally. The combination of the 4-0 silk marginal suture and 4-0 Prolene suture is used to evert the lower lid and retract it downward. Strong tension on the traction sutures highlights the lower eyelid tarsus and offers excellent exposure of the palpebral conjunctiva. The needle Bovie is used to incise the palpebral conjunctiva across the width of the lower lid at a level 1 to 2 mm beneath the inferior tarsal border to expose the capsulopalpebral fascia, a whitish fibrous tissue. Holding the tissue planes under tension, the conjunctiva is carefully dissected free from the underlying capsulopalpebral fascia (Fig. 15A). Medial and lateral relaxing incisions are made in the conjunctiva. A 4- to 5-mm rectangular block of the capsulopalpebral fascia is excised and the rest allowed to retract. The surgeon should avoid dissecting anteriorly into the orbicularis muscle layer.

At this point in the surgery, autogenous cartilage is harvested in the standard method described in Chapter 1. The edges of the elliptical autogenous cartilage graft are trimmed to avoid pointy edges. It is sometimes necessary to score one surface of the cartilage graft with a #15 blade to induce a concavity of the surface that will face the globe. A running 6-0 Vicryl suture is used to suture the cartilage graft to the inferior border of the lower eyelid tarsus (Fig. 15B). The vertical height of the cartilage graft in millimeters

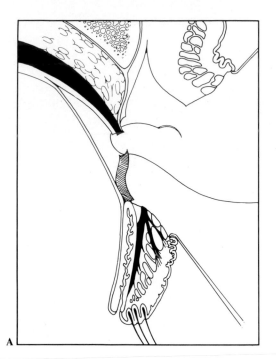

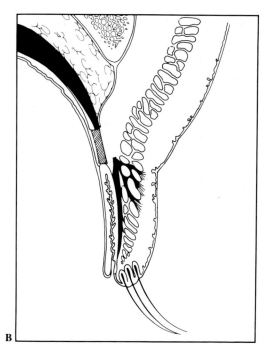

FIG. 13. Surgery for upper eyelid retraction. **A:** Cross-sectional diagram shows spacer material being sutured to the superior border of the tarsus and the cut edge of the recessed levator-Müller's muscle complex. **B:** Cross-sectional diagram shows final result with the spacer material in place and the levator-Müller's muscle recessed.

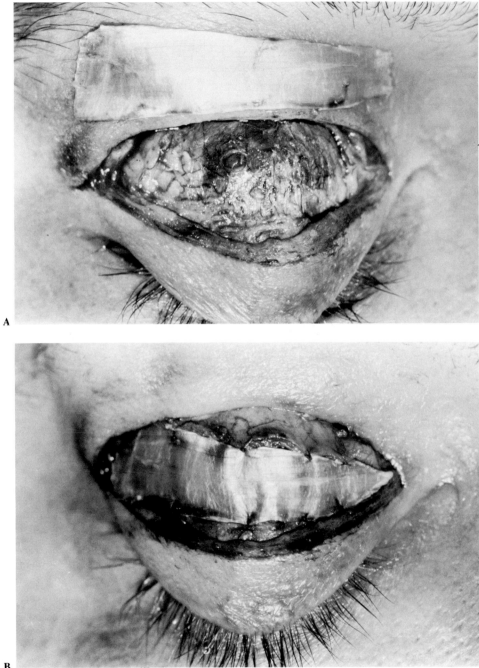

FIG. 14. Upper lid levator recession using autogenous fascia as a spacer material. **A:** The levator has been dissected to a recessed position and Müller's muscle excised. Note that the fascia is widest laterally where the greatest amount of levator recession is generally needed. **B:** The fascia serves as a spacer material as it is sutured to the cut edge of the recessed levator and to the upper lid tarsus.

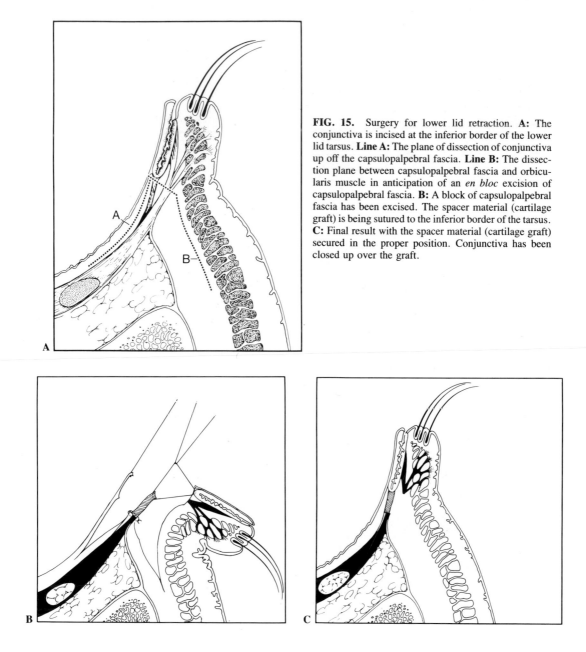

FIG. 15. Surgery for lower lid retraction. **A:** The conjunctiva is incised at the inferior border of the lower lid tarsus. **Line A:** The plane of dissection of conjunctiva up off the capsulopalpebral fascia. **Line B:** The dissection plane between capsulopalpebral fascia and orbicularis muscle in anticipation of an *en bloc* excision of capsulopalpebral fascia. **B:** A block of capsulopalpebral fascia has been excised. The spacer material (cartilage graft) is being sutured to the inferior border of the tarsus. **C:** Final result with the spacer material (cartilage graft) secured in the proper position. Conjunctiva has been closed up over the graft.

should be equal to or greater than the amount of preoperative lower eyelid retraction. The cartilage graft may be fashioned so that its greatest vertical height is laterally, a location where undercorrection is a problem. It is usually not necessary to suture the inferior border of the cartilage to the residual edge of the capsulopalpebral fascia, although one or two interrupted 6-0 Vicryl sutures can be used if the cartilage tends to rotate upward. The conjunctival layer should be adequately dissected and relaxed so that it can be advanced up over the cartilage graft and closed directly with a running 6-0 Vicryl suture (Fig. 15C). The 4-0 Prolene suture is then sutured to the periosteum inside the lateral orbital rim to achieve lateral canthal fixation. The key elements of this maneuver are to supraplace the lateral canthal tendon above the pupillary level, but avoid the tendency of tensing the lower eyelid too tightly. It may be necessary to supraplace the lateral canthal tendon 4 to 5 mm in order to reduce the eyelid retraction. If it is tensed too tightly the lower eyelid will not come up, but will tend to slide inferiorly with residual inferior scleral show.

The lateral canthotomy skin incision is closed with interrupted 6-0 nylon sutures. The prolonged use of post operative ice compresses is recommended in patients with Graves' ophthalmopathy. Oral cephalexin (Keflex®) is given for 1 week as a prophylactic antibiotic when free tissue grafts, such as cartilage, are used.

REFERENCES

1. Sisler, H. A., Jakobiec, F. A., and Trokel, S. L. (1985): Ocular abnormalities and orbital changes of Graves' disease. In: *Clinical Ophthalmology,* edited by T. D. Duane and E. A. Jaeger, Vol. 2, pp. 1–30. Harper & Row, Philadelphia.
2. Sergott, R. C., and Glaser, J. S. (1981): Graves ophthalmopathy: A clinical and immunologic review. *Surv. Ophthalmol.,* 26:1–21.
3. Riddick, F. A. (1981): Immunologic aspects of thyroid disease. *Ophthalmology,* 88:471–475.
4. Sergott, R. C., Felberg, N. T., Savino,, P. J., et al. (1981): Graves' ophthalmopathy immunologic parameters related to corticosteroid therapy. *Invest. Ophthalmol.,* 20:173–182.
5. Sergott, R. C., Felberg, N. T., Savino, P. J., et al. (1979): E-rosette formation in Graves' ophthalmopathy. *Invest. Ophthalmol.,* 18:1245–1251.
6. Sergott, R. C., Felberg, N. T., Savino, P. J., et al. (1981): The clinical immunology of Graves' ophthalmopathy. *Opthalmology,* 88:484–487.
7. Konishi, J., Herman, M. M., and Kriss, J. P. (1974): Binding of thyroglobulin and thyroglobulin-antithyroglobulin immune complex to extraocular muscle membrane. *Endocrinology,* 95:434–446.
8. Kriss, J. P. (1970): Radioisotopic thyroiodolymphography in patients with Graves' disease. *J. Clin. Endocrinol.,* 31.315–324.
9. Grove, A. S. (1981): Upper eyelid retraction and Graves' disease. *Ophthalmology,* 88:499–506.
10. Werner, S. C. (1977): Modification of the classification of the eye changes of Graves' disease. *Am. J. Ophthalmol.,* 83:725–727.
11. Fruch, B. R., Musch, D. C., and Garber, F. W. (1986): Exophthalmometer readings in patients with Graves' eye disease. *Ophthalmic Surg.,* 17(1):37–40.
12. Trokel, S. L., and Hilal, S. K. (1979): Recognition and differential diagnosis of enlarged extraocular muscles in computed tomography. *Am. J. Ophthalmol.,* 87:503–512.
13. Trobe, J. D., Glaser, J. S., and Laflamne, P. (1978): Dysthyroid optic neuropathy. Clinical profile and rationale for management. *Arch. Ophthalmol.,* 96:1199–1209.
14. Trokel, S. L., and Jakobiec, F. A. (1981): Correlation of CT scanning and pathologic features of ophthalmic Graves' disease. *Ophthalmology,* 88:553–564
15. Byrne, S. F., and Glaser, J. S. (1983): Orbital tissue differentiation with standardized echography. *Ophthalmology,* 90:1071–1090.
16. Scott, A. B. (1980): Botulinum toxin injection into extraocular muscles as an alternative to strabismus surgery. *Ophthalmology,* 87:1044–1049.
17. Trobe, J. D. (1981): Optic nerve involvement in dysthyroidism. *Ophthalmology,* 88:488–492.
18. McCord, C. D. (1985): Current trends in orbital decompression. *Ophthalmology,* 92:21–33.
19. Brenan, M. W., Leone, C. R., and Lalitha, J. (1983): Radiation therapy for Graves' disease. *Am. J. Ophthalmol.,* 96:195–199.
20. Hurbli, T., Char, D. H., Haris, J., et al. (1985): Radiation therapy for thyroid eye diseases. *Am. J. Ophthalmol.,* 99:633–637.
21. Naffzinger, H. C. (1932): Surgical treatment of progressive exophthalmos following thyroidectomy. *JAMA,* 99:638–642.
22. Kennerdell, J. S., and Maroon, J. C. (1972): An orbital decompression for severe dysthyroid exophthalmos. *Ophthalmology,* 89:467–472.
23. Wolfe, S. A. (1979): Modified three-wall orbital expansion to correct persistent exophthalmos or exorbitism. *J. Plast. Reconstr. Surg.,* 64:448–455.
24. McCord, C. D. (1981): Orbital decompression for Graves' disease; exposure through lateral canthal and inferior fornix incision. *Ophthalmology,* 88:533–541.
25. Linberg, J. V., and Anderson, R. L. (1981): Transorbital decompression. Indications and results. *Arch. Ophthalmol.,* 99:113–119.

26. Anderson, R. L., and Linberg, J. V. (1981): Transorbital approach to decompression in Graves' disease. *Arch. Ophthalmol.*, 99:120–124.
27. McCord, C. D., Putnam, J. R., and Ugland, D. N. (1985): Pressure volume orbital measurement comparing decompression approaches. *Ophthalmic Plast. Reconstr. Surg.*, 1:55–63.
28. Walsh, T. E., and Ogura, J. (1957): Transantral orbital decompression for malignant exophthalmos. *Laryngoscope*, 67:544–568.
29. Ogura, J. H., and Lucente, F. E. (1974): Surgical results of orbital decompression for malignant exophthalmos. *Laryngoscope*, 84:637–644.
30. Baylis, H. I., Call, N. B., and Shibata, C. S. (1980): The transantral orbital decompression (Ogura technique) as performed by the ophthalmologist. *Ophthalmology*, 87:1005–1012.
31. Trokel, S. L., and Cooper, W. C. (1979): Orbital decompression: Effect on motility and globe position. *Trans. Am. Acad. Ophthalmol.*, 86:2064–2070.
32. Shorr, N., Neuhaus, R. W., and Baylis, H. I. (1982): Ocular motility problems after orbital decompression for dysthyroid ophthalmopathy. *Ophthalmology*, 89:323–328.
33. Metz, H. S. (1983): Restrictive factors in strabismus. *Surv. Ophthalmol*, 28:71–83.
34. Jampolsky, A. (1979): Current techniques of adjustable strabismus surgery. *Am. J. Ophthalmol*, 88:406–418.
35. Grove, A. S. (1980): Eyelid retraction treated by levator marginal myotomy. *Ophthalmology*, 87:1013–1018.
36. Doxanas, M. T., and Dryden, R. M. (1981): The use of sclera in the treatment of dysthyroid eyelid retraction. *Ophthalmology*, 88:887–894.
37. Putterman, A. (1981): Surgical treatment of thyroid-related upper eyelid retraction. *Ophthalmology*, 88:507–512.
38. Harvey, J. T., and Anderson, R. L. (1981): The aponeurotic approach to eyelid retraction. *Ophthalmology*, 88:513–524.
39. Waller, R. R. (1978): Lower eyelid retraction: Management, *Ophthalmic Surg.*, 9(3):41–47.
40. Baylis, H. I., Perman, R. I., Fett, D. R., and Sutcliffe, R. T. (1985): Autogenous auricular cartilage grafting for lower eyelid retraction. *Ophthalmic Plast. Reconstr. Surg.*, 1:23–27.

Oculoplastic Surgery, 2nd edition, edited by
Clinton D. McCord, Jr., and Myron Tanenbaum.
Raven Press, New York © 1987.

Chapter 9

Eyelid Tumors: Diagnosis and Management

*Arthur S. Grove, Jr., **Clinton D. McCord, Jr., and †Myron Tanenbaum

*Department of Ophthalmology, Harvard Medical School, and Massachusetts Eye and Ear Infirmary,
Boston, Massachusetts 02114; **Department of Ophthalmology, Emory University School of Medicine,
Atlanta, Georgia 30308; and †Bascom Palmer Eye Institute, Department of Ophthalmology, University
of Miami School of Medicine, Miami, Florida 33101*

To appropriately treat eyelid tumors, it is first necessary to establish a diagnosis. Many tumors have a characteristic clinical appearance, but an exact diagnosis usually depends upon histological examination of tissues removed by biopsy or excision.

GENERAL PRINCIPLES OF EYELID TUMOR DIAGNOSIS

More than three-quarters of all eyelid tumors are benign. Most of these are neoplasms such as keratoses and nevi, or inflammatory lesions such as chalazions (1). Basal cell carcinoma is the most common eyelid malignancy, comprising more than 90% of all eyelid cancers and nearly 20% of eyelid tumors in general (Table 1).

History and Physical Examination

In general, eyelid lesions that have been present for many years and have not changed in appearance are usually benign (Figs. 1 and 2). However, some benign lesions may enlarge and can only be distinguished from malignancies by histological study (Figs. 3–

TABLE 1. *Incidence of eyelid tumors*[a]

Benign tumors	Malignant tumors
Keratoses/papillomas	Basal cell carcinomas
Nevi	Squamous cell carcinomas
Epidermoid cysts	Sebaceous cell carcinomas
Chalazions	Malignant melanomas

[a] Most common eyelid tumors, listed in approximate order of frequency (1).

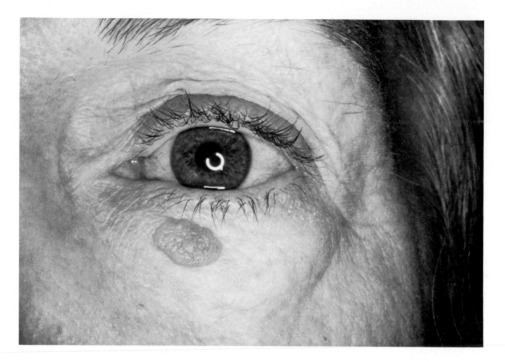

FIG. 1.   Seborrheic keratosis. Papillomatous, ''waxy,'' light brown lesion unchanged for many years.

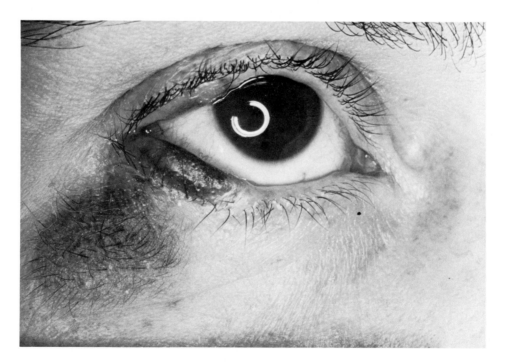

FIG. 2.   Compound nevus. Elevated, dark lesion containing many hairs, unchanged since childhood.

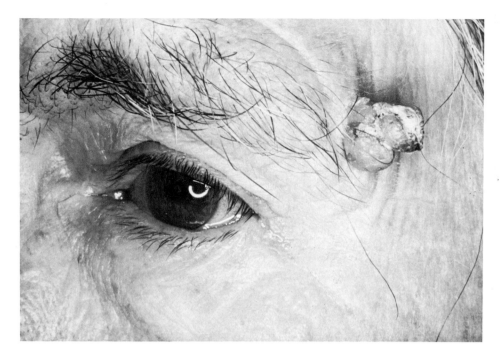

FIG. 3. Solar (actinic) keratosis. Papillomatous, hyperkaratotic lesion enlarged over a 6-month period.

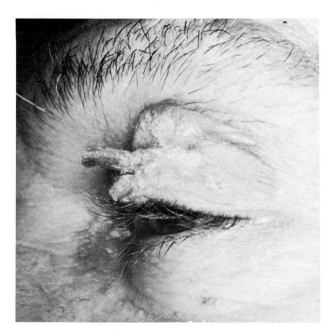

FIG. 4. Solar (actinic) keratosis. "Cutaneous horn" enlarged during previous year. Base should be completely excised, because malignancy (squamous cell carcinoma) may be present.

5). Keratoacanthomas (Fig. 6) are benign epidermal tumors that may grow very rapidly and that sometimes undergo spontaneous involution with complete disappearance. These tumors may histologically resemble squamous cell carcinomas and should be completely excised if the diagnosis is in doubt (2).

Clinical features that suggest the presence of a malignancy include loss of eyelashes and ulceration. Changes in size, contour, or color of the growth are frequent signs of malignancy. Recurrence of a lesion after previous treatment should raise the suspicion that a malignancy is present. In particular, a nodule that recurs after being treated as a chalazion should be suspected of being a sebaceous cell carcinoma arising from the meibomian glands. Sebaceous cell carcinomas sometimes spread within the conjunctival epithelium and mimic chronic blepharoconjunctivitis.

Physical examination of a patient with an eyelid tumor should include evaluation of the subcutaneous tissues to determine the clinical depth of the lesion and possible extension to the orbital bones or the globe. The entire conjunctival surface, including the palpebral conjunctiva and the fornices, should be examined when multicentric tumors such as sebaceous cell carcinomas and malignant melanomas are present. Except for basal cell carcinomas, most eyelid malignancies have the potential to spread by regional metastasis and therefore the preauricular, submandibular, and cervical lymph nodes should be examined and palpated. If possible, photographs and sketches of tumors should be made before initial biopsy or treatment.

Systemic Examinations and Diagnostic Studies

Systemic examinations other than chest X-rays, regional node evaluation, and a complete physical examination are usually not required in patients with relatively small basal cell,

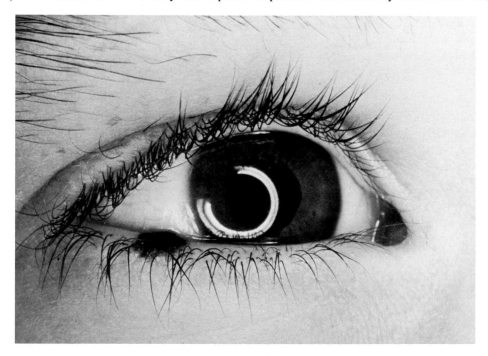

FIG. 5. Blue nevus. Highly cellular, darkly pigmented tumor enlarged over several months in a young girl. "Benign juvenile melanoma" may be histologically difficult to distinguish from malignant melanoma.

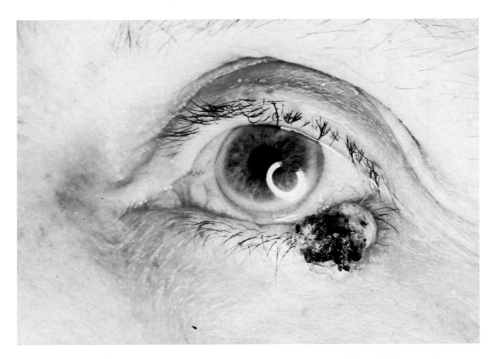

FIG. 6. Keratoacanthoma. Papillomatous tumor rapidly enlarged during several weeks. Biopsy confirmed benign keratoacanthoma, which gradually disappeared spontaneously over several months. If involution had not occurred, complete excision should have been performed.

squamous cell, or sebaceous cell carcinomas. In patients with malignant melanomas, liver scans and liver function tests should also be performed, since even small melanomas may sometimes metastasize rapidly.

In patients with large tumors, extensive recurrent tumors, or tumors that appear to extend into the deep subcutaneous tissues, it is useful to obtain plain and tomographic X-rays as well as computed tomographic (CT) scans, as described in Chapter 10. Clinical fixation of a tumor to the underlying periosteum indicates that the adjacent bone may be involved by the malignancy. In such cases bony invasion may be histologically present, even though destruction is not seen on X-rays or CT scans.

Biopsy and Tissue-Processing Techniques

If an eyelid tumor is disfiguring or is suspected of being a malignancy, it should be removed or biopsied for histological examination. A preliminary photograph and sketch should be made to document the appearance and location of the lesion. If the tumor is relatively small, excisional biopsy of the entire lesion may be performed. In most cases a wedge or plug of the tumor may be excised as a biopsy specimen. For optimal evaluation, the specimen should be representative of the clinically abnormal lesion, should be sufficiently large for histological processing, and should not be crushed or excessively traumatized. A histological diagnosis should almost always precede extensive tumor resection and reconstruction.

Most tumors can be adequately evaluated by conventional formalin fixation and histological staining with hematoxylin and eosin (H&E). However, lipids are removed from tissues during H&E staining because of alcohol immersion. Therefore, if sebaceous cell carcinoma

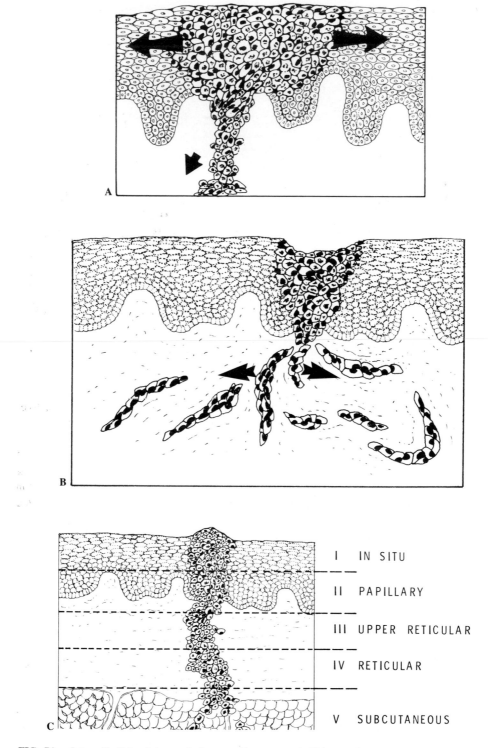

FIG. 7A. Intraepithelial radial spread of tumors (*large arrows*). This growth pattern is typical of (a) superficial basal cell carcinoma, (b) *in situ* squamous cell carcinoma, (c) pagetoid spread of sebaceous cell carcinoma, and

is suspected, the pathologist should be alerted at the time that the specimen is submitted so that fat stains can be performed. In cases when a melanoma is suspected, it is usually appropriate to request a review of the slides by a pathologist with wide experience in the examination of pigmented tumors.

Microscopic Growth Patterns

The proper choice of treatment for malignant tumors depends upon an understanding of their biological characteristics, including patterns of growth. Histological examination of excised tissue will reveal these growth patterns, although in many tumors these features will be suggested by the clinical appearance. Malignant tumors often grow beyond their apparent clinical margins. This growth may occur by local spread or by metastasis through blood vessels or lymph channels.

Local spread may be radial (intraepithelial or subepithelial) or it may be vertical (invasive into the dermis or other deep tissues) (Fig. 7) (3). Some tumors, particularly sebaceous cell carcinoma within the conjunctiva, may be multicentric with no apparent histological communication between separate neoplastic foci (3). Invasive cutaneous tumors, such as some melanomas, are classified according to the invasion level (of Clark-McGovern) (4) to which they vertically extend beneath the epidermal surface: level I—*in situ;* level II—papillary dermis; level III—upper reticular dermis; level IV—reticular dermis; and level V—subcutaneous fat.

Although the Clark-McGovern invasion levels were originally described in connection with melanomas, they are also applicable to other invasive cutaneous tumors such as squamous cell and sebaceous cell carcinomas. In general, metastasis occurs more often when tumors extend more deeply into the dermis or the subcutaneous fat. These invasion levels arc not generally used to describe conjunctival tumors, because the conjunctival epithelium is relatively thin as compared to the epidermis of the skin and because the conjunctival substantia propria is similarly much thinner than the cutaneous dermis (5,6).

MANAGEMENT OF MALIGNANT EYELID TUMORS

As previously mentioned, approximately 90% of all eyelid malignancies and 20% of all eyelid tumors in general are basal cell carcinomas. Squamous cell and sebaceous cell carcinomas are relatively uncommon and malignant melanomas of the eyelids are rare. Adequate surgical excision is the method of treatment that provides the highest cure rate of most malignant eyelid tumors. The adequacy of excision is best determined by histological examination of the margins around the resected tissue. Such microscopic evaluation can be performed either by examining tissues that are temporarily frozen (frozen sections) at the time of surgery or by examining tissues that are permanently fixed following surgery.

Frozen section examination of the margins around a resected areas allows the surgeon

(d) lentigo maligna melanoma and superficial spreading melanoma. These tumors may also spread vertically into dermis. (From McCord and Cavanagh, ref. 3, with permission.) **B:** Subepithelial radial spread of tumors (*arrows*). This growth pattern is typical of (a) invasive (nodular-ulcerative and morpheaform) basal cell carcinoma and (b) invasive squamous cell carcinoma. (From McCord and Cavanagh, ref. 3, with permission.) **C:** Vertical spread of tumors. The five invasion levels (of Clark-McGovern) shown here are used to classify vertical growth of malignant melanoma and other tumors such as invasive sebaceous cell carcinoma. (From McCord and Cavanagh, ref. 3, with permission.)

to immediately remove additional tissue if the tumor is histologically found at the edge of the incision. In the case of tumors such as basal cell carcinomas, which usually grow from a single focus, a very high cure rate can be achieved if the extent of resection is controlled by frozen section examination of the margins (7). However, this technique is not accurate in every case, and tumors may sometimes be found on permanent section review of tissue that was thought to be tumor-free on frozen section examination (8). In the case of multicentric tumors, it may not be possible to completely rely upon examination of resection margins if only one focus of the lesion is removed.

Alternatives to conventional surgical therapy include Mohs' excision (chemosurgery or lamellar excision), radiation therapy, and cryotherapy. Mohs' excision is actually a surgical technique that provides even greater reliability of complete tumor removal than conventional surgery 9–12). Radiation therapy and cryotherapy may offer some advantages over surgery, but provide lower cure rates than surgical excision with histological control of the margins (13–16). These surgical and nonsurgical treatments will be described as part of the discussion of specific tumors.

Basal Cell Carcinoma

Basal cell carcinoma is the most common eyelid cancer, arising more than 25 times as frequently as any other malignancy in this location. Most of these tumors arise on the sun-exposed lower eyelids in middle-age persons with light complexion (17). Although basal cell carcinomas often invade local tissues, they seldom metastasize. When these tumors arise near the canthi, they tend to become deeply infiltrative and may involve the eye or the lacrimal drainage system.

Most basal cell carcinomas of the eyelids grow in one of three types: (a) nodular-ulcerative, (b) morpheaform, and (c) superficial. Occasionally these tumors can be pigmented and resemble nevi or melanomas. An unusual variant is found in the basal cell nevus syndrome (Gorlin's syndrome). The margins of nodular-ulcerative tumors are usually pale, elevated, and nodular with telangiectatic vessels. The central area is often necrotic and ulcerated (Figs. 8–10,). Morpheaform tumors are characterized by indistinct margins and a smooth, leathery surface (Figs. 11 and 12). Morpheaform tumors often extend for a considerable distance beyond their clinical margins and frequently produce cicatrization of the surrounding tissues. Superficial basal cell carcinomas are relatively rare on the face and usually consist only of slightly elevated, erythematous scaling patches.

Histologically, basal cell carcinomas are composed of small, oval cells containing dark nuclei and relatively little cytoplasm. The nuclei are usually rather uniform in size with little anaplasia. Groups or clusters of cells are often surrounded by palisading columnar cells that are arranged in rows. During histological fixation, the peripheral cells often separate from the surrounding stroma to leave empty spaces or clefts, which are a useful diagnostic feature (18). Morpheaform tumors have abundant, fibrous connective tissue that produces clinical cicatrization and a smooth, leathery surface.

Surgical excision with histological control of all margins is usually the most effective treatment for basal cell carcinomas (19). Histological examination of the margins is particularly important in the case of morpheaform tumors, because of their irregular edges and microscopic extensions. Frozen section control of the margins at the time of surgery provides an opportunity to assure complete tumor removal before eyelid reconstruction is completed. Orbital exenteration may be required in patients with tumors that invade the eye, the sinuses, or the deep orbit.

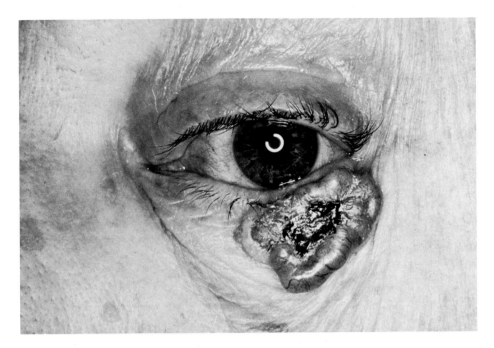

FIG. 8. Basal cell carcinoma (nodular-ulcerative type). Margin is elevated and nodular, with telangiectatic vessels. Central area is necrotic and ulcerated.

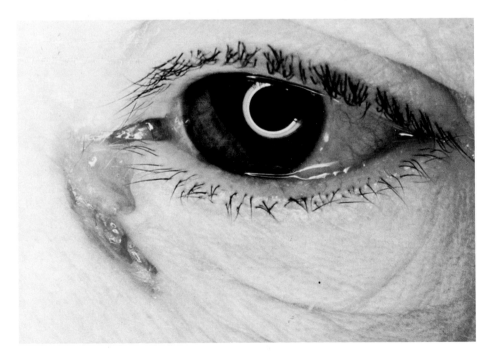

FIG. 9. Basal cell carcinoma (nodular-ulcerative type). Margin is relatively flat and central area is a smooth furrow near the medial canthus.

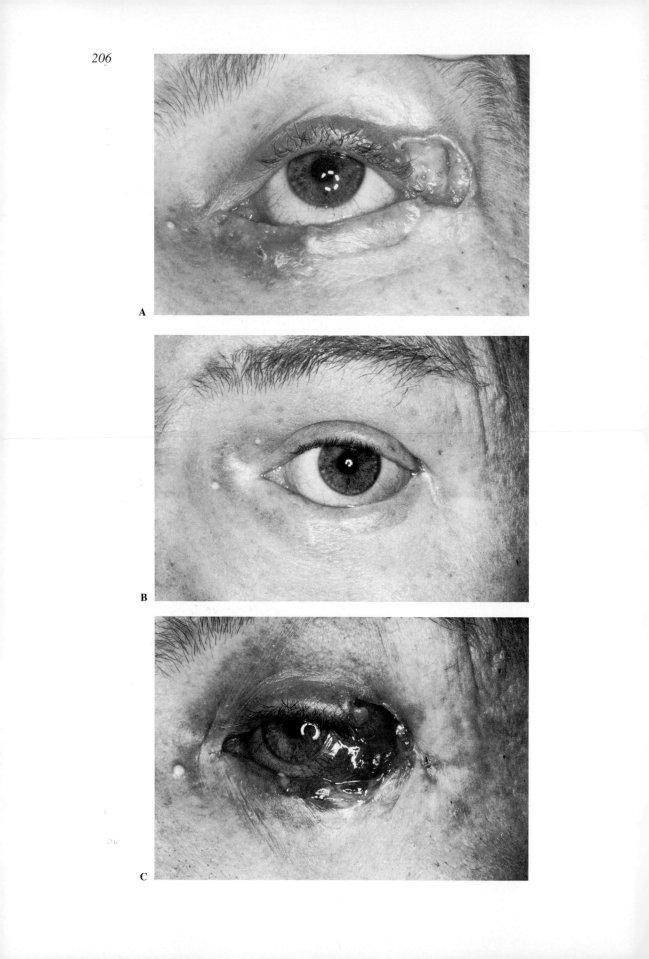

A

B

C

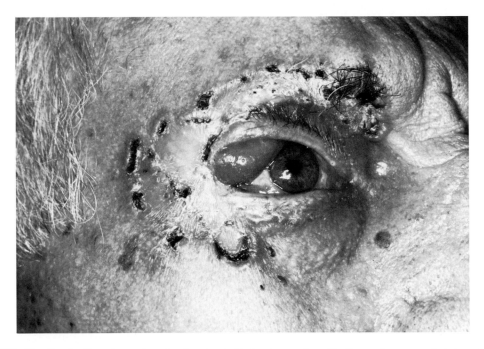

FIG. 11. Basal cell carcinoma (morpheaform type). Surface is smooth and leathery, whereas margin is irregular and indistinct. Cicatrization has produced ectropion of upper eyelid with conjunctival prolapse.

Moh's excision is a form of surgical resection in which the tumor is excised in small lamellar tissue blocks, each of which is 5 to 10 mm square and 2 to 4 mm thick. The undersurface of each lamellar block is then histologically examined, and, if tumor is present, additional lamellar blocks are excised from the adjacent tissues until all of the malignancy is removed. This procedure has also been termed chemosurgery (if the tissues are fixed *in vivo* with chemicals) or lamellar resection. Mohs' excision, or lamellar resection, is time consuming, but it is the most reliable of all procedures both to assure complete tumor removal and to preserve normal uninvolved tissues (9–12).

This procedure is particularly useful in treating deeply invasive tumors, recurrent (persistent) tumors, and extensive facial-orbital tumors. Extensive facial-orbital tumors are those lesions that involve more than 1 square inch of the skin surface near the eyelids, have tumor fixation to orbital periosteum or bone, and have tumor extending onto the inner eyelid surface or through the orbital septum (12).

Radiation therapy can destroy many basal cell carcinomas, but it is not as effective as adequate surgical excision, since the peripheral margins cannot be histologically examined to assure complete eradication of the tumor. Tumors that recur (persist) after ineffective radiation therapy are usually more difficult to control by subsequent surgery than similar

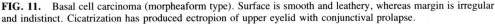

FIG. 10. Basal cell carcinoma (nodular-ulcerative type) treated initially by radiation therapy. **A:** Tumor involves lateral canthus and extends along almost entire lower eyelid margin, from which eyelashes are absent. Treatment by 5,700 rads of radiation. **B:** Six months after completion of radiation therapy, tumor is no longer clinically evident on skin surface. **C:** One year after radiation therapy much of the irradiated area has become necrotic and tumor has recurred. In order to completely remove recurrent tumor, orbital exenteration was necessary.

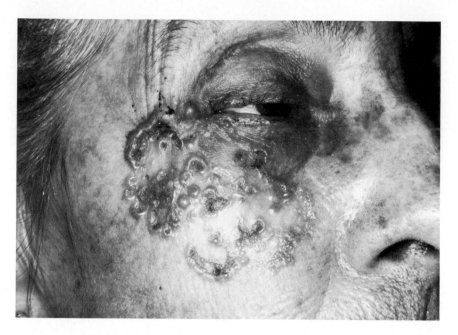

FIG. 12.   Basal cell carcinoma (morpheaform type) treated by lamellar resection (Mohs' excision). **A:** Extensive tumor has leather-like surface and irregular edges that involve the right cheek, lateral canthus, and lateral eyelids. Movement of eye was restricted by tumor growth onto conjunctiva.

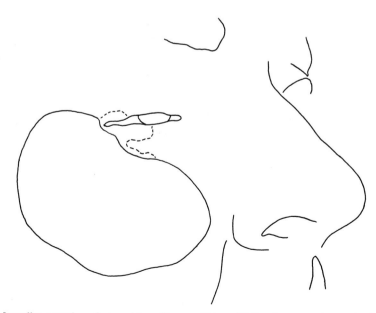

FIG. 12B.   Lamellar resection, first excision. Tissue within *solid line* is removed to a depth that includes clinically evident tumor except at lateral canthus and lid margins (*dotted lines*).

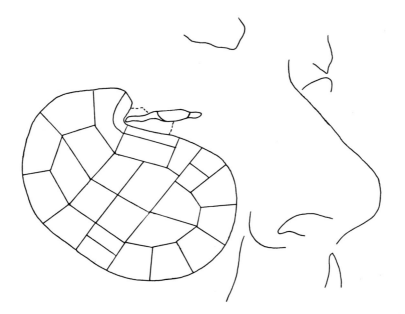

FIG. 12C. Lamellar resection, second excision. After removal of tissue shown in previous diagram, the surface and all margins surrounding the original surgical defect are removed in a group of lamellar blocks. These tissue blocks are each 2 to 4 mm thick and 5 to 15 mm wide. Each lamellar block is identified by a letter and is drawn as illustrated on a "map" of the face. Each block is histologically examined so that, if tumor is present, additional tissue can be removed from the appropriate location. Again, tumor remains at the lateral canthus and lid margins (*dotted lines*).

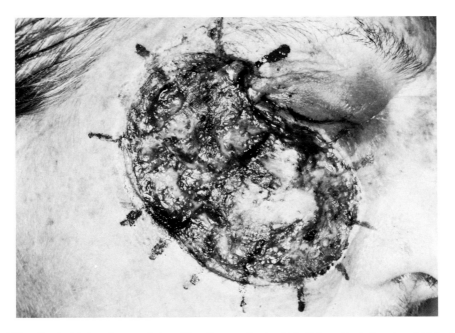

FIG. 12D. Surgical defect after completion of lamellar resection in which all tissue blocks have been histologically found to be free of tumor except at the lateral canthus and lid margins. Radial marks on skin indicate positions of tissue blocks, corresponding to lines on edge of "map."

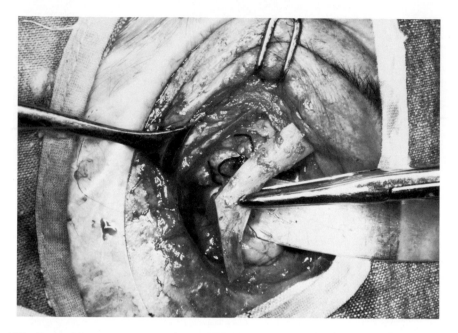

FIG. 12E. Residual tumor at lateral canthus, lid margins, and conjunctiva is then excised using frozen section control to assure complete tumor removal. Lateral orbital rim is also removed because overlying periosteum was involved by tumor.

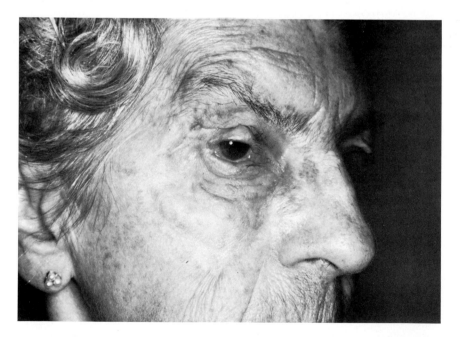

FIG. 12F. The surgical defect was reconstructed by use of a mucosal graft from the nasal septum and multiple full-thickness skin grafts. After completion of eyelid reconstruction, the lids appear relatively normal and can close completely. No tumor recurrence is evident 3 years after treatment.

tumors that were untreated (13). Radiation therapy should seldom be used when a basal cell carcinoma involves bone because such infiltrative tumors are more resistant to radiation than lesions localized to soft tissues.

Complications of radiation therapy include stenosis of the lacrimal drainage system, loss of eyelashes, skin atrophy with entropion or ectropion, and mucosal drying with conjunctival leukoplakia. Surgical excision and eyelid reconstruction in previously irradiated areas is difficult because of the presence of radiation-induced scarring and atrophy.

Cryotherapy can be used to treat basal cell carcinoma, but, as with radiation therapy, it is not possible to histologically confirm complete eradication of the tumor. Recurrence (persistence) is more frequent than with surgical excision that is adequately performed, but most patients can be treated by cryotherapy without hospitalization.

If cryotherapy is used to treat eyelid malignancies, the lesion should be carefully chosen and the cryotherapist should be skilled in the technique of treatment (16). Superficial basal cell carcinomas and tumors arising as part of the basal cell nevus syndrome are particularly suitable to treatment by cryotherapy. It is important to carefully follow patients treated by cryotherapy and to biopsy areas suspected of being persistent tumor.

Complications of cryotherapy include skin depigmentation, loss of eyelashes, and notching of the lid margin. Stenosis of the lacrimal drainage system is relatively uncommon, and subsequent surgery in an area previously treated by cryotherapy is usually not difficult.

Squamous Cell Carcinoma

Squamous cell carcinoma, or epidermoid carcinoma, is the second most common malignant skin tumor (20). Squamous cell carcinoma can arise *de novo* or from preexisting lesions (e.g., sun-damaged skin). Squamous cell carcinoma may demonstrate intraepithelial spread only, or undergo invasion of the dermis with the risk of regional lymph node metastasis and ultimately distant metastasis. Understanding of the biological behavior of squamous cell carcinoma, in the clinical settings in which it occurs, is a requisite to proper management (3,21).

Squamous cell carcinomas frequently arise from previously sun-damaged skin, typically solar keratoses or actinic keratoses. These lesions affect an older population, the greatest risk factor being sun (ultraviolet) exposure and fair complexion. The typical location of these lesions is on the face, forearm, and dorsa of the hands. Squamous cell carcinoma appears as an erythematous lesion, usually elevated and sometimes scaly (Fig. 13). Squamous cell carcinomas arising in sun-damaged skin have a low propensity to metastasize (approximately 0.5%). It is this variety of squamous cell carcinoma (excluding squamous cell carcinoma of the conjunctiva) with which the oculoplastic surgeon is usually concerned. With sun exposure a significant risk factor, it is not surprising that squamous cell carcinoma is more common on the lower eyelids than the upper eyelids. Although squamous cell carcinoma is the second most common malignant eyelid tumor, it is estimated that basal cell carcinoma is more frequent, at a rate of 40:1 (22).

Basic squamous cell carcinoma can also arise from preexisting Bowen's disease, radiation-damaged skin, chronic ulcers, burn scars, and osteomyelitic sinuses. Squamous cell carcinomas arising from these lesions metastasize at a rate of 20% to 40%. Squamous cell carcinomas arising from non-sun-exposed normal skin (e.g., the mucocutaneous junction of the lip, glans penis, or vulva) have a high rate of metastatic disease. Bowen's disease is usually a solitary lesion, commonly in non-sun-exposed skin, that slowly enlarges as a flat, erythema-

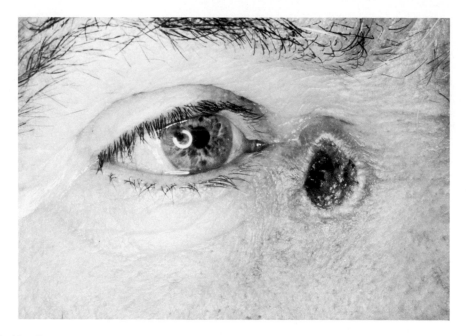

FIG. 13. Squamous cell carcinoma involving medial canthus. Central area is ulcerated, and tumor surface is more keratinized than on most basal cell carcinomas.

tous, crusted patch. Because the risk of metastasis is high, Bowen's disease or carcinoma *in situ* should be differentiated from solar or actenic keratoses.

Squamous cell carcinoma can be suspected clinically but must be biopsied for definitive diagnosis. Intraoperative, frozen section control is necessary to ensure adequate margins of excision. Histologically, squamous cell carcinomas are composed of large, pale cells with abundant cytoplasm. Cellular atypia, dyskeratoses, and loss of normal dermal cell polarity are important features. Areas of keratin pearls are seen within the masses of invading cells.

Spread of squamous cell carcinoma is often by narrow cellular strands, rather than by uniform advancement of the entire border of the tumor (23). Because of this property, and the potential to metastasize, a wider resection margin is removed from around a squamous cell carcinoma than in the case of most basal cell carcinomas. Frozen section control is mandatory when undertaking surgical excision. Radiation therapy offers less control and may be contraindicated in skin previously damaged by X-rays. The role of local chemotherapy is not well defined. Exenteration of the orbit may be necessary if the tumor is extensive or deeply invasive (Fig. 14). Lymph node removal may be appropriate if the tumor has undergone regional metastases.

Sebaceous Cell Carcinoma

Sebaceous cell carcinoma is the third most common eyelid malignancy, accounting for approximately 1% to 2% of all eyelid malignancies (20). Sebaceous cell carcinoma most commonly arises from the meibomian gland, and can arise from the glands of Zeis, hair follicle glands, and sebaceous glands of the caruncle and of the brow (24). Most of these

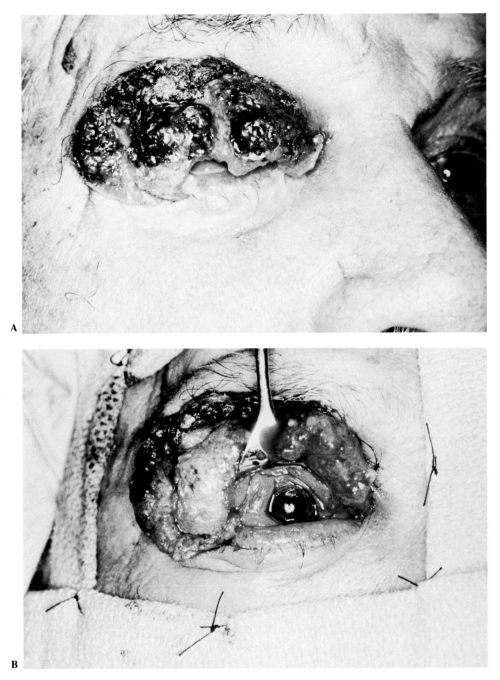

FIG. 14. Squamous cell carcinoma involving entire upper eyelid treated by orbital exenteration. **A:** Thick, keratinized tumor replaces entire upper eyelid and extends into anterior orbit. **B:** Tumor has grown onto the globe.

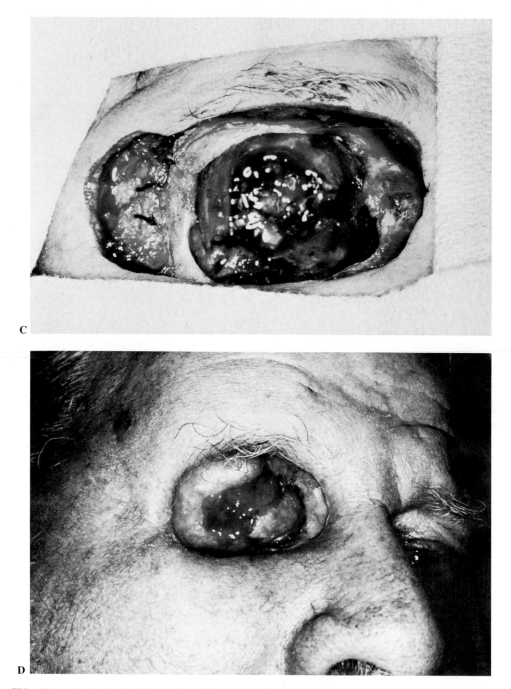

FIG. 14 (*cont.*)   **C:** Surgical defect after orbital exenteration has been performed to locally remove entire tumor. **D:** Exenteration cavity after split-thickness skin graft was placed over orbital walls.

tumors are slow-growing neoplasms, occurring in patients greater than 60 years of age. They occur in the upper eyelid with twice the frequency of occurrence in the lower eyelid, presumably because of the greater number of meibomian glands in the superior tarsus. The rarity of the lesion and its presentation as more common, benign lesions require a high index of suspicion on the part of the clinician in order to diagnose this condition.

The literature is replete with articles describing the "masquerade" syndrome presentation of sebaceous cell carcinoma (25). Sebaceous cell carcinoma may mimic symptoms of a chronic chalazion, chronic unilateral blepharoconjunctivitis, keratitis or superior limbic keratoconjunctivitis (26), localized eyelid or conjunctival inflammation, caruncular tumors or conjunctival masses, or rarely a cutaneous horn (27) or lacrimal fossa tumor (28). In its easily recognizable form, sebaceous cell carcinoma will cause a nodular induration and thickening of the eyelids, with a yellowish, erythematous coloraton. Loss of cilia and distortion of the meibomian gland orifices of the eyelid margin is typical.

It takes a high index of suspicion and a knowledgeable clinician to diagnose this condition. Surgeons must not only perform the correct type of biopsy, but also submit the specimen for the proper type of pathological exam (Fig. 15). Simple shave biopsies are often inadequate. Pagetoid spread, or intraepithelial sebaceous cell carcinoma, may be indistinguishable on a shave biopsy from squamous cell carcinoma *in situ*, superficial spreading malignant melanoma, or other lesions. It should be emphasized that a full-thickness eyelid biopsy with adequate tarsus is the definitive biopsy for diagnosing sebaceous cell carcinomas. Because of the frequently multicentric origin of these tumors, multiple biopsies are often necessary. The pathologist must be alerted to the possible diagnosis so that fat stains can be performed on fresh tissue, before alcohol processing.

Histologically, most sebaceous cell carcinomas are composed of large anaplastic cells

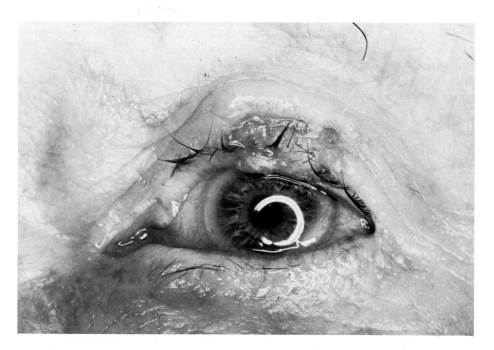

FIG. 15. Sebaceous cell carcinoma involving upper eyelid. An "inflammation" had previously been diagnosed by biopsy in the same location.

with a foamy cytoplasm. Lipid vacuoles within the cytoplasm are usually positive for fat stains. Because routine histological processing with alcohol will dissolve the lipid vacuoles, frozen sections on fresh tissues stained with oil-red-O stain must be performed. Foci of lipid in this cytoplasm and evidence of sebaceous differentiation are histopathological hallmarks of this tumor. Electron microscopy or immunoperoxidase studies can serve as useful adjuncts. Poorly differentiated tumors, with scanty cytoplasm and prominent nucleoli, have a relatively poor prognosis.

The delay in diagnosing sebacous cell carcinoma may be attributed to a number of factors: rarity of the lesion; resemblance to other more common, benign lesions; and inexperience of both the clinician and the pathologist. It should be remembered that sebaceous cell carcinoma is rare in other parts of the body and that the general pathologist may have little experience in diagnosing this malignancy of predominantly the eyelids. Zimmerman and others at the Armed Forces Institute of Pathology have found a significant correlation between the duration of symptoms of sebaceous cell carcinoma prior to excision and prognosis (29). If the duration of symptoms is between 1 and 6 months, the mortality was found to be 14%. If the duration of symptoms was greater than 6 months, the mortality was 38%. A delay in diagnosis typically correlated with larger-sized tumors, intraepithelial spread, and orbital invasion. Once the diagnosis is established, the preferred management is wide surgical excision with frozen section monitoring. Excision may include 5- to 6-mm margins of normal tissue. Even wide excisions with frozen section control may not be curative; the presence of multiple, unconnected lesion is a well-known characteristic of sebaceous cell carcinoma (30). Close clinical follow-up of every patient treated for sebaceous cell carcinoma is mandatory. Ultimately, many patients require orbital exenteration, as recurrence or multicentricity of the lesion becomes apparent during follow-up. Tumor metastases initially occur in the ipsilateral parotid gland and anterior cervical lymph nodes. Radical neck dissection is the treatment of choice for local lymph node metastatic disease. Enlarged lymph nodes must always be biopsied prior to radical neck surgery, because localized lymphadenitis without tumor metastases may occur with sebaceous cell carcinoma. Distant metastasis to the lungs, liver, and brain may occur as a later sequela. The role of radiation therapy in the treatment of sebaceous cell carcinoma remains controversial (31). Although not a primary choice of therapy, radiation treatment may be useful in selected patients who are not surgical candidates. Sebaceous cell carcinoma is radiosensitive and may regress initially, although recurrence is typical. Radiation therapy must also be questioned in that irradiation has been implicated as one of the causes of sebaceous cell carcinoma.

Malignant Melanoma

Malignant melanoma rarely involves the eyelids. Melanomas of the cheek may spread onto the eyelids, and conjunctival melanomas may extend over the lid margin onto the eyelid skin. Cutaneous melanomas are usually classified into one of three types: (a) lentigo maligna melanoma (malignant melanoma arising in Hutchinson's freckle), (b) superficial spreading melanoma, and (c) nodular melanoma. Lentigo maligna, also known as melanotic Hutchinson's freckle, is an acquired pigmentation that usually appears after the fifth decade of life on the face or on other body surfaces that have been exposed to the sun (Fig. 16). Malignant melanoma may arise within the lesion and produce an elevated nodule. Acquired melanosis is a conjunctival abnormality that is sometimes considered analogous to lentigo maligna, and malignant melanoma may similarly arise in this lesion (Fig. 17). Nodular melanoma is a tumor with a predominantly vertical or invasive growth phase (Fig. 18).

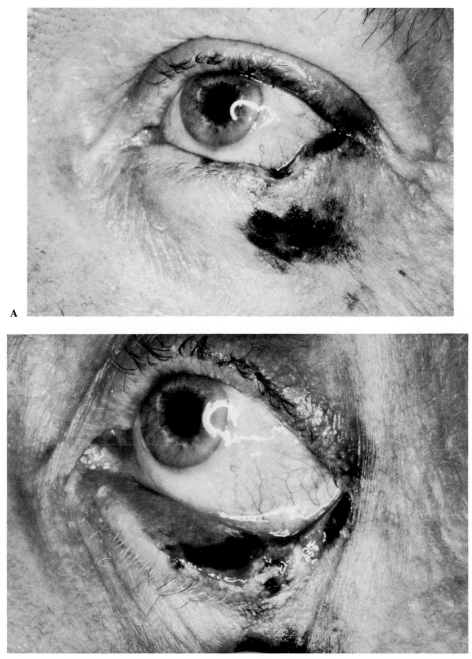

FIG. 16A. Lentigo maligna melanoma (melanotic Hutchinson's freckle) involving the skin of the lower eyelid. **B:** Lentigo maligna melanoma extending from the skin of the eyelid into the palpebral conjunctiva.

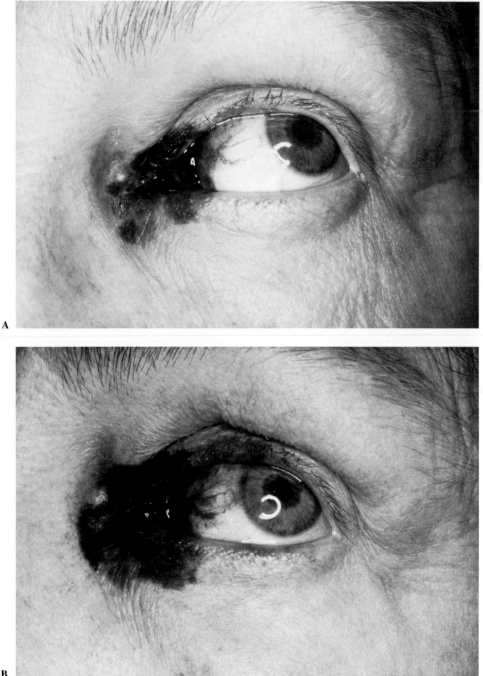

FIG. 17. Melanoma in acquired melanosis. **A:** Acquired melanosis involving bulbar conjunctiva, caruncle, and eyelid skin. Biopsy at this time showed no malignancy. **B:** Two years later, pigmented area has enlarged. Biopsy at this time showed malignant melanoma arising in acquired melanosis.

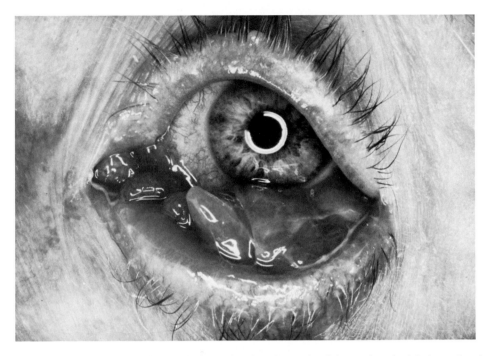

FIG. 18. Nodular melanoma. Thick, relatively amelanotic melanoma involving nearly entire inferior conjunctiva and growing onto globe. Despite orbital exenteration, patient died of metastatic melanoma.

This type of tumor usually has a relatively poor prognosis, whether it arises within the skin or the conjunctiva (5).

Histologically, malignant melanomas are composed of atypical melanocytes that demonstrate varying degrees of differentiation and tissue invasion. In both skin and conjunctiva, melanomas that measure less than 0.75 mm in thickness have a very high cure rate. In all tissues, melanomas confined to the epithelium can usually be completely removed by wide local excision (5).

Treatment of eyelid melanomas should be preceded by biopsy and histological confirmation of the diagnosis. Systemic evaluation should include not only examination of the regional lymph nodes and chest X-rays but also liver scans and liver function tests. The commonly accepted treatment for localized melanomas is surgical excision of the malignant tissue. Exenteration should be considered in patients with extensive or invasive tumors. The role of prophylactic regional lymph node dissection has not been established for patients with eyelid melanomas. Similarly, adjunctive chemotherapy, immunotherapy, and hormone therapy are of unknown value in the management of eyelid melanomas that have no evidence of metastatic spread.

Metastatic Eyelid Carcinoma

Metastatic carcinoma is perhaps the rarest form of malignant eyelid tumors (20,32,33). Forty-six cases have been reported in the medical literature, with eight of the cases also showing orbital involvement. Doubtlessly there are patients with known metastatic carcinoma who never have suspicious eyelid lesions biopsied and are never reported. In 38% of the cases in the literature, the eyelid lesion was the presenting sign of carcinoma. Thus, the oculoplastic surgeon should certainly be familiar with this condition.

Metastatic eyelid carcinoma will typically present in one of three ways (34). Approximately two-thirds of the patients will present with a solitary eyelid nodule. This nodule may be a painless growth or may be acutely inflamed and tender. Approximately one-third of the patients with metastatic eyelid carcinoma will present with diffuse eyelid induration. Less than 10% of the patients will present with a frank, ulcerative lesion. Metastatic eyelid carcinoma may be accompanied by orbital disease in patients who have proptosis or motility dysfunction. Metastatic eyelid disease should be readily differentiated from eyelid melanomas and lymphoid tumors or lymphomas, which have a different coloration and general appearance.

Metastatic eyelid disease is most commonly due to carcinoma of the breasts (65%), lungs (15%), and stomach (10%). While the eyelid lesion is the presenting sign of carcinoma in approximately one-third of the cases, two-thirds of the patients will already have known carcinoma, which stresses the importance of a thorough history. The mean time interval between the diagnosis of carcinoma and the occurrence of metastatic eyelid disease is 4 years. The late occurrence of metastatic disease is most typical of slow-growing breast carcinoma. At the time at which metastatic eyelid carcinoma is diagnosed, over two-thirds of the patients have metastatic disease elsewhere, most commonly in the liver, spleen, lymph nodes, or bones.

If feasible, the treatment of choice is excisional biopsy with eyelid reconstruction, a therapeutic and diagnostic maneuver. Palliative local radiation therapy can induce significant tumor regression, especially in metastatic breast carcinoma. The mean survival in patients with metastatic eye carcinoma is less than 10 months. The prognosis is better with slow-growing metastatic breast carcinoma, which, when presenting as a solitary eyelid nodule, has a mean survival of greater than 20 months.

REFERENCES

1. Friedman, A. H., and Henkind, P. (1976): Clinical and pathological features of eyelid and conjunctival tumors. In: *Ophthalmic Plastic Surgery*, edited by S. A. Fox, 5th ed., pp. 24–63. Grune & Stratton.
2. Schnur, P. L., and Bozzo, P. (1978): Metastasizing keratoacanthomas? The difficulties in differentiating keratoacanthomas from squamous cell carcinomas. *Plast. Reconstr. Surg.*, 62:258–262.
3. McCord, C. D., Jr., and Cavanagh, H. D. (1980): Microscopic features and biologic behavior of eyelid tumors. *Ophthalmic Surg.*, 11:671–681.
4. McGovern, V. J., Mihm, M. C., Jr., Bailly, C., Booth, J. C., Clark, W. H., Jr., Cochran, A. J., Hardy, E. G., Hicks, J. D., Levene, A., Lewis, M., Little, J. H., and Milton, G. W. (1973): The classification of malignant melanoma and its histologic reporting. *Cancer* 32:1446–1457.
5. Grove, A. S., Jr. (1980): Melanomas of the conjunctiva. *Int. Ophthalmol. Clin.*, 20(2):161–175.
6. Jakobiec, F. A. (1980): Conjunctival melanoma. Unfinished business. *Arch Ophthalmol.*, 98:1378–1384.
7. Older, J. J., Quickert, M. H., and Beard, C. (1975): Surgical removal of basal cell carcinoma of the eyelids utilizing frozen section control. *Trans. Am. Acad. Ophthalmol. Otolaryngol.*, 79:658–663.
8. Dahlin, D. C. (1980): Seventy-five years' experience with frozen sections at the Mayo Clinic. *Mayo Clin. Proc.*, 55:721–723.
9. Mohs, F. E. (1948): Chemosurgical treatment of cancer of the eyelid. A microscopically controlled method of excision. *Arch. Ophthalmol.*, 39:43–59.
10. Mohs, F. E. (1972): Chemosurgery for facial neoplasms. *Arch Otolaryngol*, 95:62–67.
11. Mohs, F. E. (1976): Chemosurgery for skin cancer. *Arch. Dermatol.*, 112:211–215.
12. Grove, A. S., Jr. (1977): Staged excision and reconstruction of extensive facial-orbital tumors. *Ophthalmic Surg.*, 8:91–109.
13. Hirshowitz, B., and Mahler, D. (1971): Incurable recurrences of basal cell carcinoma of the mid-face following radiation therapy. *Br. J. Plast. Surg.*, 24:205–211.
14. Levene, M. B. (1977): Radiotherapeutic management of carcinoma of the eyelid. In: *Controversy in Ophthal-*

mology, edited by R. J. Brockhurst, S. A. Boruchoff, B. T. Hutchinson, and S. Lessell, pp. 390–397. Saunders, Philadelphia.

15. Gladstein, A. H. (1978): Radiotherapy of eyelid tumors. In: *Ocular and Adnexal Tumors,* edited by F. A. Jacobiec, pp. 508–516. Aesculapius, Birmingham, Alabama.

16. Fraunfelder, F. T., Zacarian, S. A., Limmer, B. L., and Wingfield, D. (1980): Cryosurgery for malignancies of the eyelid. *Ophthalmology,* 87:461–465.

17. Payne, J. W., Duke, J. R., Butner, R., et al. (1969): Basal cell carcinoma of the eyelids. *Arch. Ophthalmol.,* 81:553–558.

18. Jakobiec, F. A., Rootman, J., and Jones, I. S. (1985): Secondary and metastatic tumors of the orbit. In: *Clinical Ophthalmology, Vol. 2: The Orbit,* edited by T. D. Duane and E. A. Jaeger. Harper & Row, Hagerstown, Maryland.

19. Pascal, R. R., Hobby, L. W., Lattes, R., et al. (1968): Prognosis of "incompletely excised" versus "completely excised" basal cell carcinoma. *J. Plast. Reconstr. Surg.,* 41:328–332.

20. Aurora, A. L., and Blodi, F. C. (1970): Lesions of the eyelids: A clinicopathological study. *Surv. Ophthalmol.,* 15:94–104.

21. Stroll, H. L. (1979): Squamous cell carcinoma. In: *Dermatology in General Medicine,* edited by T. B. Fitzpatrick, A. Z. Eiser, K. Wolff, H., et al., pp. 362–377. McGraw-Hill Book Company, New York.

22. Ferry, A. (1972): The eyelids. In: *Modern Ophthalmology,* edited by A. Sorsby, Vol. 4, pp. 833–853. Lippincott, Philadelphia.

23. Cottel, W. I. (1982): Perineural invasion by squamous cell carcinoma. *J. Dermatol. Surg. Oncol.,* 8:589–600.

24. Boniuk, M., and Zimmerman, L. E. (1968): Sebaceous carcinoma of the eyelid, eyebrow, caruncle and orbit. *Trans. Am. Acad. Ophthalmol. Otolaryngol,* 72:619–642.

25. Brownstein, S., Codere, F., and Jackson, W. B. (1980): Masquerade syndrome. *Ophthalmology,* 87:259–262.

26. Condon, G. P., Brownstein, S., and Codere, F. (1985): Sebaceous carcinoma of the eyelid masquerading as superior limbic keratoconjunctivitis. *Arch. Ophthalmol.,* 103:1525–1529.

27. Brauniger, G. E., Hood, I., and Worthen, D. M. (1974): Sebaceous carcinoma of the lid masquerading as a cutaneous horn. *Arch. Ophthalmol.,* 90:380–381.

28. Shields, J. A., and Font, R. L. (1974): Meibomian gland carcinoma presenting as a lacrimal gland tumor. *Arch. Ophthalmol.,* 92:304–306.

29. Rao, N. A., Hidayat, A. A., McLean, I. W., and Zimmerman, L. E. (1982): Sebaceous carcinomas of the ocular adnexa: A clinicopathologic study of 104 cases, with five-year follow-up data. *Human Pathol.,* 13:113–122.

30. Cavanagh, H. D., Green, W. R., and Goldberg, H. K. (1974): Multicentric sebaceous adenocarcinoma of the meibomian gland. *Am. J. Ophthalmol.,* 77:326–332.

31. Hendley, R. L., Reiser, J. C., Cavanagh, H. D., et al. (1979): Primary radiation therapy for meibomian gland carcinoma. *Am. J. Ophthalmol.,* 87:206–209.

32. Arnold, A. C., Bullock, J. D., and Foos, R. Y. (1985): Metastatic eyelid carcinoma. *Ophthalmology,* 92:114–119.

33. Hood, C. I., Font, R. L., and Zimmerman, L. E. (1973): Metastatic mammary carcinoma in the eyelid with histiocytoid appearance. *Cancer,* 31:793–800.

34. Riley, F. S. (1970): Metastatic tumors of the eyelids. *Am. J. Ophthalmol.,* 69:259–264.

Oculoplastic Surgery, 2nd edition, edited by
Clinton D. McCord, Jr., and Myron Tanenbaum.
Raven Press, New York © 1987.

10

Orbital Disorders: Diagnosis and Management

*Arthur S. Grove, Jr., and **Clinton D. McCord, Jr.

*Department of Ophthalmology, Harvard Medical School, and Massachusetts Eye and Ear Infirmary,
Boston, Massachusetts 02114; and **Department of Ophthalmology, Emory University School of
Medicine, Atlanta, Georgia 30308*

The appropriate management of orbital disorders must include establishing an accurate diagnosis. A systemic method of diagnostic evaluation (Table 1) should be used to determine what abnormality is present and to provide accurate localization.

GENERAL PRINCIPLES OF ORBITAL DIAGNOSIS

History and Physical Examination

A careful history and physical examination should precede laboratory and radiographic studies. The examiner should first determine if any of the most common orbital disorders are present. The incidence of orbital diseases differs in adults and children (1–5). It is also necessary to consider whether these diseases may be mimicked by conditions that produce pseudoexophthalmos, such as an enlarged globe, eyelid retraction or contralateral ptosis, extraocular muscle weakness, or asymmetric orbital sizes.

History

Among the most common symptoms of orbital disease are decreased vision, pain, and diplopia. Important features in the history of a patient with orbital disease include the duration of symptoms, the occurence of tumors elsewhere in the body, the presence of thyroid disease in the patient or his family, a report of head trauma, the presence of sinus disease, and the awareness of pulsations or bruits.

Rapidly evolving symptoms, especially if pain is a prominent feature, are usually the result of acute inflammations, such as infections or pseudotumors, or of malignant tumors. Symptoms that have been present for many months or years are most likely caused by chronic inflammations or by benign tumors. Tumors of the breast and melanomas may metastasize to the orbit years after the primary lesions have been treated. Almost any

TABLE 1. *Diagnostic evaluation of orbital disorders*

A. History and physical examination (with consideration
    of common orbital disorders and causes of pseudo-
    exophthalmos)
B. Systemic examinations (with evaluation of Graves'
    disease, which is usually thyroid related)
C. Primary diagnostic studies
    1. Plain and tomographic X-rays
    2. Ultrasonography
    3. Computed tomography
D. Secondary diagnostic studies
    1. Radionuclide scans
    2. Venography
    3. Arteriography
E. Tissue-processing techniques (after biopsy or excision)

---

systemic malignancy should be considered a possible origin for an orbital metastasis. Ophthalmic Graves' disease is the most common cause of both unilateral and bilateral exophthalmos in adults. Most patients with Graves' disease have thyroid abnormalities, and many have a family history of thyroid disorders. Head trauma may cause carotid cavernous sinus (CCS) fistulas or blood cysts and may embed foreign bodies within the orbital tissues. Fractures of the orbital floor may cause enophthalmos and thus mimic prominence of the contralateral eye. Sinus disease commonly causes orbital abnormalities as a result of spread of infection, extension of tumors, or expansion of sinus mucoceles. Dynamic abnormalities such as pulsations or bruits may result from vascular disorders or from bony defects between the orbit and the intracranial space.

Ocular Examination

A careful ocular examination should precede evaluation of the orbits. Visual acuities and visual fields should be tested and the reflective errors and intraocular pressures measured. Anterior segments must be carefully examined to locate abnormalities such as tortuous conjunctival vessels, which may indicate the presence of an arteriovenous (AV) communication. Fundus examination may reveal an intraocular tumor, papilledema, or chorioretinal folds. Pupil sizes and reactions, corneal and cutaneous sensation, and eye movements should be documented.

Orbital Examination

The findings that most often suggest the presence of orbital disease are a prominent eye, a palpable mass, or a distortion of the eyelids.

Exophthalmos is an abnormal prominence of one or both eyes, usually resulting from an orbital tumor, an inflammation, or a vascular disorder. The usual distance from the lateral orbital rim to the corneal apex is approximately 16 mm in adults. It is uncommon for an eye to normally protrude more than 21 mm beyond the orbital rim. An asymmetry of more than 2 mm between the prominence of the two eyes is suggestive of unilateral exophthalmos (1,3,4).

In adults (Table 2), unilateral exophthalmos is most often caused by ophthalmic Graves' disease. Cavernous hemangiomas are the most common benign tumors found in the orbits

TABLE 2. *Orbital disorders in adults*[a]

1.	Ophthalmic Graves' disease (usually thyroid related)
2.	Orbital cellulitis
3.	Pseudotumors (idiopathic inflammations)
4.	Lymphomas
5.	Cavernous hemangiomas
6.	Lacrimal gland tumors
7.	Meningiomas
8.	Paranasal sinus mucoceles
9.	Secondary tumors (frequently from paranasal sinuses)
10.	Metasatic tumors (frequently from breast or lung)

[a] Listed in approximate order of frequency and excluding trauma.

of adults. The most common orbital malignancies among adults are secondary tumors extending from the paranasal sinuses and metastic tumors from the breast or lung.

In children (Table 3), prominence of one eye is most frequently caused by orbital cellulitis as a complication of either ethmoid sinus disease or a respiratory infection. Dermoids and capillary hemangiomas are the most common benign orbital tumors of childhood, while rhabdomyosarcomas are the most common primary orbital malignancies in this age group.

Bilateral exophthalmos in adults is most often caused by ophthalmic Graves' disease and less often by lymphoma or by inflammations such as pseudotumor or Wegner's granulomatosis. In children, bilateral exophthalmos is most frequently caused by leukemia or metastatic neuroblastoma.

Pseudoexophthalmos is defined either as the simulation of abnormal prominence of the eye or as a truly abnormal prominence that is not due to a mass, an inflammation, or a vascular disorder. Causes of pseudoexophthalmos include an enlarged globe in patients with myopia, asymmetric eyelid positions caused by lid retraction or ptosis, extraocular muscle weakness, a shallow orbit, and contralateral enophthalmos caused by fractures or by cicatricial tumors. Even if a patient is found to have pseudoexophthalmos, it is appropriate to carefully examine the orbits clinically and to obtain orbital X-rays as a reference for future examinations.

Palpation around the globe may disclose the presence of a mass in the anterior orbit, particularly if the lacrimal gland is enlarged or if a sinus mucocele is present. Increased resistance to retrodisplacement of the globe (decreased orbital resilience) suggests the presence of a retrobulbar mass. This is a nonspecific abnormality that may occur with tumors and with inflammatory disorders.

TABLE 3. *Orbital disorders in children*[a]

1.	Cellulitis
2.	Dermoids and epidermoids
3.	Capillary hemangiomas
4.	Rhabdomyosarcomas
5.	Neurofibromas
6.	Optic nerve gliomas
7.	Lymphangiomas
8.	Pseudotumors (idiopathic inflammations)
9.	Leukemias
10.	Metastatic tumors (frequently neuroblastoma)

[a] Listed in approximate order of frequency and excluding trauma.

Eyelid distortion is characteristic of certain orbital disorders. Among the most common ophthalmic signs of Graves' disease are retraction of the lower or upper eyelids (Dalrymple's sign), lag of the upper eyelid on downgaze, and restriction of downward traction on the upper eyelid (Grove's sign). Dermoid cysts often present as firm, subcutaneous nodules beneath the brow and upper lid. Capillary hemangiomas may involve the skin of the lids during infancy and produce "strawberry birthmarks" that usually regress spontaneously within several years. Plexiform neurofibromas usually occur in patients with von Recklinghausen's disease. These tumors often cause ptosis and grow within the lateral upper eyelids as a mass that resembles a 'bag of worms.''

Dynamic orbital abnormalities are those that pulsate, that are associated with bruits, or that rapidly change in size, shape, or position. Pulsating exophthalmos may result from vascular abnormalities such as CCS fistulas and other AV communications or from bony defects between the orbit and the intracranial space. Large mucoceles can allow the transfer of intracranial pulsations to the globe or to the orbit, as can developmental abnormalities of the orbital bones in patients with von Recklinghausen's disease. Highly vascularized tumors can cause orbital pulsations on occasion. A tonometer may detect minimal pulsations that are not otherwise evident. Bruits may be objectively detected with a stethoscope or may be subjectively described by patients with AV communications. Rapid changes in the amount of exophthalmos or in the size of an orbital mass may be associated with crying, raised intrathoracic pressure, or dependence of the head. Such fluctuations in prominence or size may be caused by a varix, an AV communication, or a meningoencephalocele. This phenomenon rarely occurs with hemangiomas or lymphangiomas.

The frequency of orbital tumors will vary depending on the reporting source. Neurosurgical series most commonly list meningiomas as their most common tumors seen, radiologic series will list mucoceles as their most common orbital tumor or orbital mass, and referral institutions may have a bias toward the rare malignant processes.

In reviewing the large number of series available plus drawing on the authors' own personal experience, the recurring theme of frequency does occur. Tables 4 and 5 list the frequency of orbital tumors or tumor-like processes that occur in both adults and children. If the surgeon can learn the presenting clinical signs and symptoms of these entities, then he or she will most certainly be familiar with the setting of 90% or more of the orbital tumors that will be encountered.

Systemic Examinations

Systemic evaluation should include a hematologic examination with a complete blood count to help determine if a blood dyscrasia such as leukemia is present. Chest X-rays should be obtained to locate lung tumors that may spread to the orbit. If metastatic disease is suspected, a complete physical examination should be performed, including a breast examination and mammogram in women. Among children, tests should be considered to rule out neuroblastoma, which may metastasize to the orbit (1).

Because ophthalmic Graves' disease is the most common cause of both unilateral and bilateral exophthalmos among adults, it should be considered in the differential diagnosis of nearly every patient with orbital disease. Graves' disease is an inflammatory disorder of unknown etiology that is often, but not always, related to thyroid abnormalities such as hyperthyroidism. Thyroid function tests are of more help in guiding the management of endocrine dysfunction than in establishing the diagnosis of Graves' disease. The diagnosis of this disorder is usually made on the basis of typical clinical signs and anatomic tests that will be more completely described below under the topic of ophthalmic Graves' disease.

TABLE 4. *Orbital tumors in adults[a]*

1.	Inflammatory orbital pseudotumors
2.	Lymphoid tumors
3.	Hemangiomas, cavernous
4.	Meningioma (optic nerve or otherwise)
5.	Lymphangiomas
6.	Peripheral nerve tumors
7.	Lacrimal gland tumors (epithelial)
8.	Mucoceles
9.	Secondary or metastatic tumors
10.	Dermoid (epidermoid) cysts

[a] Listed in approximate order of frequency and excluding trauma.

Although some patients with ophthalmic Graves' disease have no thyroid abnormality, most will have elevated serum thyroxine (T_4) or serum triiodothyronine (T_3) levels. If these thyroid tests are normal or equivocal, but Graves' disease is still suspected because of clinical signs or anatomic test results, then a thyrotropin-releasing hormone (TRH) test may be ordered. This secondary test sometimes discloses a thyroid abnormality in patients whose serum T_4 or T_3 levels are normal (1,3).

Primary Diagnostic Studies

After the history and physical examination have been completed and systemic examination has been initiated, the orbits can be studied by noninvasive primary examinations that include plain and tomographic X-rays, ultrasonography, and computed tomography (3,4). Examples of some of these studies will be given under the discussion of specific orbital disorders.

Ultrasonography

Ultrasonography uses sound waves to produce echoes as they strike interfaces between acoustically different structures. The orbit can be studied most effectively by using two-dimensional (B-mode-ultrasonography with the standardized A-mode unit (6).

TABLE 5. *Orbital tumors in children[a]*

1.	Dermoid cyst (orbital rim and others)
2.	Hemangioma (capillary)
3.	Rhabdomyosarcoma
4.	Optic nerve glioma
5.	Neurofibromatosis
6.	Lymphangioma
7.	Inflammatory orbital pseudotumor
8.	Matastatic neuroblastoma
9.	Leukemia-lymphoma
10.	Optic nerve meningioma
11.	Other tumors (lipoma, Schwannoma, teratoma, sarcoma, arterio-venous malformation

[a] Listed in approximate order of frequency and excluding trauma.

This technique is particularly valuable as a screening examination since it does not utilize ionizing radiation as do X-ray studies. Ultrasonography can be considered part of an initial office examination and can be repeated without risk to the patient. Its use is limited because sound waves cannot penetrate the bony walls of the orbit and because tissues at the orbital apex and along the orbital roof are poorly visualized.

Computed Tomography

Computed tomographic (CT) scanning uses thin X-ray beams to obtain tissue density values, from which detailed cross-sectional images of the body are formed by computers. Iodine-containing contrast materials can be administered intravenously to outline blood vessels and vascular abnormalities (contrast enhancement). CT scans of the orbits visualize details of the eyes, the extraocular muscles, and the optic nerves. In addition, orbital CT scans usually visualize the orbital bones, the sinuses, and intracranial structures. These examinations are not only useful for the evaluation of orbital and intracranial tumors but can also be used to evaluate fractures and to localize foreign bodies even if they are not radiographically opaque.

Computed axial tomography (CAT) forms images that are oriented in a plane parallel to the course of the optic nerves. Computed coronal tomography (CCT) forms vertical images in a plane approximately paralleling the equator of the eye, analogous to Caldwell view X-rays. By using both CAT and CCT, structures can be localized in the orbit with three-dimensional accuracy. Extraocular muscle enlargement can sometimes be distinguished from tumors when both axial and coronal views are used to study orbital detail. This is particularly valuable in studying patients with ophthalmic Graves' disease. The horizontal length and width of objects can be determined on axial scans, and coronal scans can be used to measure vertical height and to localize the positions of tumors relative to the optic nerve. Three-dimensional CT scanning can also aid in distinguishing solid tumors from cystic lesions such as dermoids.

Orbital differential diagnosis

Through the last few years of experience with CT scan findings, lists have been compiled of differential diagnoses of anatomic abnormalities encountered. No attempt will be made to engage in extensive discussion of CT scan findings and orbital diseases, but some of the most common lists of differential diagnoses are presented in Tables 6 through 9.

As is always true, the CT scan findings must be supplemented with the signs and symptoms of the clinical setting. In the category of an enlarged optic nerve, a person presenting with acute loss of vision over a few days with pain would much more likely be considered to have optic neuritis than an optic nerve tumor. The presence of normal vision with an enlarged optic nerve would, in most cases, mitigate against an optic nerve neoplastic process. With enlarged extraocular muscles, one must differentiate a generalized enlargement of all muscles from isolated muscle involvement. In the presence of generalized enlargement of the extraocular muscles, one must most certainly look for the clinical signs and symptoms of Grave's disease.

Orbital myositis in adults usually involves a single muscle, although it may involve several in children, and the inflamed thickening of the muscle usually extends into the tendon area with an accompanying scleritis. Punched out or lytic lesions can occur from intrinsic bony disease or lesions that expand in the intramedullary space.

TABLE 6. *Differential diagnosis of enlargement of optic nerve*

Optic nerve tumor
Optic nerve sheath hematoma
Metastatic disease to the optic nerve
Arachnoid hyperplasia
Retinoblastoma invading nerve
Optic nerve sheath cyst
Optic nerve drusen
Tumor adjacent to optic nerve
Enlarged inferior rectus muscle[a]

[a] This is the most common cause of misdiagnosis of an enlarged optic nerve when CT scans are viewed in the axial plane only. This points out the value of obtaining coronal and axial views on all orbital CT scans.

TABLE 7. *Differential diagnosis of enlarged extracular muscles*

Grave's disease
Orbital myositis
Carotid or AV fistula
Metastatic disease
Lymphoma
Postorbital trauma with globe malposition

TABLE 8. *Differential diagnosis of the lytic bone lesions*

Cholesteotoma (epidermoid cysts)
Cholesterol granulomas
Dermoid
Histiocytosis X
Hematic cysts
Intrinsic bone lesions (aneurysmal bone cysts, reparative granuloma)
Cystic meningioma
Lytic neoplastic lesions

TABLE 9. *Differential diagnosis of destructive midline lesions*

Neoplastic (squamous cell carcinoma, etc.)
Midline granuloma
Wegener's vasculitis (granulomatosis)
Polymorphic reticulosis
Fungus
Mucoceles of the frontal ethmoidal sinus

Magnetic Resonant Imaging

Proton magnetic resonant imaging (MRI), with the use of surface coils, can produce high levels of resolution for imaging of the orbital tissues (7,8). MRI is rapidly becoming one of the most desirable means of imaging the orbit because of its high resolution and because it does not utilize ionizing radiation and is not harmful to biologic systems. Magnetic imaging is dependent on four tissue variables: proton density, relaxation time in modes T_1 and T_2, and motion of protons. Different radio frequency pulsing sequences are able to add or subtract the relative contributions of these variables to the final image. It has been shown that neoplastic tissue has a prolonged relaxation time (T_1, T_2) relative to normal tissue. Different contrasts are available in the T_1 mode, in which fat appears white and blood dark, and in the T_2 mode, in which fat appears dark and blood white. This method of imaging the orbital contents and other areas appears to hold great promise for the future.

Secondary Diagnostic Studies

In most patients, the localization of an orbital abnormality and a presumptive diagnosis can usually be reached after completion of the primary orbital examinations. When these studies have not provided sufficient information, and especially if a vascular abnormality or intracranial lesion is suspected, additional examinations may be performed. These secondary examinations include radionuclide scans, venography, and arteriography (1,3,4).

Venography

Venography is a relatively safe but infrequently used technique that usually involves injection of radiopaque dye into the angular, frontal, or facial veins in order to visualize veins within the orbit. Displacement or obstruction of the superior ophthalmic and other orbital veins may give a clue about the location of a mass, but such information can usually be obtained more easily with ultrasonography or CT scanning. Venography is most useful for the evaluation of varices, lymphangiomas, or lesions involving the cavernous sinus.

Arteriography

Arteriography for the evaluation of orbital disorders requires the injection of radiopaque dye into the carotid arteries. Although both orbital and intracranial arteries can be visualized, these examinations carry the low, but significant, risk of serious neurologic complications. Vascular abnormalities involving the arterial circulation, such as AV communications and aneurysms, are best evaluated by arteriography. Maximum information can be obtained from these studies by use of selective internal and external carotid injections, magnification, and radiographic subtraction.

Tissue-Processing Techniques

Except in some patients with inflammations, vascular abnormalities, and clinically distinctive tumors, it is usually necessary to either biopsy or excise an orbital lesion to establish a definite diagnosis. If fresh tissue is obtained, a specimen should be submitted for examination by light microscopy. Frozen section examination of most orbital tumors should be performed while the patient is in the operating room. However, in most cases, radical or mutilative surgery should not be carried out solely on the basis of a frozen section diagnosis.

Before the excised tissue is placed into formalin, consideration should be given to reserving some of the specimen for study by other techniques. Features seen with electron microscopy and growth patterns in tissue culture may help to diagnose poorly differentiated tumors such as childhood sarcomas. Immunologic identification of cell-surface markers on lymphocytes can be used to type lymphocytic tumors as containing primarily B or T cells and as being monoclonal or polyclonal in origin. Such immunologic classification can be used to help distinguish benign lymphocytic pseudotumors from malignant lymphomas. If metastatic breast cancer is found at the time of orbital exploration, fresh tissue can be submitted for assay of estrogen and progesterone receptor activity. Hormone therapy is most likely to be of value in patients whose tumors are receptor-positive. Some of these tissue-processing techniques will be additionally described in conjunction with the discussion of specific orbital disorders (1,3,4).

MANAGEMENT OF COMMON ORBITAL DISORDERS

To illustrate the usefulness of the diagnostic studies that have been described, the features of the most common orbital disorders in both adults and children will be described and their management will be discussed.

Inflammations

Ophthalmic Graves' Disease

Graves' disease is an inflammatory disorder that occurs more frequently in adults than in children and is usually associated with a thyroid abnormality. Many patients with Graves' disease have hyperthyroidism, but it has not been established that an etiologic relationship exists between these disorders. Some patients wtih Graves' disease have no thyroid abnormality that can be detected even after repeated examination.

A wide variety of clinical abnormalities, such as exophthalmos, eyelid edema, and epibulbar vascular congestion have been described in association with ophthalmic Graves' disease (9). However, these findings are nonspecific and may be found with many orbital disorders. Eyelid abnormalities, which are among the most common ophthalmic signs of Graves' disease, have already been mentioned: retraction of the lower or upper eyelids (Dalrymple's sign), lag of the upper eyelid on downgaze, and restriction of downward traction upon the upper eyelid (Grove's sign) (Figs. 1A and 1B).

The downward traction test is useful in distinguishing ophthalmic Graves' disease from other disorders that cause a similar, wide palpebral fissure, such as exophthalmos resulting from an orbital tumor. When Graves' disease has produced a contracture of the levator muscle and levator aponeurosis, resistance is met as downward traction is applied to the upper eyelid by pulling upon the lashes. An accentuated upper eyelid crease is often seen in such patients (Fig. 1C). When a widened palpebral fissure is caused by other conditions, the downward traction test is usually negative and no resistance is met when the eyelid is pulled inferiorly (Fig. 1D).

Another common abnormality in Graves' disease is strabismus (Fig. 2). Eye movements are most often limited because of contracture and fibrosis of the medial rectus or inferior

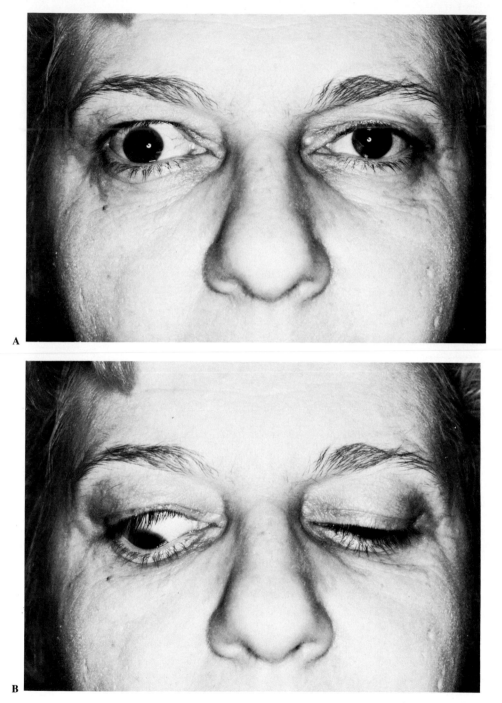

FIG. 1. Eyelid abnormalities in patient with Graves' disease. **A:** Retraction of right upper eyelid (Dalrymple's sign). **B:** Lag of right upper eyelid in downgaze.

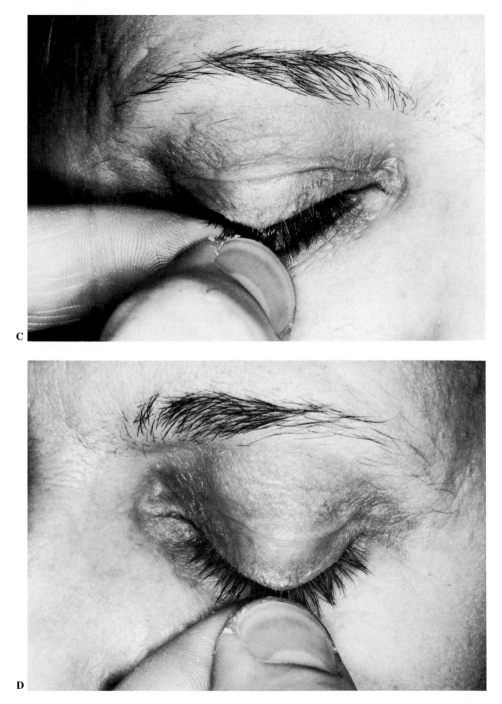

FIG. 1 (*cont.*)   **C:** Restriction of downward traction upon right upper eyelid (Grove's sign). Traction is applied by grasping eyelashes and gently pulling downward. Lid crease is accentuated. **D:** Downward traction test performed upon uninvolved left upper eyelid. Downward traction is not restricted and lid crease is not accentuated.

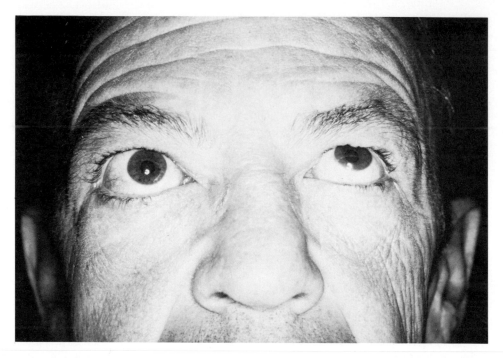

FIG. 2. Strabismus and restricted elevation of right eye in patient with Graves' disease. Right hypotropia was present in primary gaze and inferior rectus muscle appeared enlarged on CT scans.

rectus muscles. A forced traction test, performed by grasping the insertion of the involved muscle with forceps and attempting to move the eye, usually shows that motion is mechanically restricted.

Histologically, the orbital tissues become swollen by edema that may involve the extraocular muscles, the retrobulbar fat, and the lacrimal gland. This edema is usually accompanied by infiltration of plasma cells and lymphocytes, many of which initially group near blood vessels. As the inflammation becomes chronic, fibrosis may develop within the extraocular muscles and produce restrictive myopathy.

As previously mentioned, ophthalmic Graves' disease is usually diagnosed on the basis of characteristic clinical findings and changes in the orbital anatomy. Although orbital X-rays do not show abnormalities resulting from Graves' disease, X-rays should usually be obtained to exclude other orbital disorders. Radionuclide scans have been found to show characteristic changes in patients with Graves' disease, but these tests are seldom used unless other examinations are equivocal. The most important anatomic tests in patients with Graves' disease are CT scans and ultrasonography, which often demonstrate enlargement of multiple extraocular muscles. Because enlarged muscles near the orbital apex can sometimes resemble neoplasms on CT scans, abnormalities in this area must be very carefully studied and correlated with clinical findings before performing orbital surgery. Muscle enlargement can be best confirmed by three-dimensional computed tomography, using both axial and coronal views (Figs. 3 and 4).

Thyroid function tests, including serum T_4 and T_3 levels, will usually be abnormal in patients with Graves' disease. If these examinations are normal or equivocal and if Graves' disease is suspected on the basis of clinical findings or anatomic test results, then a TRH test may be used to discover more occult forms of thyroid dysfunction (1,3,9,10).

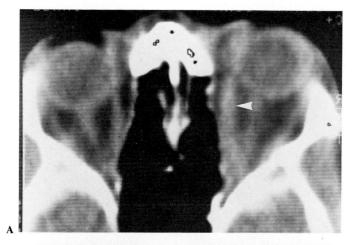

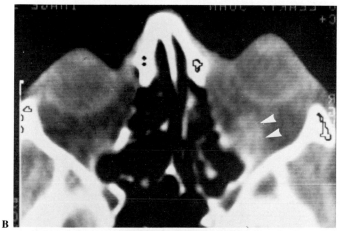

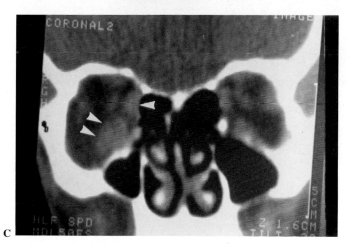

FIG. 3. Patient with Graves' disease. **A:** Computed axial tomogram (CAT) through middle orbit shows thickened right medial rectus muscle (*single arrow*) right exophthalmos, and right hypotropia. **B:** CAT through lower orbit shows enlarged right inferior rectus muscle (*double arrows*), which resembles a tumor. **C:** Computed coronal tomogram (CCT) shows enlarged medial rectus (*single arrow*) and inferior rectus (*double arrows*) muscles in right orbit.

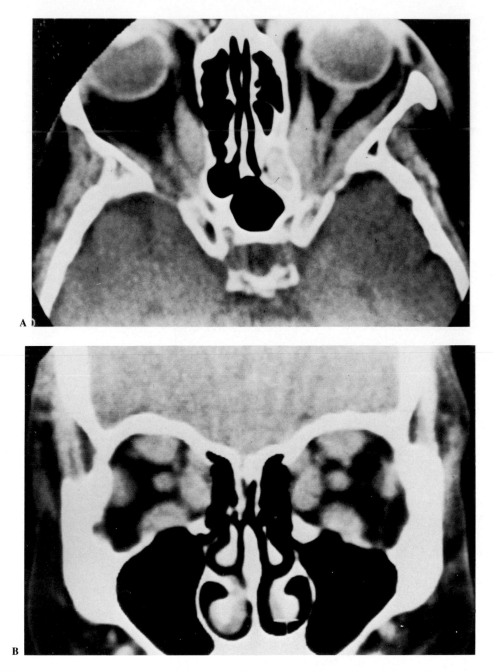

FIG. 4. Computed tomography findings in Graves' disease. **A:** Computed axial tomogram (CAT) demonstrates the classical findings—enlargement of the extraocular muscle bellies with sparing of the tendinous insertions. **B:** Computed coronal tomogram (CCT) demonstrates the ''hamburger patty'' appearance of the enlarged recti muscles in cross-section.

Treatment of ophthalmic Graves' disease should usually be as conservative as possible because of the unpredictable development of eyelid malpositions, motility disorders, and orbital congestion. Some of these abnormalities will improve after treatment of thyroid dysfunction, but occasionally they will become more severe following control of hyperthyroidism. In many instances, the orbital disease will be self-limited, with resolution of the acute inflammatory changes after a period of months or years.

Early ophthalmic Graves' disease is usually treated by topical lubricants to prevent corneal drying. When possible, thyroid abnormalities should be stabilized for seveal months before corrective eyelid or muscle surgery is performed. If corneal damage becomes severe because of lid retraction or exophthalmos, the palpebral fissure may be narrowed by elevating the lower lid or lowering the upper lid (11).

If orbital congestion becomes very severe, and particularly if optic neuropathy occurs, the use of high-dose systemic steroids should be considered. Radiation therapy may sometimes be used in the treatment of severe inflammation, especially in debilitated patients (12). Surgical decompression of the orbit can provide dramatic reduction of exophthalmos and congestion, especially if portions of the orbital floor and medial wall are removed to allow prolapse of the congested tissues into the maxillary and ethmoid sinuses (13).

In patients with both exophthalmos and eyelid retraction, corneal protection and cosmetic improvement may be provided by eyelid surgery alone (11). Surgical decompression is usually, indicated when visual function is impaired by optic neuropathy and steroid therapy either cannot be used or fails to improve vision.

The reader is referred to Chapter 8 for a more thorough discussion of the diagnosis and management of Graves' ophthalmopathy.

Cellulitis

Orbital cellulitis is probably the most common cause of exophthalmos in young children, but is considerably less common in adults. Cellulitis is usually the result of a bacterial infection that spreads from the nasopharynx or the paranasal sinuses (14). In children, most orbital infections extend through the lamina papyracea, from the ethmoid sinus. Cellulitis may occasionally result from an eyelid infection, from dacryocystitis, or from hematogenous dissemination. Clinical features of orbital cellulitis include fever, pain, exophthalmos, lid edema, and restricted ocular movements.

Orbital X-rays often show sinus opacification if the cellulitis is caused by sinus disease. CT scans and ultrasonography may visualize either diffuse inflammatory changes or a focal abscess cavity if the infection is localized.

In young children, *Haemophilus influenzae* is a common cause of orbital cellulitis, and initial treatment with ampicillin should be considered. In adults, most orbital cellulitis is caused by *Staphylococcus aureus* or *Streptococcus*. When cellulitis is suspected, cultures should be obtained from the nasopharynx and conjunctiva, after which initial treatment usually involves the systemic administration of a penicillinase-resistant drug such as methicillin. Most patients with orbital cellulitis respond to medical therapy alone. Sometimes an infected sinus must be drained if a pyocele is present. It is rarely necessary to surgically explore an infected orbit unless an abscess cavity is present.

Cavernous sinus thrombosis may result from orbital cellulitis. This life-threatening complication often produces rapidly progressive exophthalmos, ophthalmoplegia with pupillary abnormalities, and diffuse neurologic disorders. Meningitis may develop, in which case the cerebrospinal fluid obtained by lumbar puncture often contains acute inflammatory cells and organisms that may grow in culture.

Fungal infection of the orbit is usually caused by fungi of the genuses *Rhizopus* or *Mucor,* in which case the infection is termed mucormycosis. These fungi belong to the class Phycomycetes, which gives rise to the more general diagnosis of phycomycosis. Phycomycosis usually results from extension of the organisms from the nasal cavity or the sinuses. The fungi often invade blood vessels with resultant thrombosis and intracranial extension. Almost all patients with phycomycosis are systemically debilitated and many have metabolic acidosis. The majority of such patients have diabetes or have been treated with antimetabolites and steroids.

Orbital X-rays often show sinus opacification, whereas CT scans and ultrasonography may visualize inflammatory changes in the orbit. The diagnosis of phycomycosis is made by biopsy of the involved tissues and demonstration of nonseptate-branching hyphae.

Treatment of phycomycosis usually involves control of any underlying metabolic disorder, the administration of amphotericin B, and local surgical excision of the infected tissues, which are frequently necrotic. Exenteration may be necessary if the infection involves tissues near the orbital apex, especially if vision has been destroyed.

Pseudotumors

Orbital pseudotumors are idiopathic inflammations that are unrelated to a specific local or systemic disorder. These inflammatory disorders are common in both adults and children (15,16). Orbital pain, restricted eye movements, and exophthalmos are common clinical findings in patients with pseudotumors. The inflammatory changes can be diffuse within the orbit or may involve a specific structure such as an extraocular muscle or the lacrimal gland. Although the presentation of orbital pseudotumors is usually acute, idiopathic inflammations may become chronic and produce scarring with fibrosis of the orbital periosteum, the retrobulbar fat, or extraocular muscles.

It is clear that inflammatory orbital pseudotumor is a collection of orbital inflammatory processes, which may not be homogeneous in etiology or effect. The Tolosa-Hunt syndrome, or idiopathic painful ophthalmoplegia, is a form of pseudotumor in which the inflammatory process probably involves the cavernous sinus, or the superior orbital fissure and optic canal. Orbital pain and restriction of all eye movements are the most common features of this disorder, and visual acuity may be reduced as well.

Histologically, orbital pseudotumors may range from a vasculitis to a granulomatous process. Most idiopathic orbital inflammations are composed of a mixture of lymphocytes, plasma cells, and eosinophils. Some pseudotumors may histologically be granulomas or may be heavily infiltrated by fibrous tissue. When lymphocytes predominate, the process is frequently described as lymphoid hyperplasia (see following section on lymphoid tumors).

Ultrasonography and CT scans may show thickened extraocular muscles, enlargement of the lacrimal gland, or a ring of tissue around the globe that enhances with contrast (Fig. 5). Sometimes older focal masses may be seen around the optic nerve, within the retrobulbar fat, or near the orbital periosteum. The diagnosis of pseudotumor is made by excluding other causes of orbital mass lesions such as neoplasms and other causes of orbital inflammation such as Graves' disease and infections.

Treatment of orbital pseudotumors usually involves the use of high-dose systemic steroids. Sometimes this therapy can be given after establishing a presumptive diagnosis based upon clinical findings and diagnostic studies. Often it is necessary to perform surgical exploration

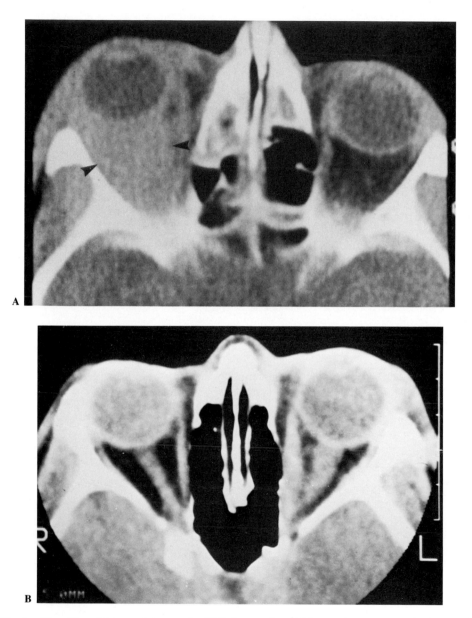

FIG. 5. Idiopathic orbital pseudotumor. **A:** CAT shows enlarged left superior rectus muscle (*arrows*) in a patient with myositis. **B:** CAT shows enlarged left medial rectus muscle and contiguous optic nerve swelling in patient with myositis.

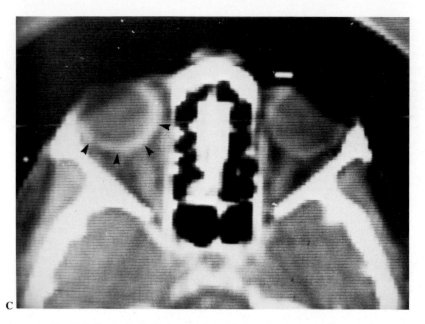

C

FIG. 5. (*cont.*)   **C:** CAT shows ring of increased tissue density surrounding left eye (*arrows*) in patient with episcleritis.

and obtain tissue for histologic examination. When a pseudotumor fails to respond to these measures, radiation therapy may sometimes be effective (17).

Benign or Malignant Tumors

Lymphoid Tumors

Lymphoid tumors are probably the most common tumor of the orbit in adults. The presenting signs of the lymphoid tumors are usually of very slow onset and occur in middle-age patients, with a peak incidence at age 60 (18). Clinically, the patients present with a gradual proptosis of the eye with some displacement and have a motility disturbance with diplopia in some field of gaze. Visual loss is uncommon. The lids may assume a doughy, puffy appearance and there may be some pinkish subconjunctival change. A mass is palpable in at least 50% of the cases.

Lymphomas commonly arise in the superior orbit and have characteristic CT scan findings (19). They often appear as a mass that may simulate an extraocular muscle (Fig. 6). They generally cause no bone erosion and have ill-defined borders with a frayed contour and a knobby, excrescent appearance. The lymphoma tissue will insinuate itself into potential spaces and fascial planes, producing streaky trails. Many lymphomas will arise from lymphoid tissue within the lacrimal gland and present as a lacrimal gland mass (Fig. 7). There is no means of differentiating benign lymphoid hyperplasia from a malignant lymphoma on the basis of the CT scan findings. Lymphoma tumors may also occur in the lacrimal sac.

Classifying lymphoid lesions with light microscopy, grouping them as reactive lymphoid hyperplasia, atypical lymphoid hyperplasia, and malignant lymphoma, has not been entirely successful in determining whether or not a patient will get systemic involvement over a 5-year period. Some patients diagnosed as having benign reactive lymphoid hyperplasia

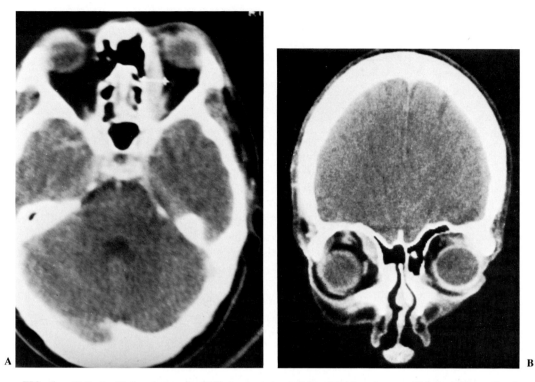

FIG. 6. Patient with lymphoma. **A:** CAT demonstrates a right orbital lymphoma, which is easily confused with the medial rectus muscle when viewed axially. **B:** CCT clearly defines the lymphoma as a distinct superonasal orbital mass. The recti muscles are normal.

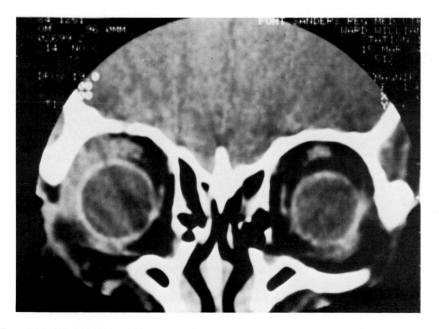

FIG. 7. CCT demonstrates a lymphoma within the lacrimal gland fossa. It is typical that the lymphoma conforms to the shape of the globe and that there is no erosion of bone.

have shown as high as 20% systemic involvement in 5 years, whereas patients diagnosed initially as having malignant lymphoma may not get systemic involvement in a high number of cases (20–30%).

There seems to be a much better ability to predict the occurrence of systemic spread using the technique of analysis with surface immunoglobins, although at the time of this writing there is no absolute prognostic indicator. Very probably, all lymphoid tumors should be considered to have a malignant potential or a potential for signs of systemic involvement at some time in the future.

Benign lymphoid hyperplasia cannot always be distinguished from malignant lymphomas on the basis of histologic criteria alone. Therefore, immunologic identification of cell-surface markers on lymphocytes has been used to help classify lymphocytic tumors (20,21). Most human lymphocytes can be categorized as B or T cells. B lymphocytes chiefly originate in the bone marrow. These cells are primarily responsible for antibody production, as a consequence of which immunoglobulins are located upon their surface membranes. These B lymphocytes tend to localize in lymph nodes and the spleen, and can transform into plasma cells. T lymphocytes are predominately derived from the thymus and are primarily responsible for cell-mediated immunity. These cells comprise most of the circulating lymphocytes in the blood.

The origin of groups of B lympocytes can be determined by analysis of the classes of immunoglobulins found on their cell surfaces. A monoclonal proliferation is one in which a single immunoglobulin class predominates in a tumor. Polyclonal proliferations are those in which multiple classes of immunoglobulins are found.

Benign lymphoid hyperplasia is usually composed of T cells or of B cells of polyclonal origin. Malignant lymphomas are commonly composed of B cells of monoclonal origin. Some lymphomas of T cell origin do exist, such as Hodgkin's disease, but these are less common than B cell lymphomas and they rarely involve the orbit. If a lymphoid tumor is found at the time of surgery, some fresh tissue should be submitted for cell-surface immunologic analysis to aid in diagnosis and classification.

At present, many experts feel that a systemic work-up is indicated in the patient with an orbital lymphoid tumor, regardless of whether it appears to be a "malignant" lymphoma or simply "benign" lymphoid hyperplasia. A relatively noninvasive systemic evaluation may include: examination for lymphadenopathy and liver or spleen enlargement, complete blood count (CBC) and serum protein electrophoresis, chest roentgenogram, abdominal CT scan, and bone marrow aspiration/biopsy. It must be emphasized that these patients should be evaluated over a lengthy follow-up period of several years.

The present treatment of choice of orbital lymphoid tumors and orbital lymphomas is low-dose radiation therapy (22). The patient is usually treated with 2,500 to 3,000 rads of supravoltage radiation in divided doses over a 10-day period. These tumors generally regress within 1 month following the radiation treatment. Just as there is difficulty classifying these tumors and determining their prognosis, questions regarding the long-term response of lymphoid tumors and lymphomas to radiation therapy remain to be answered.

Hemangiomas and Lymphangiomas

Cavernous hemangiomas, capillary hemangiomas, and lymphangiomas are the most common vascular abnormalities that involve the orbit. The majority of these lesions are not considered to be neoplasms but instead are thought to be benign developmental hamartomas.

Hamartomas are growths arising from tissue elements that are usually found at the position in which the tumor is located.

Cavernous hemangiomas are the most common benign tumors of the orbit in adults. Although a rudimentary lesion may be present at birth, symptoms do not usually occur until the hemangioma enlarges during the second to fourth decades of life. These tumors are usually located within the muscle cone behind the eye, but they may also lie against an orbital wall and cause bone displacement. Exophthalmos and chorioretinal folds are commonly caused by these abnormalities.

Histologically, cavernous hemangiomas are composed of large vascular channels that are lined by endothelial cells and are separated by fibrous septa. These tumors are usually well circumscribed with a firm capsule and few significant feeding arteries or draining veins.

Orbital X-rays may show fossa formation caused by chronic pressure against the orbital walls. Ultrasonography commonly demonstrates multiple high-amplitude internal echoes. CT scans usually show smooth surfaces around a discrete tumor that enhances after contrast administration (Fig. 8).

Cavernous hemangiomas should usually be surgically removed, most often by a lateral orbital exploration, because they are most frequently located within the muscle cone. Complete excision is usually facilitated because of the presence of a firm capsule and the relative lack of significant feeding or draining vessels. These tumors rarely undergo spontaneous involution.

Capillary hemangiomas are among the most common benign tumors of the orbit in children. These lesions typically appear as elevated red nodules within or near the eyelids

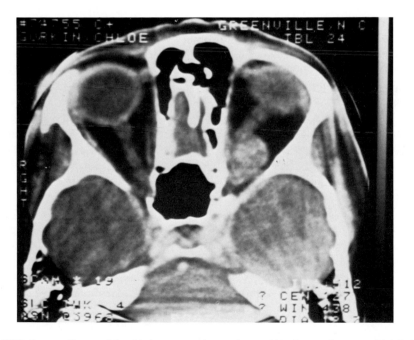

FIG. 8. CAT shows a discrete, left orbital cavernous hemangioma within the muscle cone, which is indenting the optic nerve. The mottled appearance of the tumor with contrast enhancement is typical.

during the first month after birth. The surface of the lesion may be dimpled, giving rise to the name "strawberry birthmark." A mass is often found within the deep lids and the anterior orbit. In addition, lesions may arise elsewhere in the head and neck or in other locations on the body. Displacement of the eye, astigmatism, and ptosis may be caused by eyelid involvement.

Histologically, these tumors are typified by a proliferation of capillaries and endothelial cells with a rare mitoses. Large feeding vessels are common and the margins of the tumors are relatively indistinct.

Because capillary hemangiomas have such a typical clinical appearance, the diagnosis can usually be made without resorting to elaborate tests. Orbital X-rays may show enlargement of the bony orbit. CT scans and ultrasonography may be considered if a deep lesion cannot be distinguished from other orbital lesions of childhood such as dermoids, rhabdomyosarcomas, or meningoceles.

Treatment of capillary hemangiomas should be delayed if possible because these tumors usually undergo partial or complete involution by 5 years of age. Even after regression of the tumor, however, the patient may be left with crêpe-like skin and ptosis that require surgical correction. Amblyopia should be combated by correction of significant refractive errors. If the tumor is so large or disfiguring that some treatment must be initiated, intralesional steroid injections may hasten resolution of the tumor (23). Steroid responsiveness is often greatest in young children. Low-dose radiation therapy may cause reduction in tumor size, and surgical excision can sometimes be used to remove portions of particularly large lesions (24).

Lymphangiomas are benign vascular tumors that most often appear during childhood. These tumors may be found in the conjunctiva, the eyelids, the orbit, or elsewhere in the head and neck.

One of the most common manifestations of orbital lymphangiomas is spontaneous hemorrhage that may cause sudden exophthalmos and limited eye movement. The hemorrhage usually subsides without treatment, but a chronic blood cyst may form and require surgical drainage or removal. Lymphangiomas may rapidly enlarge during acute respiratory infections, probably because of lymphoid hyperplasia.

Histologically, these tumors consist of cystic spaces filled with clear fluid and lined by flattened endothelial cells. Smooth muscle cells are usually absent in the vascular walls of lymphangiomas. Lymphoid follicles may be found within the interstitial stroma. Chronic lymphangiomas may contain phleboliths and calcified nodules.

Orbital X-rays are usually normal, although a blood cyst may sometimes produce enlargement of the orbit and calcifications are occasionally seen in chronic lesions. CT scans and ultrasonography usually show irregular internal densities and may demonstrate cystic spaces that can contain blood. Lymphangiomas are commonly infiltrative with irregular outlines.

Treatment of lymphangiomas may involve surgical excision of disfiguring portions of the tumors or drainage of blood cysts that fail to spontaneously resolve. Since these tumors may infiltrate irregularly into the orbit, complete excision is often difficult or impossible (25). Extensive surgery is usually avoided. When performing surgery, the carbon dioxide laser is a valuable tool that can maintain hemostasis while debulking the tumor (26). The vaporizing/cutting action of this laser depends on water content of the tissue, rather than tissue color. Systemic steroids may reduce the size of the lymphoid nodules and the amount of inflammation. Radiation therapy by external sources or implantation has sometimes been recommended, but this has not been found to be of significant value in the control of most lymphangiomas.

Dermoids and epidermoids are benign lesions that can be found in nearly all age groups, although they produce symptoms in children more frequently than in adults. Most dermoids and epidermoids are cystic, but some may have solid components as well. These lesions are usually not considered to be neoplastic but instead are thought to be benign developmental choristomas. Choristomas are growths arising from tissue elements that are not usually found at the position in which the tumor is located.

Dermoids are usually caused by developmental sequestrations of surface epidermis, often adjacent to bony suture lines. One of the most common locations of dermoid cysts is the superior-temporal quadrant of the orbit, where they are commonly fixed to periosteum near the zygomatic-frontal suture. Solid epibulbar dermoids with a fatty component are described as lipodermoids or dermolipomas. These lesions are usually smoothly elevated white or yellow nodules that are most commonly located beneath the conjunctiva on the superior-temporal surface of the globe.

Histologically, dermoids are composed of epidermal tissue together with one or more dermal adnexal structures and skin appendages such as hair follicles, sebaceous glands, and sweat glands. The cystic component is lined by keratinizing epidermis and may be filled with keratin, hairs, and fatty material. If these contents are relased into the orbit either spontaneously or during surgery, an inflammatory reaction may result.

Dermoids can be anatomically classified into three groups: (a) superficial subcutaneous dermoids, (b) subconjunctival dermoids, and (c) deep orbital dermoids. Superficial dermoids are usually discovered during childhood, when they appear as painless subcutaneous nodules that are most often beneath the lateral brow. Subconjunctival dermoids or lipodermoids are usually located on the temporal surface of the globe and may extend into the posterior orbit. Deep orbital dermoids are most often found in adults after a long period of slow growth. Many deep dermoids may resemble lacrimal gland tumors when they are located in the superior-temporal orbit.

Orbital X-rays are usually normal in patients with superficial subcutaneous dermoids and subconjunctival dermoids or lipodermoids. Deep orbital dermoids often cause sharply marginated defects in the orbital bones adjacent to the cyst. Ultrasonography and CT scans usually demonstrate a cystic lesion, frequently with an adjacent solid component that may represent chronically inflamed and organized orbital fat (Fig. 9).

Superficial subcutaneous dermoids can usually be removed through a skin incision directly over the cyst. The deep surface of the tumor is nearly always adherent to periosteum, from which it must be sharply divided. The diagnosis of these lesions can commonly be made from their clinical appearance, and excision may be delayed when the abnormality is discovered in young infants.

Subconjunctival dermoids or lipodermoids can also be recognized by their location and appearance in most instances. These tumors are usually solid and may lie near the levator and extraocular muscles. Excision of lipodermoids may be complicated by ptosis, restricted ocular motility, or damage to the eye. Because of this potential for complications, excision of subconjunctival dermoids and lipodermoids should usually be avoided if possible. If excision is necessary because of enlargement, cosmetic deformity, or irritation, then surgery should be performed with great care.

Deep orbital dermoids are usually best approached by a lateral orbital exploration. Excision of the cyst is made easier if it is preliminarily decompressed by careful removal of the contents before dissection of the cyst wall (27). Some deep orbital dermoids extend through the orbital bones and involve the intracranial space, in which case they should usually be removed through a neurosurgical approach.

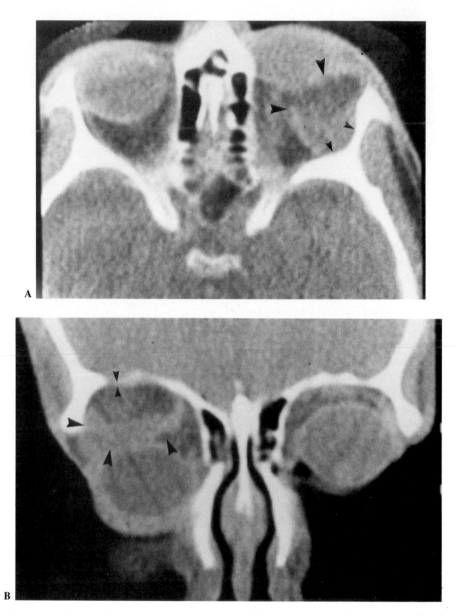

FIG. 9. Patient with dermoid cyst. **A:** CAT shows retrobulbar dermoid cyst (*large arrows*) that displaces lateral wall (*small arrows*) of right orbit. **B:** CCT shows dermoid cyst (*large arrows*) above right eye and thinned roof (*small arrows*) of right orbit.

Epidermoids are benign cystic choristomas that differ from dermoids in that they are composed of only tissues without adnexal structures or skin appendages. The cyst may be filled with cholesterol crystals and epithelial debris such as keratin. X-rays frequently show bony defects with sharp margins similar to those produced by deep dermoid cysts. Treatment consists of incision and aspiration of the cyst contents followed by removal of the cyst wall.

Peripheral Nerve Tumor (Neurilemoma, Schwannoma)

Neurilemomas are one of the more common orbital tumors, and are well-encapsulated nerve sheath tumors occurring anywhere along the course of the peripheral, cranial, or sympathetic nerves. Usually benign, these do occur in the orbit and cause proptosis and possible reduction in vision if adjacent to the optic nerve, where they produce a compressive effect (Fig. 10). Neurilemomas develop in approximately 10% of the patients with neurofibromatosis. There are two types of histology: the Antonioni type A, which is solid, consisting of Schwann cells, and the type B, which has cystic spaces. Ultrasound of these lesions as well as CT scan findings may mimic that of an orbital hemangioma. The well-encapsulated tumors can be generally shelled out with blunt dissection, but in many cases there is much vascularity of the capsule and brisk bleeding can be encountered following excision of these lesions (Fig. 11). Sarcomatous degeneration has been reported in some cases of initially benign tumors.

Lacrimal Gland Tumors

Most mass lesions in the superior temporal quadrant of the orbit arise within the lacrimal gland, but other tumors such as dermoids may also be found in this location. Of the tumors that involve the lacrimal gland, approximately half are nonepithelial and half are epithelial in origin.

Nonepithelial lacrimal gland lesions include idiopathic inflammatory pseudotumors that may present in a variety of histologic forms, especially lymphocytic proliferations (lymphoid hyperplasias) and granulomas. Sjögren's syndrome and sarcoidosis may cause lacrimal gland enlargement that is sometimes bilateral. Malignant lymphomas may involve the lacrimal gland, and these tumors may be difficult to distinguish from benign lympocytic pseudotumors.

Epithelial lacrimal gland lesions are approximately half benign and half malignant. Almost all of the benign epithelial lesions, totaling nearly one quarter of all lacrimal gland tumors,

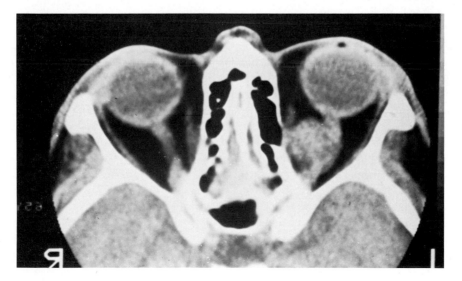

FIG. 10. CAT demonstrates compression of the left optic nerve by an intraconal neurilemoma (peripheral nerve tumor).

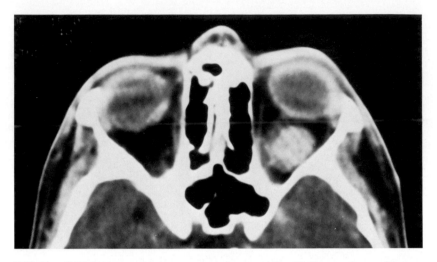

FIG. 11. CAT demonstrates strong contrast enhancement in a highly vascular neurilemoma.

are mixed tumors. These benign mixed tumors usually produce a slowly enlarging mass beneath the lateral upper lid with no significant pain or inflammation. These lesions are usually discovered during the third through sixth decades of life. Although a mass and symptoms are usually present for at least 12 months, the duration often cannot be accurately determined by history alone (28).

Histologically, mixed tumors are composed primarily of epithelial tissue. In addition, they contain mesenchymal elements, some of which appear to be formed by metaplastic transformation of myoepithelium. Malignant epithelial tumors include adenocystic carcinomas, malignant forms of mixed tumors, and uncommon lesions such as squamous cell carcinomas.

Orbital X-rays are usually normal in patients with nonepithelial lacrimal gland lesions such as pseudotumors or lymphomas. Because benign mixed tumors are usually painless and slow growing, they often produce localized pressure erosion of the bone overlying the lacrimal gland. These tumors are variable, however, and some benign mixed tumors may have a relatively short duration of symptoms and no bony changes. Although bone destruction, which is irregular, is frequently due to a malignancy, some benign mixed tumors, dermoids, and inflammatory lesions sometimes produce similar changes. Ultrasonography will usually detect tumors arising from the lacrimal gland, but CT scans are generally more useful for visualizing the extent of lacrimal gland tumors (Fig. 12).

Treatment of lacrimal gland tumors involves some of the most important decisions in orbital surgery. Benign mixed tumors should be completely removed without preliminary biopsy whenever possible, since if their contents are spilled or seeded within the orbit, they can recur as widely infiltrative and even truly malignant lesions.

Surgical excision of small lacrimal gland tumors can sometimes be accomplished through a superiororbital incision without bone removal. However, since it is desirable to remove the entire lesion *en bloc* when a mixed tumor may be present, a lateral orbital exploration is usually the most satisfactory approach for lacrimal gland tumor excision. If a lacrimal gland tumor has invaded bone so that a malignancy is very likely, a biopsy through an

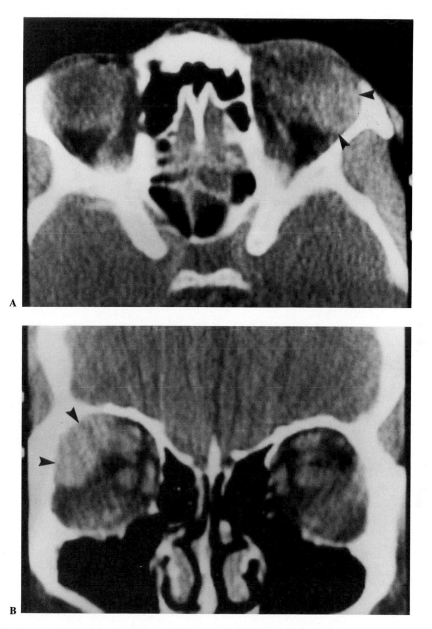

FIG. 12. Patient with benign mixed tumor. **A:** CAT shows enlarged right lacrimal gland caused by growth of tumor (*arrows*). **B:** CCT shows benign mixed tumor (*arrows*) of right lacrimal gland.

anterior incision is justified. The management of malignant lacrimal gland tumors will be considered separately under the topic of malignant tumors.

Malignant Tumors

Secondary and Metastatic Tumors

Secondary tumors are those that extend directly into the orbit from adjacent regions such as the eye, the eyelids, the paranasal sinuses, or the intracranial space. Most secondary tumors are malignant, although some benign tumors may also involve the orbit secondarily. The most common of all malignant tumors that involve the orbit in adults extend directly from the adjacent paranasal sinuses or the nose. Squamous cell carcinoma, sebaceous cell carcinoma, and malignant melanoma extend from the eyelids into the orbit less frequently.

Orbital X-rays are almost always abnormal in patients with sinus tumors that involve the orbit. CT scans are useful for the study of secondary tumors because they demonstrate details of both soft tissue and bones.

Treatment of secondary orbital tumors is essentially based upon treatment of the primary lesion. Eradication of many such tumors involves orbital exenteration in addition to surgery upon the sinuses or eyelids.

Metastatic tumors in adults most commonly spread from primary sites in the breast or lung (29). In children, neuroblastoma and Ewing's sarcoma are the most common tumors that cause orbital metastases.

Breast carcinoma is the most frequent primary source of orbital metastasis in women (29,30). Metastases may occur many years after the primary lesion has been removed. The findings of exophthalmos, ophthalmoplegia, and bone destruction should raise the suspicion of a metastatic tumor. Metastatic breast carcinoma may elicit a fibrous response that produces cicatrization and enophthalmos. Because lung carcinoma frequently metatasizes to the orbit, a chest X-ray should be performed in most patients with an orbital disorder. Less commonly, tumors such as malignant melanoma may metastasize to the orbit.

Neuroblastoma is a malignant tumor that usually arises in the retroperitoneal area and almost always occurs in patients younger than 7 years of age. Metastatic orbital neuroblastoma typically produces abrupt exophthalmos and eyelid ecchymosis that may be bilateral (31).

Histologically, neuroblastomas are composed of primitive neuroectodermal cells that originate in the adrenal medulla, sympathetic ganglia, or peripheral nervous system. An intravenous pyelogram often demonstrates adrenal abnormalities, and bone defects may be found on X-rays. Increased urinary excretion of vanillylmandelic acid is common, and bone marrow examination shows tumor cells in many patients with neuroblastoma (1).

Ultrasonography and CT scans may demonstrate either a focal mass (Fig. 13) or a diffuse infiltrative lesion in patients with metastases (Fig. 14). Although bone destruction is common in patients with metastatic tumors, the lesion may be confined to the soft tissues and orbital X-rays may appear normal.

Treatment of metastatic tumors is usually palliative, consisting of local radiation therapy, systemic chemotherapy, or immune therapy. Since hormone therapy may be useful in the treatment of some patients with metastatic breast carcinoma, tissue removed at the time of orbital exploration can be submitted for assay of estrogen and progesterone receptor activity (32). Occasionally, metastatic tumors should be treated by aggressive local therapy such a exenteration, since patients with some primary lesions such as carcinoids may survive for many years after their metastasis is controlled.

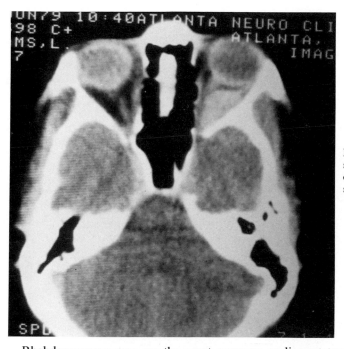

FIG. 13. CAT demonstrates metastatic breast carcinoma to the right orbit as a focal mass causing proptosis.

Rhabdomyosarcomas are the most common malignant tumors of the orbit in children. More than three-quarters of these tumors are found in patients under 15 years of age. On rare occasions, rhabdomyosarcomas have been found in newborn infants and sometimes they arise in adults. The most common clinical manifestation of these tumors is exophthalmos that becomes rapidly progressive over several days or weeks. Although any portion of the orbit can be involved, many of these tumors arise above or medial to the globe. Sometimes a palpable nodule may appear beneath the eyelids or conjunctiva. Pain is usually not an early symptom, and bone involvement is variable.

Histologically, rhabdomyosarcomas are composed of malignant mesenchymal cells that frequently resemble immature striated muscle. They have been traditionally classified according to their degree of cellular differentiation and histologic pattern into three types: (a) embryonal, (b) pleomorphic, and (c) alveolar. Embryonal rhabdomyosarcoma is the most common type, and is usually composed of poorly differentiated cells called rhabdomyoblasts arranged in a loose syncytial pattern. Pleomorphic rhabdomyosarcoma is a relatively well-differentiated type of tumor that is frequently found in older patients. Cells are arranged in a disorganized pattern but may contain multiple nuclei in the form of straps. Cross-striations are found easily in most of these tumors. Alveolar rhabdomyosarcoma is found in all age groups. Cells are poorly differentiated and are arranged in a distinctive alveolar pattern, with connective tissue trabeculae. Among these three types of tumors, alveolar rhabdomyosarcomas generally have the worst prognosis and pleomorphic rhabdomyosarcomas seem to have the best prognosis (33).

Orbital X-rays may be normal when rhabdomyosarcomas are confined to the soft tissues. Bone destruction suggests that a rhabdomyosarcoma may be present when rapidly evolving exophthalmos occurs in childhood. Tomographic X-rays sometimes detect focal areas of bone destruction that are not apparent on any other diagnostic studies. Ultrasonography and CT scans usually demonstrate a solid tumor that may have well-circumscribed margins or may infiltrate into adjacent tissues and destroy bone (Fig. 15).

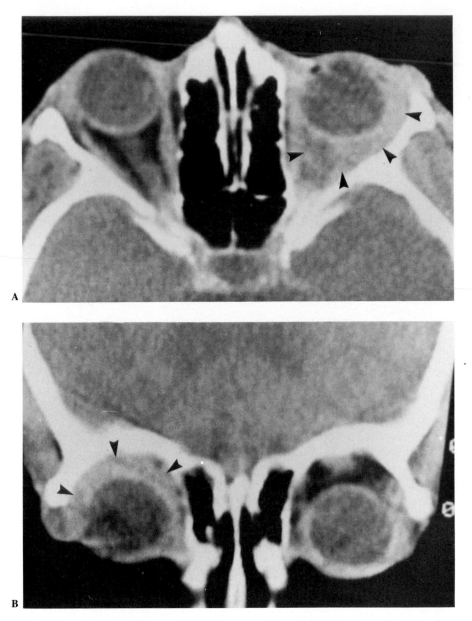

FIG. 14. Patient with infiltrative tumor. **A:** CAT shows tumor (*arrows*) behind right eye of patient with cicatricial enophthalmos caused by metastatic breast cancer. **B:** CCT shows infiltrative tumor (*arrows*) above right eye.

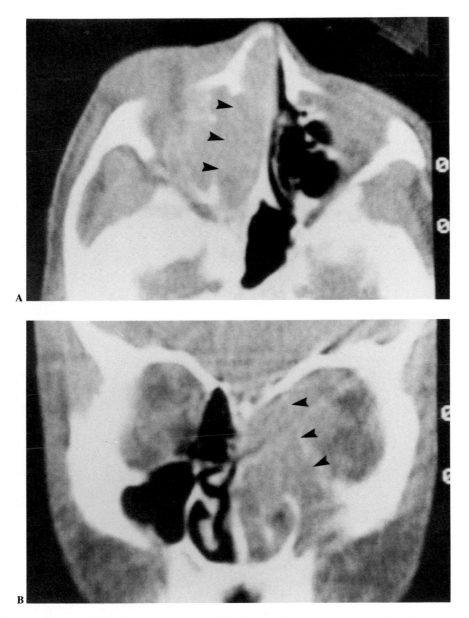

FIG. 15. Patient with rhabdomyosarcoma. **A:** CAT shows rhabdomyosarcoma extending into nose through destroyed bones (*arrows*) of medial wall of left orbit. **B:** CCT shows rhabdomyosarcoma extending through destroyed bones (*arrows*) of medial wall and floor of left orbit.

The preauricular and cervical lympyh nodes should be palpated to locate regional metastases, and a chest X-ray as well as a bone marrow aspirate should be obtained to locate more distant metastases. The diagnosis of rhabdomyosarcoma is established by biopsy as soon as possible. If the lesion presents in the anterior orbit, an anterior approach through the conjunctiva or eyelid is preferred. When a retrobulbar tumor is present, it is usually necessary to perform a lateral orbital exploration. Surgery should be performed with minimal trauma and the tumor should not be excessively manipulated to minimize the chance of dissemination.

In addition to routine histologic examination of the tumor, a specimen should be submitted for electron microscopy, preferably after fixation in glutaraldehyde. Some poorly differentiated rhabdomyosarcomas may not be diagnosed by light microscopy, and characteristic cross-striations may only be found by electron microscopy. In children, rhabdomyosarcomas may be confused with a number of rare, poorly differentiated neoplasms such as neuroblastomas, lymphomas, and soft tissue sarcomas. Electron microscopy, selective histologic staining, and growth patterns seen in tissue culture may help to distinguish among these tumors (1,3,4).

The treatment of orbital rhabdomyosarcomas usually consists of local radiation therapy with the total dose reaching 5,000 to 6,000 rads. If the tumor extends beyond the orbit, the sinuses and neck may also be treated with radiation. Systemic chemotherapy with a combination of drugs such as cyclophosphamide (Cytoxan®), vincristine, and dactinomycin is usually given as an adjunct to radiation treatment. Orbital exenteration, which in the past was the preferred treatment of these tumors, is rarely indicated. The survival rate using combined radiation therapy with systemic chemotherapy is nearly 70% compared to less than 50% when exenteration was the treatment of choice. By using such combination therapy, some patients have been cured of their disease even when bone involvement and cervical metastases were present (34). High-dose local radiation therapy may cause orbital hypoplasia and ocular damage, including keratopathy and cataract formation.

Malignant Lacrimal Gland Tumors

Approximately 50% of lacrimal gland tumors are nonepithelial and 50% are epithelial. Most nonepithelial malignant lacrimal gland tumors are lymphoid in origin. As previously mentioned, it is often difficult to distinguish benign lymphoid hyperplasia from malignant lymphoma. The identification of malignant lymphomas can sometimes be aided by the immunologic study of cell-surface markers on lymphocytes. Lymphomas and other nonepithelial malignant tumors are usually treated by local surgical excision or biopsy, followed by orbital radiation or systemic chemotherapy. Since many cases of lymphoma are multifocal, a systemic evaluation should be performed, including a general physical examination, chest X-ray, and serum immunoprotein electrophoresis for the detection of abnormal immunoglobulins. When malignant lymphoma is found in the orbit, bone marrow aspiration, abdominal CT scans, and lymphangiography for the detection of involved retroperitoneal lymph nodes should be considered. Periodic follow-up examinations of patients with lymphocytic tumors is appropriate because systemic lymphoma can appear years after the presentation of an orbital lesion.

Approximately half of all epithelial lacrimal gland tumors are malignant. Most of the remaining epithelial tumors are benign mixed tumors, which have already been discussed. Most of the epithelial malignancies are adenoid cystic carcinomas, with squamous carcinomas and malignant mixed tumors arising less frequently. Orbital X-rays usually show evidence of bone destruction overlying the lesion.

Malignant epithelial tumors of the lacrimal gland are among the most lethal tumors of the orbit (35). Even if exenteration is performed, local recurrence in the orbital bones or metastatic spread is relativly common. For this reason, radical exenteration with removal of portions of the superior and lateral bony walls of the orbit has been recommended as treatment of these tumors. Radiation therapy is sometimes used in addition to exenteration (28). Because of the mutilative nature of such surgery, the diagnosis of a malignant lacrimal gland tumor should be based upon permanent section histologic evaluation rather than frozen section examination.

REFERENCES

1. Grove, A. S., Jr. (1975): Evaluation of exophthalmos. *N. Engl. J. Med.*, 292:1005–1013.
2. Jones, I. S., Jakobiec, F. A., and Nolan, B. T. (1985): Patient examination and introduction to orbital disease. In: *Clinical Ophthalmology Vol. II: The Orbit*, edited by T. D. Duane and E. A. Jaeger. Harper & Row, Hagerstown, Maryland.
3. Grove, A. S., Jr. (1979): Orbital disease: Examination and diagnostic evaluation. *Ophthalmology*, 86:854–863.
4. Grove, A. S., Jr. (1979: Orbital diagnosis. *Head Neck Surg.*, 2:12–24.
5. Shields, J. A., Bakewell, B., Ausburger, J. J., et al. (1986): Space-occupying orbital masses in children. A review of 250 consecutive biopsies. *Ophthalmology*, 93:379–384.
6. Byrne, S. F., and Glaser, J. S. (1983): Orbital tissue differentiation with standardized echography. *Ophthalmology*, 90:1071–1090.
7. Zimmerman R. A., Bilaniuk, L. T., Yanoff, M., et al. (1985): Orbital magnetic resonance imaging. *Am. J. Ophthalmol*, 100:312–317.
8. Haik, B. G., Saint Louis, L., and Smith, M. E. (1985): Nuclear magnetic resonance imaging in orbital disease. *Ophthalmic Forum* 3(1):31–34.
9. Sergott, R. C., and Glaser, J. S. (1981): Graves' ophthalmopathy. A clinical and immunologic review. *Surg. Ophthalmol.*, 26:1–21.
10. Kaplan, M. M., and Utiger, R. D. (1978): Diagnosis of hyperthyroidism. *Clin. Endocrinol. Metab.*, 7:97–113.
11. Grove, A. S., Jr. (1980): Levator lengthening by marginal myotomy. *Arch. Ophthalmol.*, 98:1433–1438.
12. Brenan, M. W., Leone, C. R., and Lalitha, J. (1983): Radiation therapy for Graves' disease. *Am. J. Ophthalmol.*, 96:195–199.
13. McCord, C. D., (1985): Current trends in orbital decompression. *Ophthalology*, 92:21–23.
14. Weiss, A., Friendly, D., Eglin, K., et al. (1983): Bacterial periorbital and orbital cellulitis in childhood. *Ophthalmology*, 90:195–203.
15. Chavis, R. M., Garner, A., and Wright, J. E. (1978): Inflammatory orbital pseudotumor. A clinicopathologic study. *Arch. Ophthalmol.*, 96:1817–1822.
16. Mottow, L. S., and Jakobiec, F. A. (1978): Idiopathic inflammatory orbital pseudotumor in childhood. I. Clinical characteristics. *Arch. Ophthalmol.*, 96:1410–1417.
17. Sergott, R. C., Glaser, J. S., and Charyulu, K. (1981): Radiotherapy for idiopathic inflammatory orbital pseudotumor. *Arch. Ophthalmol.*, 99:853–856.
18. Jakobiec, F. A., Iwamoto, T., and Knowles, D. M., II. (1982): Ocular adnexal lymphoid tumors. Correlative ultrastructural and immunologic marker studies. *Arch. Ophthalmol.* 100:84–98.
19. Yeo, J. H., Jakobiec, F. A., Abbott, G. F., and Trokel, S. L. (1982): Combined clinical and computed tomographic diagnosis of orbital lymphoid tumors. *Am. J. Ophthalmol.*, 94:235–245.
20. Cooper, M. D. (1980): Immunologic analysis of lymphoid tumors. *N. Engl. J. Med.*, 302:964–965.
21. Knowles, D. M., II, and Jakobiec, F. A. (1983):Identification of T-lymphocytes in ocular adnexal neoplasms by hybridoma monoclonal antibodies. *Am. J. Ophthalmol.*, 95:233–242.
22. Kennerdell, J. S., Johnson, B. L., and Deutsch, M. D. (1976): Radiation treatment of orbital lymphoid hyperplasia. *Ophthalmology*, 86:942–947.
23. Kushner, B. J. (1982): Intralesional corticosteroid injection for infantile adnexal hemangioma. *Am. J. Ophthalmol.*, 93:496–506.
24. Hiak, B. G., Jakobiec, F. A., Ellsworth, R. M., and Jones, I. S. (1979): Capillary hemangioma of the lids and orbit: An analysis of the clinical features and therapeutic results in 101 cases. *Ophthalmology*, 86:760–789.

25. Iliff, W. J., and Green, W. R. (1979): Orbital lymphangiomas. *Ophthalmology,* 86:914–929.
26. Wesley, R. E., and Bond, J. B. (1985): Carbon dioxide laser in ophthalmic plastic and orbital surgery. *Ophthalmic Surg.,* 16:631–633.
27. Grove, A. S., Jr. (1979): Giant dermoid cysts of the orbit. *Ophthalmology,* 86:1513–1520.
28. Stewart, W. B., Krohel, G. B., and Wright, J. E. (1979): Lacrimal gland and fossa lesions: An approach to diagnosis and management. *Opthalmology,* 86:886–895.
29. Ferry, A. P., and Font, R. L. (1974): Carcinoma metastatic to the eye and orbit. A clinicopathologic study of 227 cases. *Arch. Ophthalmol.,* 92:276–286.
30. Bullock, J. D., and Yanes, B. (1980): Ophthalmic manifestations of metastatic breast cancer. *Ophthalmology,* 87:961–973.
31. Mortada, A. (1967): Clinical characteristics of early orbital metastatic neuroblastoma. *Am. J. Ophthalmol.,* 63:1787–1793.
32. Lippman, M. E., and Allergra, J. C. (1978): Receptors in breast cancer. *N. Engl. J. Med.,* 299:930–933.
33. Jones, I. S., Reese, A. B., and Krout, J. (1965): Oribtal rhabdomyosarcoma: An analysis of 62 cases. *Trans. Am. Ophthalmol. Soc.,* 63:223–255.
34. Abramson, D. H., Ellsworth, R. M., Tretter, P., Wolff, J. A., and Kitchin, J. A. (1979): The treatment of orbital rhabdomyosarcoma with irradiation and chemotherapy. *Opthalmology,* 86:1330–1335.
35. Henderson, J. W., and Farrow, G. M. (1980): Primary malignant mixed tumors of the lacrimal gland. Report of 10 cases. *Ophthalmology,* 87:466–475.

Oculoplastic Surgery, 2nd edition, edited by
Clinton D. McCord, Jr., and Myron Tanenbaum.
Raven Press, New York © 1987.

Chapter 11

Surgical Approaches to Orbital Disease

Clinton D. McCord, Jr.

Department of Ophthalmology, Emory University School of Medicine, Atlanta, Georgia 30308

The need for surgical entry into the orbit occurs in a variety of clinical situations. Surgical exploration of the orbit is commonly used to remove an orbital tumor or to biopsy an orbital mass, in order to obtain a histologic diagnosis. Surgical entry into the orbit is also needed in some cases of intraorbital foreign bodies, fractures of an orbital wall, or to decompress the orbit in Graves' disease. Orbital decompression may also be needed in other clinical situations in which expanding orbital tissue compromises optic nerve function, such as posttraumatic hematomas, and those in which known benign orbital lesions cause intractable proptosis, such as lymphangiomas and dermoids, which may not be completely excisable.

With the great advances in the technology of computerized tomography and diagnostic ultrasound, "diagnostic exploratory surgery" of the orbit no longer occurs in most cases. In the large majority of cases, the exact location and, many times, the histologic nature of an orbital tumor can be diagnosed preoperatively, allowing the surgeon to approach the orbit surgically in a more specific manner to give better anatomic exposure and to avoid any unnecessary morbidity as the result of surgery. The diagnostic approach to a patient with proptosis and/or an orbital mass and consideration of therapeutic modalities has been discussed in Chapter 10.

The basic surgical techniques that will be emphasized in this chapter are the lateral orbitotomy (Berke modification) (1), the lateral orbitotomy for lacrimal gland lesions (Wright modification) (2–4), the superior nasal orbitotomy (5–7), the combined inferior and lateral orbitotomies, and the combined medial and lateral orbitotomies (9). The surgical technique of the inferior orbitotomy is presented in detail in Chapter 6, and orbital decompression is extensively covered in Chapter 8.

Good exposure is a key principle of successful orbitotomy. The bicoronal forehead flap can offer useful exposure of lacrimal gland lesions and other diseases of the superior orbit. This technique is discussed briefly in this chapter and is detailed in Chapter 18.

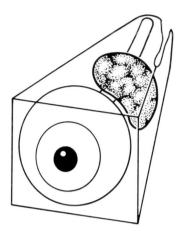

FIG. 1.   Lesion located in the lateral orbit or muscle cone area.

LATERAL ORBITOTOMY

Lesions that are most amenable to the lateral orbitotomy approach are those lying within the muscle cone or within the lateral portion of the orbit, including those that extend posteriorly (Fig. 1). The best exposure obtainable for this area remains the classic Berke modification of the Kronlein procedure (1) and this technique is superior to other techniques.

Surgical Technique

The preferred general anesthetic is enthrane anesthesia because it seems to induce less bleeding. Unless there are specific contraindications, the lateral canthal area and the temporalis muscle are injected before the surgeon scrubs with lidocaine (red label Xylocaine®) containing 1:100,000 epinephrine mixed with 1 ml of hyaluronidase (Wydase®) to a total of 10 ml. Patients are given oral steroids (adult dosage prednisone 80 mg p.o.) preoperatively and intravenous steroids (adult dosage dexamethasone 10 mg i.v.) intraoperatively. The head of the operating table is elevated 15°, which decreases venous congestion of the head and orbit.

A protective contact lens is inserted over the cornea and a malleable retractor is inserted inside the lateral canthus. A complete canthotomy is performed down to the lateral orbital rim and the skin incision is extended for 5 to 6 cm horizontally (Fig. 2A). The upper and lower limb of the lateral canthal tendon are detached from the lateral orbital rim with sharp dissection (Fig. 2B) and the skin edges are undermined from the temporalis fascia. There is a good cleavage plane in this area. The upper and lower canthal tendons and the skin edges are retracted with 4-0 silk sutures (Fig. 2C). An incision is then made through the periosteum from the outer surface of the bone. Two horizontal relaxing incisions are made in the periosteum so that it peels away from the rim and is reflected easily (Fig. 2D). The inner layer of the periosteum is then dissected from inside the lateral bony wall with the sharp Tenzel periosteal elevator along the entire edge of the lateral wall and 2 cm posteriorly. Care is taken to preserve its integrity. A malleable retractor is then inserted between the inner layer of the periosteum and the bony orbital wall and, with the use of the Stryker oscillating saw, cuts are made above the frontozygomatic suture and below, just above the body of the zygoma (Fig. 2E). The distance between the two cuts is usually about 3 to 3.5 cm. Wide exposure is necessary for safe exploration of the orbit. The bone

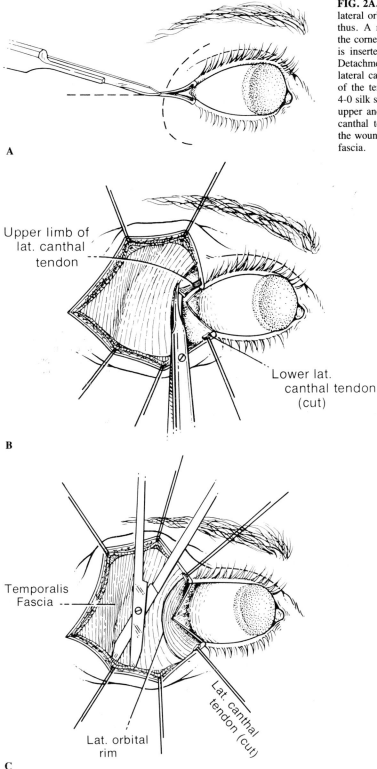

FIG. 2A. Initial incision for Berke lateral orbitotomy at the lateral canthus. A moist Gelfoam disc covers the cornea, and a malleable retractor is inserted to protect the globe. **B:** Detachment of the upper and lower lateral canthal tendon and retraction of the tendons and skin edges with 4-0 silk sutures. **C:** Retraction of the upper and lower limb of the lateral canthal tendon and undermining of the wound edges over the temporalis fascia.

A

Upper limb of lat. canthal tendon

Lower lat. canthal tendon (cut)

B

Temporalis Fascia

Lat. canthal tendon (cut)

Lat. orbital rim

C

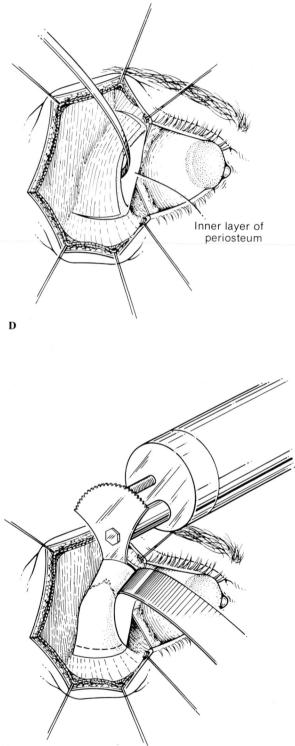

D

E

FIG. 2 (*cont.*) D: Reflection of the inner layer of the periosteum with the sharp periosteal elevator. Relaxing incisions have also been made in the outer periosteal layer of the lateral wall. **E:** Bony cuts made in the lateral orbital wall with the Stryker oscillating saw. The inferior cut should be just above the body of the zygoma and the superior cut above the frontozygomatic suture approximately 3 to 3.5 cm in vertical distance to give accurate exposure. The inner layer of the periosteum is protected with a malleable retractor.

Inner layer of
periosteum

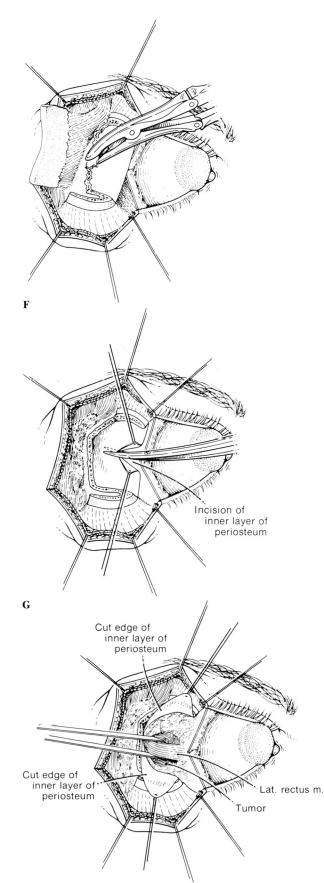

F

G

FIG. 2 (*cont.*) F: Excision of the remaining thin portion of the lateral orbital wall with the Rongeurs in a piecemeal manner, preserving the inner layer of the periosteum. **G:** A longitudinal incision is made in the intact inner layer of periosteum, tagging the cut edges with 4-0 silk sutures for retraction and subsequent identification. **H:** Retraction of the periosteal edges and of the lateral rectus muscle with umbilical tape, exposing the muscle cone area.

Incision of
inner layer of
periosteum

Cut edge of
inner layer of
periosteum

Cut edge of
inner layer of
periosteum

Lat. rectus m.

Tumor

H

flap is then grasped with a large Rongeur and fractured outwardly; it usually breaks at a thin area behind the rim, about 12 mm posteriorly to the edge of the rim, although this is variable from person to person. With the bone flap retracted outwardly, a Bovie with a cutting current is used to excise the bone flap from its attachment to the temporalis muscle.

The use of the cutting current greatly facilitates the avoidance of bleeding in the temporalis muscle, which is the major source of bleeding, and it provides excellent exposure. About another 10 to 12 mm of thin bone is still present in the posterior section of the lateral wall of the orbit; it is excised in a piecemeal manner while the temporalis muscle is retracted laterally, giving more posterior exposure (Fig. 2F). The inner layer of the periosteum, which is still intact, is then incised horizontally, tagging the corner and edges with 4-0 silk sutures in order to preserve it and also for retraction (Fig. 2G). The lateral rectus muscle is then identified and looped with umbilical tape. With finger palpation, the mass located in this area can usually be identified easily (Fig. 2H). In rare cases the lateral rectus muscle may be disinserted and retracted; however, it can be reattached during closure with few aftereffects.

When the lesion is encountered, its nature must be determined with regard to its adherence to surrounding structures. If the lesion is encapsulated and not adherent to surrounding structures, it can be removed *in toto;* however, it is usually advisable to determine the nature of the lesion at the time of surgery with frozen sections. If the lesion is infiltrative or adherent to vital structures that must be preserved, frozen sections at the time of surgery will determine the course of the orbitotomy (i.e., lymphomas and other lesions, such as metastatic lesions, are best treated by irradiation or chemotherapy; they are not surgical diseases). The key words for successful and atraumatic orbital exploration are ''adequate exposure.'' The use of a fiberoptic headlight is recommended, and an operating microscope with a 150-mm lens should be present if the preservation of small vessels and other structures is required. A special orbital retractor and microsurgical instruments have been described by Kennerdell and Maroon (10). The use of the bipolar cautery and cottonoid sponges greatly facilitates hemostasis. If a large venous vascular lesion with feeder vessels is encountered, it can be shrunk with a bipolar cautery with bayonet forcep tips and ligated. However, if the lesion is arterial (pulsatile) in nature, the feeder vessels (which should have been identified preoperatively) should be ligated alone. After the orbital procedure has been carried out, the orbitotomy may be closed.

Closure

Reapproximation of the edges of the inner layer of the periosteum is the key element in repair of the orbitotomy. These edges must be approximated meticulously since they furnish the basis for reformation of the canthal angle and also the replacement of the multiple extensions of the lateral rectus muscle and levator aponeurosis, which adhere to the lateral periosteum, as demonstrated by Koorneef (11). This is performed with interrupted sutures of 5-0 Dexon (Fig. 3A). The bony flap may be replaced at this point, if desired, with drill holes and 32-gauge stainless steel wire, although postoperatively it is cosmetically acceptable if the bone flap is not replaced, and an added decompressive effect is obtained to counteract postoperative edema if it is not replaced. The edges of the upper and lower canthal tendons are then sutured to the anterior edge of the inner layer of the periosteum with 4-0 Prolene sutures, reconstructing the canthal angle (see Fig. 3A). The reformation of the inner layer of the periosteum and reattachment of the limbs of the canthal tendon are the key steps in closure of the lateral orbitotomy. The skin is then closed with spanning

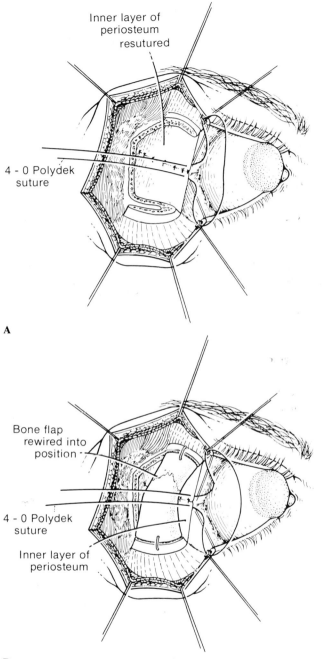

Inner layer of
periosteum
resutured

4 - 0 Polydek
suture

A

Bone flap
rewired into
position

4 - 0 Polydek
suture

Inner layer of
periosteum

B

FIG. 3A. Closure of the lateral orbitotomy showing reattachment of the upper and lower limb of the lateral canthal tendon to the edge of the inner layer of periosteum, which has been resutured. This essential step re-forms the lateral canthal angle. **B:** Closure of the lateral orbitotomy showing the lateral canthal fixation to the inner layer of the periosteum as well as replacement of the bone flap.

mattress sutures of 4-0 silk tied over cotton bolsters, and routine skin closure with 6-0 nylon is carried out. A split Penrose drain may be inserted if necessary at the extreme lateral limits of the incision.

If the bone flap is to be replaced, small drill holes at the edges of the flap and at the edges of the osteotomy are made with a dental burr and 32-gauge stainless steel wires can then be placed to wire the flap back into position. Replacement of the bone flap should be done only after closure of the periosteum and placement of the canthal sutures to the periosteum have been accomplished (Fig. 3B).

Postoperatively no compression bandages are used, but continuous ice compresses are used. All patients are placed on postoperative steroids (a Medrol Dosepack®) after 40 mg of methylprednisone sodium succinate (Solu-Medrol®) are given intramuscularly. Systemic antibiotics are used for 5 days postoperatively. In most cases the patients have only mild puffiness of the lids and slight bruising using this method.

LATERAL ORBITOTOMY FOR LACRIMAL GLAND LESIONS

Although statistically the majority of lesions occurring in the lacrimal gland fossa are not infiltrative epithelial tumors, one does not know the nature of these lesions ahead of time in many cases (Fig. 4). In the approach to the lacrimal gland lesion, one must be prepared to resect the entire lateral wall and part of the orbital roof, including the lateral inner periosteum, in order to cure these patients. Stewart et al. (12) have systematized the approach to surgical decisions in the management of the ''knotty'' problem of masses occurring in this area. Since the inner layer of the periosteum is usually excised in these patients, postoperative repair of this orbitotomy requires a different surgical approach to reconstruct the angle; the Wright style lateral orbitotomy (2) is used for lesions in this area.

Surgical Technique

The patient is prepared in a manner similar to the Berke lateral orbitotomy. An outline using methylene blue is then made in an S shape according to the method of Wright (Fig. 5A). An incision is carried down to the periosteum and the wound edges are retracted with 4-0 silk sutures or rake retractors (Fig. 5B). The periosteum is incised in the same manner as previously described and reflected from the outer surface of the orbital rim. The Stryker oscillating saw is then used to excise the lateral wall bone flap as in the lateral orbitotomy technique. If one has a low index of suspicion of an epithelial tumor, the lacrimal gland mass, which is encountered at this point, may be biopsied for frozen

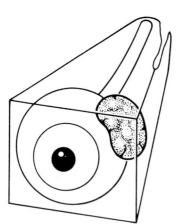

FIG. 4.   Lesion located in the lacrimal gland fossa area.

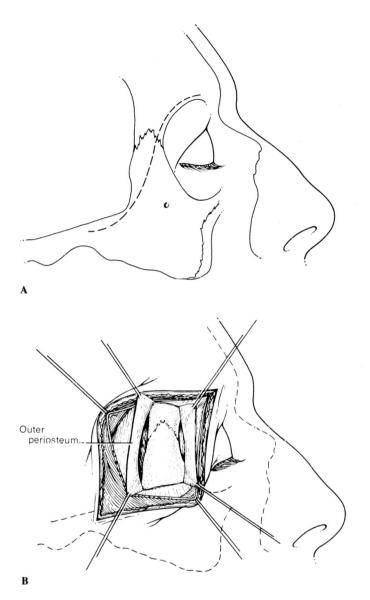

A

B

Outer
periosteum

C

Additional area of
bone removed

FIG. 5A. Outline of the skin incision to be made for the Wright lateral orbitotomy. **B:** Reflection of the inner and outer layer of the periosteum showing the area of bone to be incised with the right lateral orbitotomy. **C:** The area of bone removal that is required with the radical resection of an invasive lacrimal gland tumor (benign mixed tumor).

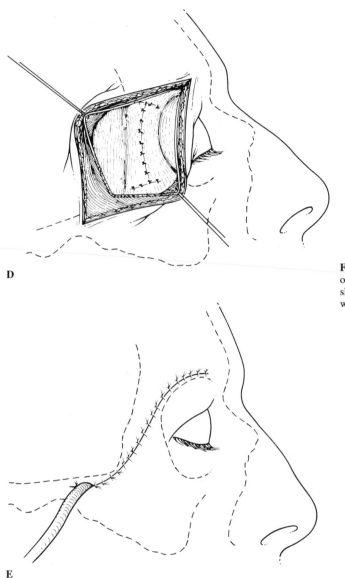

D

E

FIG. 5 (*cont.*) D: Closure of the outer layer of periosteum. **E:** Final skin closure in right lateral orbitotomy with drain inserted.

sections. The nature of the disease, whether it be surgical or nonsurgical, can be determined at this time.

If there is a high index of suspicion of an epithelial lacrimal gland tumor, then the lesion must be excised *in toto,* including the entire inner layer of the periosteum, the outer table of the roof of the orbit and, in many cases, a portion of the temporal eyelid, depending on the size of the lesion (Fig. 5C). Frozen sections of this mass will then determine initially the nature of the lesion; permanent sections will determine any possible subsequent treatment, such as exenteration, at a later date in the case of malignant epithelial tumors. Closure of the outer layer of the periosteum, which has remained intact, is then performed with a 5-0 chromic catgut suture (Fig. 5D) and the skin is closed with conventional skin closure (Fig. 5E); a drain may be inserted if necessary.

This surgical approach provides excellent exposure for lacrimal gland lesions and excellent information of the contour in spite of large areas of bone excision and the loss of the inner layer of the lateral periosteum. This author uses this technique primarily for lacrimal gland fossa masses and believes that the conventional Berke lateral orbitotomy gives better exposure for muscle cone and deeper orbital lesions that may be encountered laterally. Many surgeons, however, use the Wright orbitotomy as their universal lateral orbital approach.

SUPERIOR NASAL ORBITOTOMY

The superior nasal orbitotomy approach is ideal for lesions occurring most commonly in the superior orbit and superior nasal orbit (Fig. 6). Mucoceles of the frontal sinus, dermoids, and hemangiomas are common in the superior nasal orbit; this is also a common location of peripheral nerve tumors. Mucoceles occurring in this area must be studied closely with the use of computerized tomography to determine the integrity of the posterior wall of the frontal sinus. If erosion of the posterior wall is present, one will encounter exposed dura, and a neurosurgical colleague must be present to repair any dural defects that may be present. Other orbital lesions may erode the roof of the orbit, and preoperative evaluation of the integrity of the orbital roof or possible exposure of the anterior cranial fossa must be done so that necessary preparations can be made.

Surgical Technique

Mucoceles of the Orbit

The superior orbital rim and nasal canthal area are infiltrated with lidocaine 2% with epinephrine 1:100,000 and hyaluronidase. Methylene blue is used to outline the area of the incision (Fig. 7A). An incision down to the superior nasal orbital rim is made, in many cases initially encountering the eggshell-like, rounded-shaped mucocele that may be isolated to the frontal sinus or may have extended downward, forming a frontoethmoidal mucocele (Fig. 7B). The periosteal incision must be made along the superior rim and bridge of the nose and reflected so that proper preservation will allow replacement of the periosteum and trochlear function. The thin-walled mucocele is usually easily penetrated,

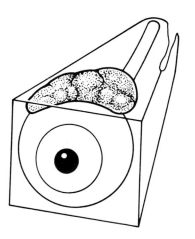

FIG. 6. Superior or superionasally located orbital lesion.

and the mucoid material present is suctioned out. After the mucoid or mucopurulent contents of the mucocele are evacuated, the thin-bone-lined lesion is then excised together with the mucous membrane in a piecemeal manner with front biting forceps. All of the floor of the mucocele is removed and the orbital rim is trimmed to a smooth contour with Rongeurs. The mucous membrane is curetted from the sinus lining (Fig. 7C). Since the formation of mucoceles is due to an obstructive sinus process, adequate drainage of the sinus must be reestablished into the intranasal cavity and communication from the frontal sinus must be made through the ethmoids into the intranasal cavity either through a surgical passage or through the nasofrontal duct itself, if it can be identified. This is done with the use of a hemostat introduced intranasally that penetrates into the mucocele cavity. The infranasal wall of the mucocele, particularly if it extends into the ethmoidal area, must be excised, and intranasal drains must be left in position for at least 2 to 3 weeks. This usually takes the form of one or two large French catheters that may be left in position either with sutures or with nasal packing (Fig. 7D). The periosteum of the orbital rim is then closed with 5-0 chromic sutures, and subcuticular 4-0 plain sutures with inverted knots are used in the dermis. The skin is then closed meticulously with interrupted 6-0 nylon sutures or a running 6-0 silk vertical mattress suture. For recurrent or bilateral muco-

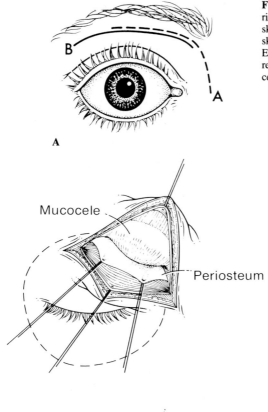

FIG. 7A. Outline of skin incisions made for the superior nasal approach to the orbit. *Dotted line A* shows skin incision for mucocele exposure. *Solid line B* shows skin incision for superior orbital tumor exposure. **B:** Exposure of the superior nasal orbit with periosteum retracted with 4-0 silk sutures showing the intact mucocele.

A

Mucocele

Periosteum

B

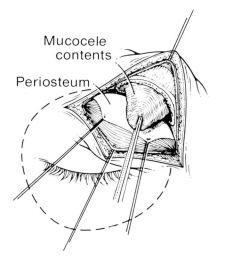

C

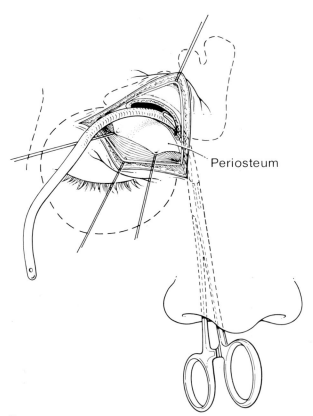

FIG. 7 (*cont.*) C: Aspiration of mucocele contents. **D:** Insertion of the intranasal drain into the frontal sinus or frontoethmoidal area after the inferior wall and mucous membrane lining have been excised.

D

celes, the osteoplastic flap operation with adipose obliteration of the sinus should be performed by a surgeon familiar with the procedure (6).

Superior Orbital Tumors

In the case of a tumor mass in the superior orbit, a similar incision is made; however, the incision may extend from the superior nasal portion of the orbit through the entire

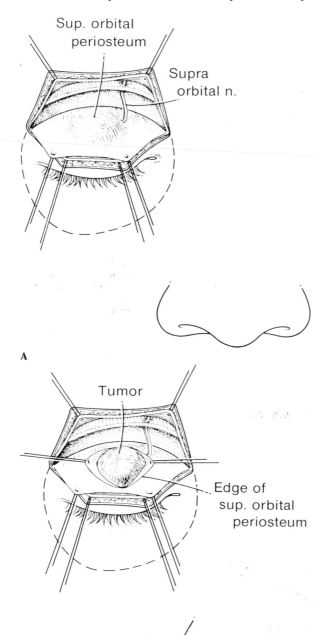

FIG. 8A. Superior orbital exposure for superior orbital tumors. Retraction of the periosteal edge with 4-0 silk sutures gives excellent exposure of the superior orbit and allows the superior orbital tumor to be approached in the extraperiosteal space. **B:** Incision of the periosteum in the superior orbit longitudinally over the area of the superior orbital tumor.

superior orbital rim inferior to the brow (see Fig. 7A). When the bony edge of the brow has been exposed, the skin edges are retracted with 4-0 silk sutures and rake retractors. When the superior orbital rim has been exposed, an incision is made through the periosteum along the superior orbital rim. Traction sutures are then placed in the edge of the orbital periosteum with 4-0 silk sutures, pulling the periosteal lid complex downward (Fig. 8A). This is a key step in exposure of the superior orbit. Small rake retractors may also be used to accomplish this downward traction that is essential for exposure. The supraorbital nerve will be encountered in penetrating the periosteum at this point, and can be preserved by nasal retraction. Dissection of the periosteum from the roof of the orbit is carried out, taking care not to fracture the orbital roof. With this surgical approach, the plan of exposure is to remain in the extraperiosteal space until the lesion can be palpated; then a longitudinal incision can be made in the periosteum, thus exposing the lesion. Confining the surgical procedure as much as possible to the extraperiosteal space is a basic principle or orbital exploration that minimizes orbital morbidity. The lesion is then extracted with blunt dissection through the periosteal incision (Fig. 8B). After removal of the lesion, the periosteal edges at the rim incision are then reapproximated with 5-0 chromic sutures and the thick dermis is reapproximated with inverted 5-0 plain subcuticular sutures; then skin sutures are placed in position. With careful dissection the procedure can be carried out with little or no sequelae.

INFERIOR ORBITOTOMY

Many lesions that occur inferiorly can be palpated easily through the inferior fornix. Lymphomas are common in this area (Fig. 9A). The lesions can best be approached directly, avoiding bone excision or additional periosteal dissection in many cases.

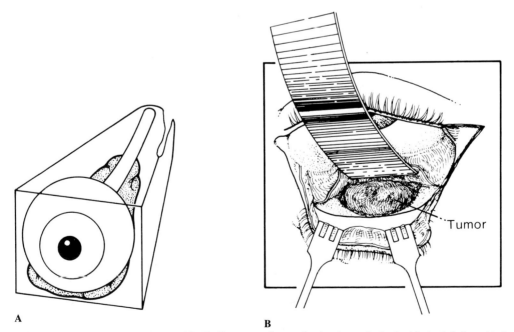

A **B**

FIG. 9A. Mass located in inferior orbit. **B:** Exposure of mass that has been obtained with the inferior orbital exposure as described in Chapter 6. This exposure consists of a lateral cantholysis and canthotomy of the lower canthal tendon, rotating the eyelid outward, followed by an incision in the lower fornix down to the inferior orbital rim. The periosteum has been reflected, exposing the inferior orbital tumor.

Surgical Technique

The best exposure for lesions lying in the inferior orbit or inferior nasal orbit is one that bypasses the eyelid proper; it involves an inferior orbitotomy through a fornix incision with a lateral cantholysis with complete severance of the lower limb of the lateral canthal tendon, thus allowing downward rotation of the eyelid. This surgical technique of exposure of the inferior orbit is described in Chapter 6. In patients with orbital inferior tumors, the periosteum may not need to be incised or elevated after inferior exposure is obtained if the lesion presents itself directly in the orbital fat. A biopsy for frozen sections can be obtained at this time. If the lesion is more extensive or posteriorly located, an incision is made in the periosteum; the inferior periosteum is elevated from the floor of the orbit and palpation is carried out posteriorly (Fig. 9B). After the nature of the lesion is diagnosed by frozen sections and excised, if indicated, closure of this exposure is then performed. This inferior fornix approach has the advantage of bypassing the lid proper and avoiding lengthy skin incisions and any possibilities of skin shrinkage, and gives better cosmesis.

BICORONAL FOREHEAD FLAP FOR ORBITAL SURGERY

The bicornal forehead flap is widely used to gain exposure for sinus surgery, neurosurgery, and craniofacial reconstruction. Although the coronal flap offers excellent exposure of the superior orbit, it has yet to gain widespread popularity among orbital surgeons. This is evidenced by the complete omission of this technique from recent "comprehensive" reviews of orbital surgery techniques (13,14).

The basic surgical technique involves a bicoronal forehead incision at or behind the hairline. The coronal flap of scalp skin and galea aponeurotica is then "turned down" and bluntly dissected to expose the superior orbital rim. This surgical technique is described in detail in Chapter 18.

The coronal flap can be dissected past the superior orbital rim. Elevation of periorbita from the superior orbit can be readily performed with excellent exposure. This approach is applicable to superior orbital and orbital apex tumors. The wide exposure is also well suited for the excision of bone and periorbita performed with resection of lacrimal gland tumors. Frontal sinus mucoceles can also be approached directly through the coronal flap exposure.

COMBINED APPROACHES

Inferior and Lateral Orbitotomy

Many large lesions can occupy both the muscle cone and the inferior nasal portion of the orbit (Fig. 10). For complete excision, more exposure must be obtained, which can be acquired by either lateral orbitotomy or inferior orbitotomy. An example of a lesion in which this exposure would be needed is a large benign lesion, such as a dermoid, which requires total excision. With this situation a Berke lateral orbitotomy combined with inferior orbitotomy with a fornix incision gives excellent exposure.

Surgical Technique

If preoperative evaluation with a CT scan demonstrates that the lesion indeed occupies these portions of the orbit, then an initial Berke lateral orbitotomy, as described in the

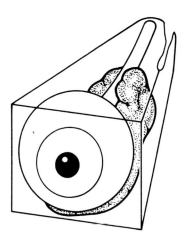

FIG. 10. A large lesion occupying the inferior and lateral orbit and extending somewhat into the nasal orbit.

first section, is carried out with removal of the bone flap and incision and retraction of the inner layer of the lateral periosteum. Palpation can then determine the lateral extent of the lesion. In many cases the bulk of the lesion can be detected with this exposure; however, in some cases one must "get around" behind the lesion for dissection, and this can be accomplished only by combining this lateral approach with the inferior orbitotomy. One then proceeds as follows. The lower limb of the lateral canthal tendon, which has already been detached from the orbital rim, is reflected outward and an incision is carried through the inferior conjunctival fornix (Fig. 11A). A further incision is then made in the lower fornix down to the periosteum of the inferior orbital rim and the periosteum is elevated, exposing the inferior and nasal orbit (Fig. 11B). With this exposure large lesions occupying the lateral, inferior, and nasal orbit can then be excised (Fig. 11C). Closure of this combined lateral and inferior approach requires first a closure of the inferior fornix conjunctiva, which also reapproximates the inferior capsulopalpebral fascia. Then the lateral periosteum is closed, reforming the inner layer of the periosteum of the lateral orbital wall. The canthal tendons of the upper and lower lid that have been detached are then reattached to the edge of the reformed inner layer of the periosteum; this restores the lateral canthal angle as described with lateral orbitotomy. The lateral orbitotomy is then closed in the manner previously described.

Medial and Lateral Orbitotomy

Lesions occurring in the nasal apex of the orbit or nasal to the optic nerve, in the deep orbit are basically unapproachable by any anterior or lateral approach (Fig. 12). With any lateral orbitotomy, one must transgress the sphenoidal fissure to approach the nerve at this level. Conjunctival incisions on the nasal portion of the orbit can allow some visualization posteriorly; however, adequate exposure for surgical purposes cannot be obtained with this nasal conjunctival incision alone. The need for wider exposure of the nasal apex occurs when an adequate biopsy or excision of optic nerve lesions, such as gliomas and meningiomas, is required. This approach may also be utilized in indicated cases for optic nerve sheath decompression. Other lesions that may nestle in the posterior orbit nasal to the nerve are peripheral nerve tumors and in some cases hemangiomas. To approach this area with adequate surgical exposure, the lateral orbitotomy is first performed, with removal

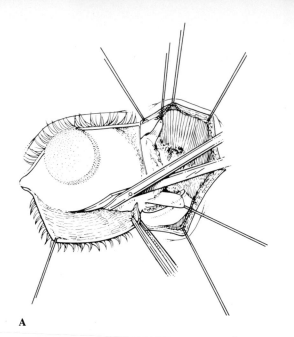

A

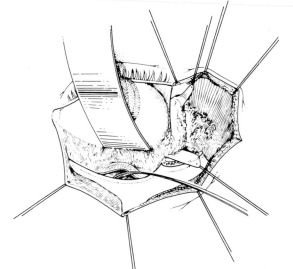

B

FIG. 11A. The combined lateral and inferior orbitotomy. The lateral orbitotomy has been performed with removal of the bone flap and retraction of the lateral periosteal edges. An incision is being made in the lower fornix down to the inferior orbital rim so that the periosteum may be elevated from the floor of the orbit. **B:** The elevation of the periosteum from the floor of the orbit and the combined lateral and inferior orbitotomy. **C:** Exposure of the large tumor that occupies the lateral inferior orbit and extends somewhat nasally into the orbit. The inferior periosteum has not yet been incised.

Outline of
large tumor

C

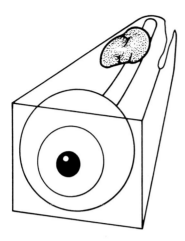

FIG. 12. A lesion located in the nasal apex of the orbit.

of a bone flap and opening of the lateral periosteum. The surgeon then performs a nasal conjunctival peritomy with relaxing incisions and detaches the medial rectus muscle so that the globe can be displaced temporally, exposing the nasal apex of the orbit (Fig. 13).

Surgical Technique

The lateral orbital area and nasal orbital area are infiltrated with lidocaine 2% with 1:100,000 epinephrine and hyaluronidase. The lateral orbitotomy (Berke) is performed first in the usual manner with excision of the bone flap, ensuring that a wide enough bone flap is excised to allow the globe to be displaced as previously described. The surgeon then moves from the lateral position of the operating table to the superior position. A

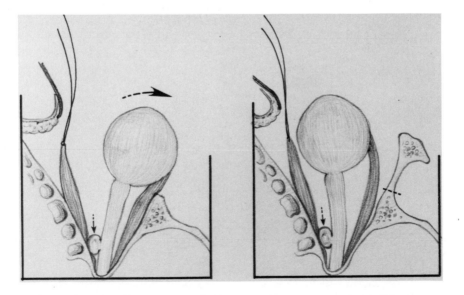

FIG. 13. Diagrammatic representation of the technique of combined lateral orbitotomy with removal of the lateral wall with medial orbitotomy. Outward rotation of the globe exposing the optic nerve and optic apex is obtained. A diagrammatic lesion nasal to the optic nerve is depicted.

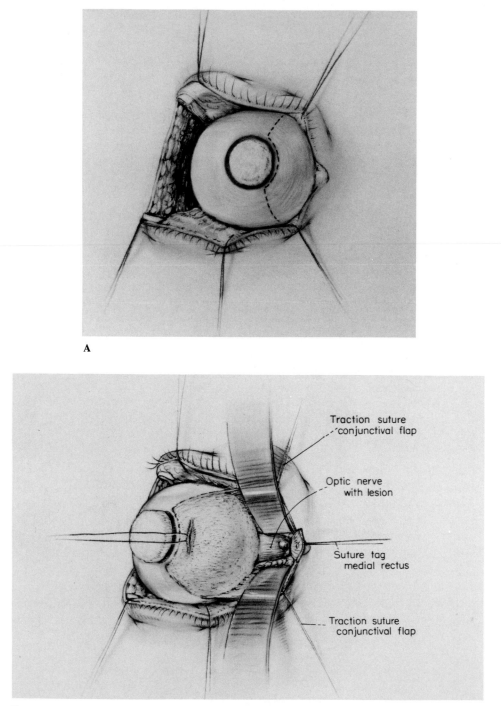

A

B

FIG. 14A. The operative field view from above the head of a patient showing the nasal conjunctival peritomy of 180° with relaxing incisions extending into the upper and lower fornices. The lateral wall to the left of the globe has been previously removed. **B:** The operative field of nasal orbitotomy viewed from above showing the exposure of the optic nerve and orbital apex after the globe has been retracted temporally, with a diagrammatic lesion of the optic nerve.

nasal limbal peritomy of 180° is performed with relaxing vertical incisions into the superior and inferior fornix (Fig. 14A). The conjunctival flap is then retracted and tagged with 6-0 silk sutures and with serrafin clamps. The medial rectus muscle is detached and tagged with a 6-0 Vicryl suture and retracted with an additional clamp. The stump of the medial rectus muscle is then lock stitched with 4-0 silk suture; the use of this traction suture allows the globe to be rotated and displaced laterally, angulating 30° to 40°, and displaced 3 to 4 cm. Exposure of the optic nerve is then obtained by the insertion of three thin malleable retractors. Two retractors are placed superiorly and inferiorly, retracting billowing orbital fat away from the optic nerve trunk. The third retractor is placed nasally in front of the medial rectus muscle. Three retractors are necessary to ensure exposure, and an extra surgical assistant may be necessary (Fig. 14B). At this point an operating microscope with a 150-mm lens can be brought into position to view the fine detail of the optic nerve or any lesions adjacent to it. Dissection and removal of a mass lesion, controlled excision of the optic nerve itself, or decompression of the nerve sheath with removal of dura can be carried out at this point. Hemostasis is obtained with bipolar cautery and cottonoid sponges. Closure of this surgical procedure is then carried out. The medial rectus muscle is reattached to its stump tendon with 6-0 Vicryl and the conjunctival flap is reapproximated to the edge of the limbus. Attention is then directed to the closure of the lateral orbitotomy, where the periosteum of the inner layer is first resutured and the canthal angle is reapproximated as described in the section on lateral orbitotomy. Again, the bone flap may be replaced or discarded as desired, and the skin is then closed.

PREOPERATIVE COMPLICATIONS OF ORBITAL SURGERY

Preoperative discontinuation of aspirin for 2 weeks and identification and treatment of clotting deficiencies will prevent excessive bleeding during surgery. No blood replacement has ever been necessary to date. Hypotensive anesthesia and head elevation are also helpful.

POSTOPERATIVE COMPLICATIONS OF ORBITAL SURGERY

Orbital Edema

Proper hemostasis during surgery and the use of postoperative steroids and diuretics will allow the surgeon to reduce any unusual postoperative orbital edema. Most pain and morbidity in the postoperative period is due to severe edema, and its prevention is emphasized. If during the course of the surgical procedure it is noted that there is an unusual amount of oozing or bleeding, it is advisable to leave a Penrose drain in position to allow drainage to occur through the wound postoperatively.

Diplopia

Excessive traction or trauma to the extraocular muscles during surgery can produce a temporary weakness or indeed a permanent paresis. However, if the trauma is minimal the paresis will resolve in a few weeks. Permanent paralysis or paresis is exceedingly rare. The muscle most commonly involved is the lateral rectus muscle.

Ptosis

Ptosis does not occur with any frequency except with the surgical excision of lacrimal gland lesions. If an aggressive excision of a lacrimal gland lesion is performed, including the lateral horn of the levator muscle, a ptosis will occur; however, this can be corrected by appropriate surgery at a later date.

Visual Loss

Visual loss is a rare complication of orbital surgery except when dealing with optic nerve lesions, which produce this inherent possibility. Traumatic manipulation of the optic nerve or its blood supply during surgery or severe postoperative edema causing an ischemic neuropathy can result in visual loss. Although extremely uncommon, this possibility does exist and the patient should be so informed.

REFERENCES

1. Berke, R. M. (1954): A modified Kronlein operation. *Arch. Ophthalmol.*, 51:6096–6132.
2. Wright, J. E. (1976): Surgery of the orbit. In: *Operative Surgery*, edited by S. Miller, 3rd ed. Butterworth and Co., London.
3. Callahan, A. (1978): Wright's lateral orbitotomy. In: *Ocular and Adnexal Tumors*, edited by F. A. Jakobiec, pp. 893–897. Aesculapius, Birmingham, Alabama.
4. Leone, C. R. (1979): Surgical approaches to the orbit. *Trans. Am. Acad. Ophthalmol.*, 86:930–940.
5. Illif, C. (1973): Mucoceles of the orbit. *Arch. Ophthalmol.*, 89:392–395.
6. Montgomery, W. W. (1979): Surgery of the frontal sinus. In: *Surgery of the Upper Respiratory System*, 2nd ed., Vol. 1, pp. 162–165. Lea & Febiger, Philadelphia.
7. Henderson, J. W. (1973): The anterior surgical approaches and lateral surgical approaches. In: *Orbital Tumors*, edited by J. W. Henderson. W. B. Saunders, Philadelphia.
8. McCord, C. D., and Moses, J. L. (1979): Exposure of the inferior orbit with fornix incision and lateral canthotomy. *Ophthalmic Surg.*, 10:59–63.
9. McCord, C. D. (1978): A combined lateral and medial orbitotomy for exposure of the optic nerve and orbital apex. *Ophthalmic Surg.*, 9:58–66.
10. Kennerdell, J. S., and Maroon, J. C. (1976): Microsurgical approach to intra-orbital tumors. *Arch. Ophthalmol.*, 94:1333–1336.
11. Koorneef, L. (1977): *Spatial Aspects of Orbital Musculo-Fibrous Tissue in Man.* Sweetz and Zeitlinger, Amsterdam.
12. Stewart, W. B., Krohel, G. B., and Wright, J. E. (1979): Lacrimal gland and fossa lesions, an approach to diagnosis and management. *Ophthalmology*, 86:886–894.
13. Nowinski, T., and Anderson, R. L. (1985): Advances in orbital surgery. *Ophthalmic Plast. Reconstr. Surg.*, 1:211–217.
14. Linberg, J. V., Orcutt, J. C., and Van Dyk, H. J. L. (1985): Orbital surgery. In: *Clinical Ophthalmology*, edited by T. D. Duane and E. A. Jaeger, Vol. 5, Chpt. 14, pp. 1–46. Harper & Row, Philadelphia.

Oculoplastic Surgery, 2nd edition, edited by
Clinton D. McCord, Jr., and Myron Tanenbaum.
Raven Press, New York © 1987.

Chapter 12

Eyelid Malpositions: Entropion, Eyelid Margin Deformity and Trichiasis, Ectropion, and Facial Nerve Palsy

*Clinton D. McCord, Jr., **Myron Tanenbaum, †Robert M. Dryden, and §Marcos T. Doxanas

*Department of Ophthalmology, Emory University School of Medicine, Atlanta, Georgia 30308;
**Bascom Palmer Eye Institute, Department of Ophthalmology, University of Miami School of
Medicine, Miami, Florida 33101; †Department of Ophthalmology, University of Arizona Medical
School, Tucson, Arizona; and §Department of Ophthalmic Plastic Surgery, Greater Baltimore Medical
Center, Baltimore, Maryland 21204*

This chapter considers together those disorders that affect the eyelid margin and lashes, and the eyelid margin position. The major sections of this chapter are: entropion, eyelid margin deformity and trichiasis, ectropion, and facial nerve palsy. The pathology and pathophysiologic mechanisms are presented so that the reader may better understand the cause, classification, and surgical treatment of these disorders. The importance of a thorough patient evaluation is stressed, because this will decide the surgical treatment modality.

ENTROPION[1]

Entropion of the eyelids is characterized by inturning of the eyelid margin [such that] the margin, the lashes, and sometimes the external skin surface turn inward, causing irritation of the eye and corneal [epithelial abrasion].

Some conditions simulate entropion, although they are not true entropion because the eyelid margin position is normal. These include:

Epiblepharon, an abnormal fold of skin occurring in young children that retracts over the lower lid, pressing the lashes inward; epicanthal folds occurring in children and orientals, which may produce the same effect as epiblepharon; aberrant lash position; and [distichiasis] and trichiasis, in which the lid margin is normally positioned [while the] lashes or extra rows of lashes are pointed inward, abrading the cornea and eye. [There may be other cases] in which the margin of the lid has been destroyed from a disease process so that it is difficult to see if the margin is actually turning in or not. It may nevertheless contain lashes, scar tissue, and epidermalized

---

[1] Extracted portions of this chapter are modified from McCord, ref. 1, with permission. © 1985 Lippincott/
Harper & Row.

tissue that abrade the cornea. [It is] important to differentiate true entropion from some of these other conditions [because the] treatment may vary . . .

Classification and Etiologies

Congenital Entropion

Congenital entropion is [very] rare and must be differentiated from epiblepharon. It may occur in the upper and lower lids, and spasm of the orbicularis muscle is a striking feature of this condition. Fox has stated that the underlying cause is hypertrophy of the pretarsal [orbicularis fibers] and a deficiency or absence of the tarsal plate. Congenital entropion may be accompanied by some epiblepharon, although the margin itself is rolled inward. It has been treated by canthotomy and full-thickness mattress sutures to maintain eversion of the lid and by excision of the thickened pretarsal orbicularis fibers.

Transient Spastic Entropion

An acute swelling of the eyelid accompanied by orbicularis spasm can cause a temporary inturning of the eyelid. It [frequently] occurs after prolonged patching and inflammation of the eye. Although some underlying laxity of the eyelid may be present, [often there is none]. Temporary spastic entropion can occur in young persons. It generally resolves as the eyelid edema goes down. . . . [The physician should be aware, however, that] this type of entropion may be an early sign of involutional entropion.

Involutional Entropion

Involutional or laxity entropion is entropion that occurs at an advancing age; in the past, it has been called *senile entropion,* although it is not equated with senility. It has also been given the misnomer of *spastic entropion* because a certain element of spasm is present, but true involutional entropion is not of a transient nature. There has been much study of the pathogenesis [and biomechanics of involutional entropion (2–6)].

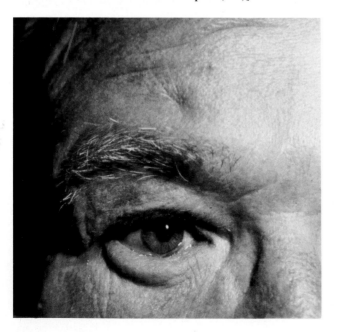

FIG. 1. Clinical picture of a patient with entropion showing inversion of the lid margin and spasm of the preseptal orbicularis fibers overriding the pretarsal fibers.

TABLE 1. *Mechanics of lower lid entropion*

1. Relaxation of inferior eyelid retractors capsulopalpebral fascia (Jones)
2. Horizontal laxity of eyelid tissue at lower tarsal border and canthus
3. Enophthalmos
4. A. Spasm and migration of preseptal orbicularis fibers upward.
   B. Outward rotation of lower tarsal border; inward rotation of lower eyelid margin

. . . Most patients with entropion will present with the eyelid margin rolled in and the orbicularis muscles in spasm, accompanied by a red, watery, scratchy eye. Occasionally a person will present with symptoms resembling entropion without the inturning. Entropion in its early stages may be intermittent, and incipient entropion can be elicited by asking the patient to squeeze the eyelids tightly and look downward; generally, this will precipitate entropion in those who have a strong tendency. When the lower eyelid margin rolls inward, the lower border of the tarsal plate swings outward. The preseptal orbicularis fibers migrate upward into the preseptal area, forming a tight band of muscle tissue on the surface of the tarsus [Fig. 1]. This outward swinging of the lower tarsal border in what by necessity causes an inward turning of the eyelid margin. The underlying anatomic defects that have been implicated in this process are horizontal lid laxity, with laxity of the tarsoligamentous sling, and laxity or disinsertion of the capsulopalpebral fascia in the lower lid. A factor that may cause an entropion rather than an ectropion in older patients with loose lids is excessively vertically mobile preseptal orbicularis fibers. In entropion patients these fibers bunch up and migrate superiorly and evert the lower border of the tarsus. Sisler and colleagues, [in a histopathology study, demonstrated] that patients with entropion usually have more hypertrophy of the orbicularis and Riolan's muscle and fewer ischemic changes than do patients with ectropion [7]. Another factor that can aggravate an entropion is enophthalmos of an acquired or constitutional nature [Table 1]. Through the years there have been many approaches to the correction of involutional entropion to correct these anatomic problems [Table 2]. Elements of all of these procedures as they affect the eyelid anatomy have been incorporated in the newer procedures [6–8].

Cicatricial Entropion

Cicatricial entropion is inward turning of the eyelid margin caused by shortening of the internal [lamella] of the eyelid, forcing the margins of the eyelid and lashes against the globe. It can occur in the upper and lower eyelids and can be caused by trauma, chemical injuries, and inflammatory processes, including . . . ocular pemphigoid and Stevens-Johnson syndrome. [Rarely seen in the United States is severe trachoma, although it is probably the most common cause of cicatricial upper lid entropion worldwide.] Usually accompanying these cicatricial pro-

TABLE 2. *Historic entropion procedures*

Anatomic correction	Procedure
1. Vertical musculocutaneous shortening	Ziegler cautery
2. Horizontal tightening of lid at lower tarsal border	Fox procedure
	Schimek suture
	Bick procedure
3. A. Barricading of orbicularis fibers	Wies procedure
	Jones procedure
B. Tightening of orbicularis fibers	Wheeler procedure
4. Repair or tightening of inferior retractors (capsulopalpebral fascia)	Jones procedure

cesses is epidermalization of the mucosal surface of the inner eyelid margin and tarsoconjunctiva, causing [chronic epithelial irritation of the cornea (8)]. The findings of scarring of the eyelid margin and internal surface combined with a clinical history . . . are . . . sufficient to make a diagnosis of cicatricial . . . entropion. Many patients who have had surgical procedures for involutional laxity entropion can re-present with a recurrent entropion that has been converted from a laxity involutional type to a cicatricial type because of the previous surgical procedures. It [is very] important to recognize this particular situation.

Marginal Entropion and Trichiasis

Marginal entropion together with trichiasis is a variant of cicatricial entropion in which the disease process has primarily affected the eyelid margin, causing destruction of marginal architecture and [inturning] of the margin with abrasion of the cornea from normal and abnormal cilia and epidermalized tissue. It can result from some of the usual causes of cicatricial entropion, but [is more commonly the] result of a chronic meibomianitis or rosacea. The treatment of marginal entropion and trichiasis is best accomplished by reconstruction of the eyelid margin with mucous membrane grafting, [combined] with excision of the diseased tissue.

Complex or Positional Entropion

In damaged eyelids a complex entropion can occur in which the entropion process is a combination of the above mechanisms. The elements of laxity or involutional entropion may be combined with those of cicatricial changes, particularly following previous surgery . . . or multiple trauma to the eyelids. The eyelid structures may be fused or the retractor fascia attached in an unusual way to cause an entropic position that may require additional procedures for correction. It is important to recognize this type of entropion [because] it may be unresponsive to the standard procedures.

Before considering surgical correction in a patient presenting with ''entropion,'' one must attempt to categorize the entropion into one of the above categories. Special attention must be given to ''problem entropion'' patients. These patients may . . . have been previously operated on and had portions of tarsus excised, or they may have combined laxity and cicatricial components. The entropion itself may be combined with trichiasis and epidermalization, and simple restoration of the eyelid margin to a normal position may not [cure] the patients' symptomatology. Patients who have coexistent severe enophthalmos may require correction of the enophthalmos before an entropion procedure can be successful. Other coexisting problems such as epiblepharon, epicanthal folds, and margin deformities following tarsorrhaphy must be [noted. Other] anatomic anomalies such as unusual adhesions between the inferior rectus muscle and the capsulopalpebral fascia and the oblique muscle following inferior orbital trauma must be detected and corrected to prevent continued abnormal traction on lower lid structures.

Nonsurgical Correction Procedure

[In the Quickert-Rathbun three-suture technique, three 4-0 silk mattress sutures are placed full thickness through the lower lid [Fig. 2], at the lower border of the tarsus or, in some cases, deeper into the fornix [9]. This procedure can be used in the office in cases of congenital entropion and involutional laxity entropion as a temporizing procedure.

Surgical Correction Procedures

Congenital Entropion

Many cases of congenital entropion are temporary, and with the use of adhesive tape or temporizing mattress sutures in the eyelid they will resolve in a period of time. Cases

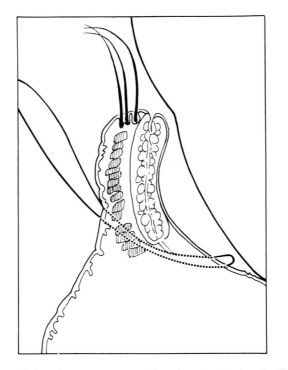

FIG. 2. The three-suture technique for temporary correction of acute entropion. **A:** Three 4-0 silk mattress sutures are introduced in a double-armed manner from the inner surface of the lid beneath the lower tarsal border and tied anteriorly. The suture may be brought out on the skin higher up and closer to the lashes for rotation. This is generally a bedside or office technique and may be used as such.

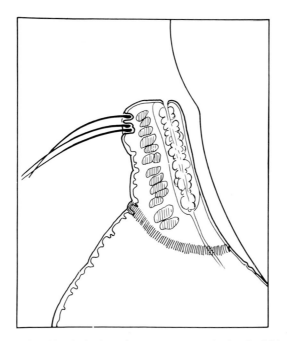

FIG. 2B. Scar produced by the horizontal mattress suture maintains the lid in correct position.

that are untreatable by temporizing procedures and have more obviously thickened orbicularis fibers can be corrected by excision of the skin fold and pretarsal orbicularis fibers in combination with a Wies procedure. Such a procedure can also be helpful in some cases of congenital epiblepharon.

Involutional Laxity Entropion of the Lower Lid

Many procedures described in the literature to correct an involutional entropion have attacked only one of the three major elements that combine to cause involutional entropion; these are horizontal laxity, stretching of the capsulopalpebral fascia (inferior retractors), and the vertical mobility of the preseptal orbicularis fibers. [Other] procedures, [however,] have been described that remedy at least two of those elements; these are procedures that have generally been most successful in terms of percentage of cure and absence of recurrence [10–12]. To date there have probably been no procedures that are 100% successful in [preventing a] recurrence.

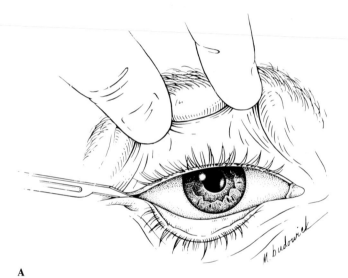

A

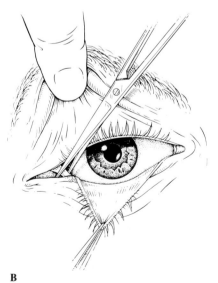

B

FIG. 3. The primary steps involved in the repair of laxity entropion and ectropion with the procedure preformed at the lateral canthus. **A:** A horizontal canthotomy is performed. (From McCord, ref. 1, with permission. © 1985, Lippincott/Harper & Row.) **B:** The tarsoligamentous sling is severed at its insertion at the lateral orbital rim, and lysis of the lateral canthal tendon is performed so that the lower lid rotates outward. (From McCord, ref. 1, with permission. © 1985, Lippincott/Harper & Row.)

. . . The following procedure is one that has stood the [test of time in the authors' experience. This technique directs] itself to the repair of two of the anatomic defects and possibly has a beneficial effect on the third. The procedure is a horizontal tightening procedure combined with plication of the preseptal orbicularis fibers and also probably some tightening of the capsulopalpebral fascia. . . . As opposed to an ectropion procedure, this entropion procedure is accomplished by tightening the tarsoligamentous sling at the lower tarsal border, and extra plication sutures are placed into the preseptal orbicularis fibers before the closure of the incision [Fig. 3].

The surgeon should observe that the extra plication sutures tense the orbicularis muscle and capsulopalpebral fascia of the lower lid.

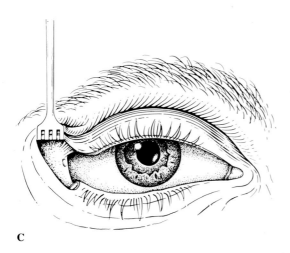

FIG. 3 (*cont.*) C: The lid rotates outward, having been detached from the lateral orbital rim. (From McCord, ref. 1, with permission. © 1985, Lippincott/Harper & Row.) **D:** The resection of the lax tarsoligamentous sling and a portion of the tarsal plate is made temporally in a wedge-shaped manner. (From McCord, ref. 1, with permission. © 1985, Lippincott/Harper & Row.)

C

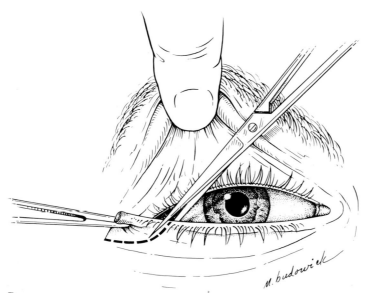

D

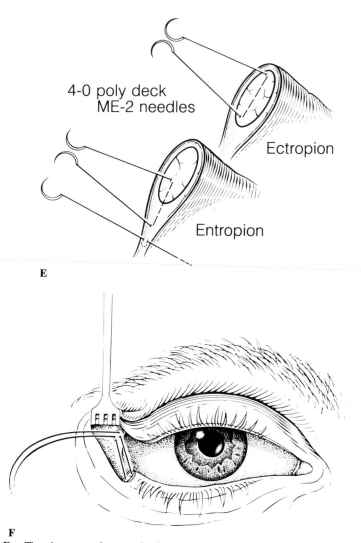

E

F

FIG. 3 (cont.) E: The placement of sutures for the entropion repair, a double-armed 4-0 nonabsorbable suture (4-0 Prolene with a semicircular needle) is used to attach the edge of the tarsal plate at its lower border and the bite in the capsulopalpebral fascia to the periosteum inside the lateral orbital rim. This double-armed suture is used in the half-circle needle and enables one to introduce the suture inside the rim of the periosteum. An additional suture is taken below the tarsal plate in the capsulopalpebral fascia to tighten it to the lateral rim, as well as to stiffen the lower border of the tarsus. The figure also shows the suture placement in the case of laxity ectropion, in which the double-armed 4-0 nonabsorbable suture is introduced into the tarsal plate higher up, so that the superior limb of the double-armed suture exits just inside the cut edge beneath the eyelid margin. (From McCord, ref. 1, with permission. © 1985, Lippincott/Harper & Row.) **F:** The two arms of this double-armed suture are then introduced into the lateral orbital rim at a horizontal level about on the plane of the midpupillary axis and then tightened, correcting the entropion. The skin is then closed. The lower edge of the skin may be somewhat redundant, and a small dog ear may be excised before closure. (From McCord, ref. 1, with permission. © 1985, Lippincott/Harper & Row.)

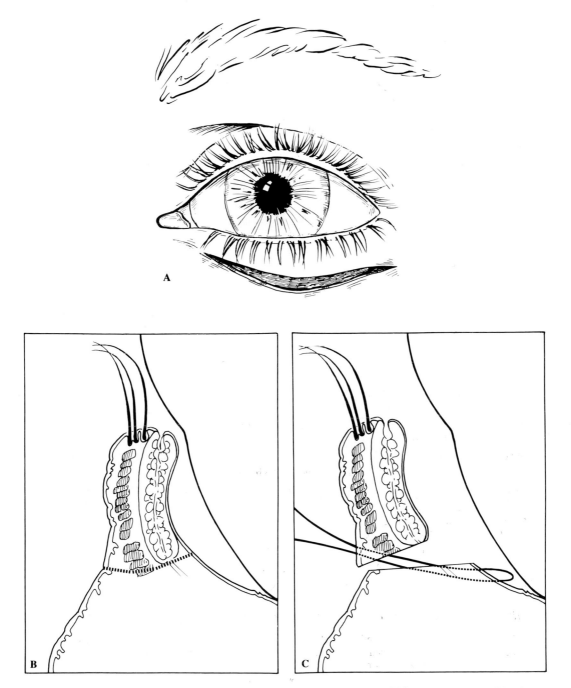

FIG. 4. Wies procedure for entropion. **A:** Front view. **B:** Side view. A full-thickness, horizontal incision is created at the base of the tarsus. **C:** Front view. **D:** Side view. An absorbable suture unites conjunctiva inferiorly to skin superiorly.

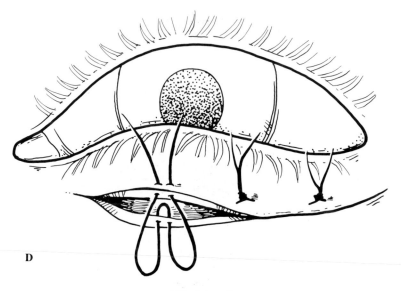

D

FIG. 4 (*cont.*)

Cicatricial Entropion

The soundest surgical principle that one can use to correct cicatricial entropion is to replace the deficient tissue in the lid with a graft in the proper anatomic area of deficiency. There are some short-cut procedures that are valuable and may be used to supplement one's armamentarium. The transverse tarsotomy, or Wies procedure (13), has been used very frequently to correct mild cases of cicatricial entropion of the lower lids. The shortcoming of this procedure is that it produces a vertical shortening of the lid, even though it does rotate the lashes satisfactorily. In very severe cases with deficient tissue, this must be replaced with a graft. Proposed sources of graft tissue have included eye bank sclera, autogenous buccal mucous membrane, nasal chondromucosa, and autogenous ear cartilage (14,15). In the upper lid, since the tarsal plate is much wider than the lower lid, a rotational procedure can be used there for milder cases. However, many cases must be corrected with grafting and commonly, in cases of margin destruction, a reconstructive procedure to the margin itself.

Mild cicatricial entropion of the lower lids (transverse tarsotomy of wies procedure)

[The authors] do not frequently use the transverse tarsotomy, but [it is presented] here for completeness [Fig. 4]. [It can be used on occasion] in combination with a horizontal tightening procedure and in some cases of mixed laxity and cicatricial entropion. It was described initially for laxity entropion but has become widely used for mild cases of cicatricial entropion.

Mild entropion of the upper lid (modified Tenzel procedure)

A procedure to rotate the upper lid margin without grafts has been described by Tenzel. [16]. It can be used in milder cases in which the tarsus is healthy. Some lid retraction can occur [Fig. 5]. It should not be used in severe cases of cicatricial entropion because in these cases it will produce a vertical shortening of the eyelid.

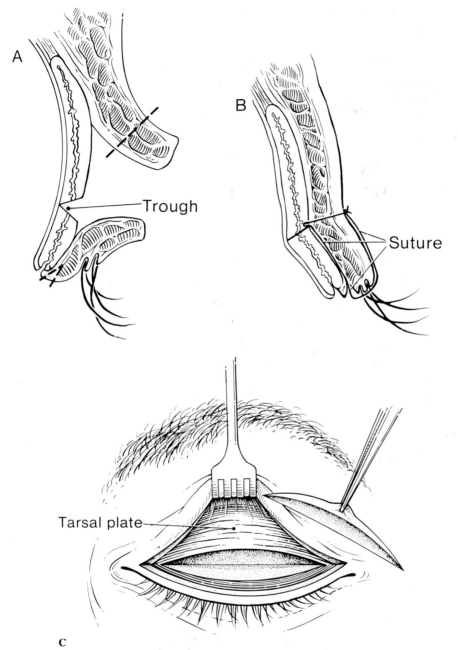

FIG. 5. Repair of cicatricial entropion of the upper lid (modified from Tenzel's procedure). **A:** A lid crease incision is made with elevation of the musculocutaneous layer from the tarsal plate. A trough or wedge is cut in the tarsal plate; try not to make a full-thickness incision. An incision is also made in the margin separating the skin and muscle from the tarsal plate in that area. Some redundant skin and muscle is excised from the upper edge of the skin incision. **B:** Sutures are placed through the musculocutaneous area and through the two cut edges of the tarsal trough and then through beneath the musculocutaneous layer to exit at the eyelid margin. The sutures from a large loop or circle, which on tying everts the skin edges and closes the superior musculocutaneous incision. Separate sutures may be placed in the musculocutaneous closure. This procedure is a tarsal rotation of the upper lid, which can be used in mild cases of cicatricial entropion of the upper lid. **C:** Anterior view of skin and tarsal incision. (From McCord, ref. 1, with permission. © 1985, Lippincott/Harper & Row.)

In severe cases, the deficient posterior lamella must be restored with tissue grafts (e.g., autogenous ear cartilage).

Severe cicatricial entropion (*replacement of the posterior lamella with graft*)

When the posterior lamella of the eyelid, the tarsoconjunctiva, and the forniceal conjunctiva [are] contracted, the only procedure that can be used successfully is lengthening of the posterior lamella by grafted material [16].

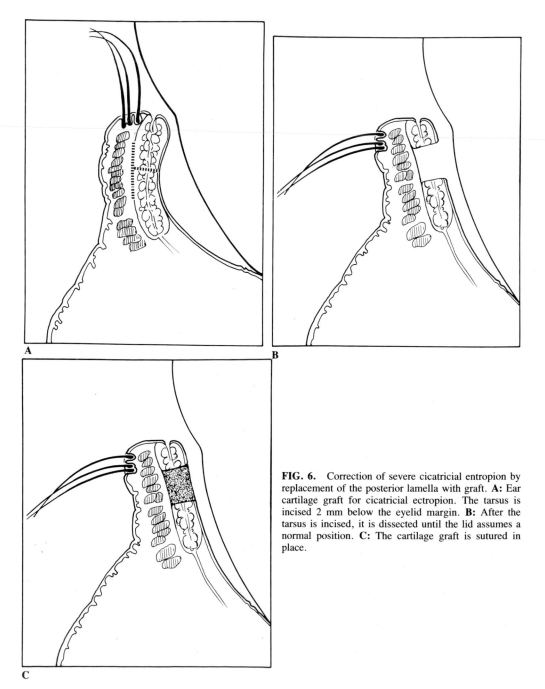

FIG. 6. Correction of severe cicatricial entropion by replacement of the posterior lamella with graft. **A:** Ear cartilage graft for cicatricial ectropion. The tarsus is incised 2 mm below the eyelid margin. **B:** After the tarsus is incised, it is dissected until the lid assumes a normal position. **C:** The cartilage graft is sutured in place.

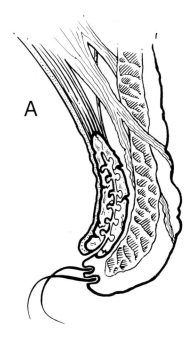

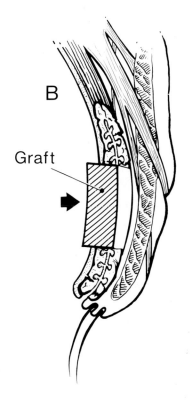

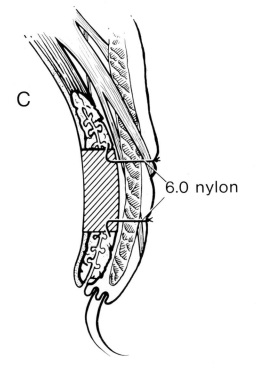

FIG. 7A. Correction of cicatricial entropion of upper lid, with loss of tarsoconjunctiva requiring replacement. Many cases of cicatricial entropion of the lids with trichiasis cannot be treated with other described procedures because of a tarsal shortage. In these cases a graft must be placed on the posterior lamella of the eyelid. The available materials are ear cartilage, naso-chondromucosa, and eyebank sclera. At present, the graft material of choice is autogenous ear cartilage. **B:** The residual tarsal plate or scar tissue is then incised with a transverse incision throughout the entire width of the lid, and the dissection is carried out, creating space in which to put the graft. **C:** The graft is then fixed in position with sutures that are brought externally through the lid and tied on the anterior surface. In the case of ear cartilage, approximately 3 to 4 weeks are required for it to gain a mucosal surface. The use of nasochondromucosa may have an advantage; the nasal septal cartilage is more difficult to work with, but it carries its own mucous membrane. Eyebank sclera can be used and will ultimately epithelialize but will contract and absorb to varying degrees. Any graft not lined with mucosa has the potential of abrading the cornea in the early postoperative period. (From McCord, ref. 1, with permission. © 1985, Lippincott/Harper & Row.)

The grafting technique used in lower lid surgery is shown in Fig. 6. It should be remembered that the average normal vertical height of the lower lid tarsus is 3.8 mm (17). Figure 7 details the upper lid surgical technique.

> . . . [We have] successfully used autogenous full-thickenss buccal mucous membrane and occasionally ear cartilage. . . . Nasochondromucosa can be used; however, because the nasal septal cartilage is very brittle and thick and the nasal mucous membrane is also very thick, there is excessive mucoid discharge. Donor eye bank sclera has been used and left bare on the internal lamella of the lid; however, it promotes an inflammatory response, and before it is reepithelialized with conjunctiva will shrink significantly. If adequate tarsal plate is a problem with cicatricial entropion in either the upper or lower lid, one may consider an eyelid reconstructive procedure. Autogenous ear cartilage may be used in certain cases with good results, and the surface will completely epithelialize in 4 to 6 weeks.

The use of steroid/antibiotic eye drops will reduce ocular irritation in the immediate postoperative period.

EYELID MARGIN DEFORMITY AND TRICHIASIS

Disorders of the margin of the eyelid arise from a variety of causes, including inflammation, trauma, and surgery, and may manifest themselves in different anatomic situations. Regardless of the etiology or the specific anatomic changes, any change in the eyelid margin has significant impact on the integrity of the cornea because of the constant movement of the eyelid margin against its surface.

Three basic processes can occur pathologically in the eyelid margin that have adverse effects on the cornea: trichiasis, margin destruction and entropion with trichiasis, and epidermalization of the margin and palpebral conjunctiva. Some patients will manifest all three of these changes, whereas in others one aspect will predominate. It is useful to try to group these patients in this manner for treatment. Insofar as possible, one must determine clinically the specific underlying problem and treat it accordingly.

Trichiasis

Trichiasis refers to the misalignment of lashes, with their direction inward against the conjunctiva and cornea. If these lashes are adjacent to the conjunctiva, a foreign body sensation occurs and conjunctival infection may result. However, if the lashes are directed against the cornea, pain, corneal epithelial irregularities, and even corneal ulceration may occur. Although it would seem that these lashes could be easily destroyed, management of trichiasis requires a systematic and persistent approach. Patients and physicians are frequently annoyed by the recalcitrant nature of this problem.

Classification and Etiology

The eitiology of trichiasis is varied. The classifications include trichiasis resulting from the following situations: (a) mechanical disruption of the eyelid margin, (b) cicatricial changes in the eyelid that produce an inversion of the lid margin (cicatricial entropion) with or without metaplastic changes of the meibomian glands, (c) congenital misdirected lashes (distichiasis or epiblepharon), (d) involutional entropion, and (e) idiopathic. This classification is effective in gaining an appreciation of the etiology of trichiasis; however, treatment considerations are based on physical features of trichiasis.

Mechanical disruption of the eyelid margin may produce trichiasis. Laceration of the eyelid margin requires careful repair. Faulty approximation of the wound edges may result in notching of the eyelid and trichiasis. Block resections of the eyelid for tumor excision or lid-shortening procedures may also produce notching and trichiasis. Even with careful anatomic reapproximation, trichiasis may result from disruption of follicles. Trichiasis may be observed following shave excision of nevi of the eyelid margin or may result from the mechanical disruption of the tumor itself. Trichiasis resulting from lacerations or surgical manipulation of the eyelid margin tends to be local in nature. Lid swelling or malposition may direct the hairs against the cornea. Multiple fine lanugo hairs may be the result of eyelid reconstructions such as the Mustarde cheek rotation. Diffuse trichiasis is more apt to be present in the latter conditions.

Cicatricial changes of the eyelids may be a manifestation of chronic inflammatory conditions, including cicatricial pemphigoid ("benign" ocular pemphigoid), erythema multiforme (Stevens-Johnson syndrome), chemical injury, trachoma, chronic blepharitis, acne rosacea, and chronic allergic reactions. These conditions have a common feature in that a chronic inflammatory infiltrate produces cicatricial changes in the eyelid. The posterior lamella of the eyelid, consisting of the tarsus and conjunctiva, is shortened, causing inversion of the eyelid margin to produce an entropion of varying degrees. In addition, the chronic inflammatory changes of the meibomian glands produce a metaplasia of the glands and fine hairs emerge from the orifices of the gland. There may be an associated irritating epidermalization of the conjunctiva. These abnormal lashes and cicatricial changes of the eyelid aggravate the inflammation of the eyelid tissues. A cycle is then created. Trichiasis persists and even worsens, causing more inflammation and scarring. Trichiasis may be the initial complaint of patients with cicatricial pemphigoid. A slit-lamp examination may reveal blunting of the cul-de-sacs and symblempharon to confirm this diagnosis.

Congenital trichiasis may be associated with distichiasis, epiblepharon, or tarsal kink. Distichiasis is an extra one or two rows of lashes. Epiblepharon consists of lashes rolled against the cornea by an infralash fold of skin. This defect frequently occurs in Orientals or is associated with epicanthal folds. Distichiasis is usually a dominant congenital anomaly. The accessory row of lashes comes from the meibomian gland openings. These accessory cilia may produce irritation.

The last two categories are involutional entropion and idiopathic. Senile, involutional entropion involves an unstable eyelid with the lashes directed against the cornea when the lid rolls inward. Trichiasis that does not have apparent etiology is termed idiopathic. Idiopathic aberrant lashes are usually localized in nature but may affect the entire eyelid margin. These patients may sometimes represent an early manifestation of cicatricial pemphigoid.

Sullivan (8) reported 72 patients with trichiasis. Numerous etiologies of trichiasis were noted (Table 3). The most common single class of trichiasis encountered was idiopathic aberrant lashes, accounting for approximately 30% of cases encountered.

Treatment

Multiple treatment modalities are employed for the management of trichiasis. Management is based upon the diagnosis, the degree, and the extent of the abnormal lash involvement. A localized area of abnormal lashes following eyelid laceration would be approached differently from a trichiasis associated with cicatricial pemphigoid. Fine lanugo hairs are more difficult to erradicate than normal-appearing cilia, so their presence should be noted. Associated ocular features characteristic of inflammation or cicatrization should be observed.

TABLE 3. *Trichiasis etiology*

	Type	Total
Idiopathic		31
Idiopathic aberrant lashes	23	
Misdirected normal lashes	8	
Inflammatory—cicatricial		27
Pemphigoid	10	
Inflammatory metaplastic	7	
Trachoma	4	
Chemical injury	3	
Erythema multiforme	3	
Mechanical traumatic and postoperative		7
Traumatic and postoperative	7	
Congenital		3
Congenital misdirected	2	
Distichiasis	1	

Adapted from Sullivan (18) with permission.

Cicatricial pemphigoid may have progressive scarring of the eyelids and mucous membranes of the eyelid. The resulting dry eye syndrome produced by obliteration of goblet cells (mucin secretion), meibomian glands (lipin secretion), and accessory lacrimal glands (Krause, Wolfring) personifies the damaging effects of trichiasis. All attempts at the correction of this condition may be futile in that approximately 30% of eyes affected with this condition become blind (19).

Surgical approaches

The surgical approach to trichiasis should be tailored to the individual and clinical situation. Management of trichiasis will vary based on its localized or generalized nature. One or several lashes may be epilated, but persistent recurrences should be treated with electrolysis. A local anesthetic agent may be used. The lash follicle is impaled with the electrolysis needle. Current is applied until bubbles exude from the follicle (Fig. 8). Approximately 15 to 20 sec of treatment is required for each lash. All the lashes in a localized area are treated. If lashes are effectively treated, they can easily be extracted from their follicle. Fine lanugo hairs respond poorly to treatment with electrolysis (18,20). It has been stated that electrolysis has a success rate of 30% to 50%. It should be noted that electrolysis does produce localized scarring of the eyelid and may accentuate entropion. Therefore, it should be used with caution because of the cicatricial and metaplastic changes it may produce.

Localized trichiasis associated with notching or scarring or involving a localized segment of the eyelid should be resected by removing a pentagonal block of the eyelid (procedure outline in Chapter 4).

Cryotherapy

If widespread trichiasis or fine lanugo hairs are present, local resection is not possible. If trichiasis is diffuse and entropion is not present, cryotherapy is usually the treatment of choice (20). It should be noted that cryotherapy of the upper eyelid may produce a total loss of lashes and may be cosmetically undesirable. Additionally, loss of pigment is to be expected. Cryotherapy has been utilized in diffuse trichiasis resulting from inflammatory or cicatricial eyelid disorders, including postsurgical problems.

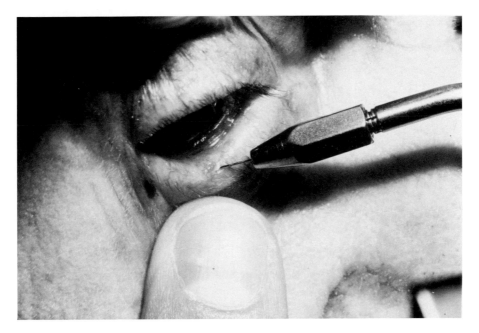

FIG. 8. Electrolysis of aberrant lashes.

Cryotherapy of the eyelid for trichiasis should begin with injection of an anesthetic containing epinephrine. The epinephrine produces a vasoconstriction that facilitates tissue freezing. Thermocouples to monitor tissue temperature are crucial to ensure adequate but not excessive freezing. Two freeze-thaw cycles to $-20°C$ are recommended for ablation of lashes. A nitrous oxide–cooled cryoprobe (Krymed) is utilized as the heat sink in the procedure. The thermocouple needle probe is placed in the skin side of the eyelid so that the monitoring point is near the follicles. An opaque scleral contact lens is inserted to protect the globe. A small amount of ophthalmic ointment is applied to the area of eyelid margin to be treated. The tip of the cryoprobe is then lightly held against the ointment. The eyelid is pulled away from the globe at the commencement of freezing with the thermocouple. Once the ice ball reaches $-20°C$, the freeze is halted. After the tissues have thawed slowly, the freeze is reapplied. Most effective results are obtained with a rapid freeze and a slow thaw (Fig. 9).

Sullivan and co-workers (21) have found that tissue temperatures to $-10°C$ are ineffective in destroying lashes. However, the authors have utilized this temperature successfully in pemphigoid. Probes utilizing carbon dioxide will not freeze the eyelid tissues to the required $-20°C$. Treatment failures are most likely attributed to inadequate tissue freezing. Correct freezing technique significantly reduces recurrences and postoperative complications. Success has been reported at 70% with one freeze-thaw cycle and 90% with a double freeze-thaw cycle. Localized or occasional lashes could be easily treated with electrolysis following cryotherapy (20). If treatment is administered by applying the freezing probe to the anterior surface of the eyelid, the globe should be protected by placing a plastic plate between the lid and the globe. Corneal perforation has occurred from inadvertent corneal freezing.

Cryotherapy is usually tolerated by the eyelid, but the procedure is not innocuous. Eyelid structures have varying sensitivities to cryogens. As previously stated, the hair follicle is

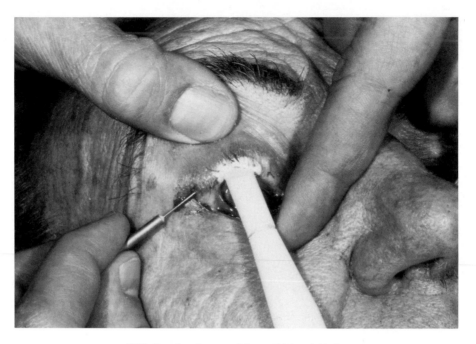

FIG. 9.   Cryotherapy of the eyelid for trichiasis.

destroyed at temperatures of −20°C. Fortunately, the tarsus and lacrimal outflow system are relatively resistent to freezing and require tissue temperatures of −40° to −70°C (21,22) before destruction occurs. Because of this discrepancy in sensitivity to cryotherapy, the eyelid usually displays little sequelae of treatment. Cicatricial changes of the eyelids, particularly in pemphigoid, may be aggravated by cryotherapy, thus causing significant progression of damage to the lids and the eye. Therefore, we are very reluctant to freeze pemphigoid lids unless it is absolutely necessary because of lack of a better procedure. In these cases, repeated treatments at −10°C are safer than those at −20°C in our experience.

Complications are minimized by correct freezing techniques. The thermocouple plays an essential role in the surgical technique. Monitoring of tissue temperatures ensures a correctly applied freeze to maximize the destruction of lashes and minimize the damage to the eyelid. Double freeze-thaw cycles may produce considerable postoperative pain and edema. Dermal melanocytes are sensitive to temperatures ranging from −15° to −20°C. A localized area of depigmentation results from treatment and may persist. Cryotherapy should therefore be used with reservation in darkly pigmented individuals. Eyelid sloughing has been reported following therapy. Such loss is more likely to occur in patients with neuroparalytic eyelids (20). However, most individuals do have some thinning and alteration of eyelid thickness with the use of cryotherapy.

> . . . Patients who have borderline tear film are noted to be more symptomatic following freezing than before freezing, even though the lashes are ablated; hence, it is implied that freezing of the tarsal glands reduces the integrity of the precorneal tear film. [I]n many cases patients with ocular pemphigoid seem to have an exacerbation of their disease following cryopexy, presumably due to inciting of the autoimmune reaction. In general, the patients who will benefit from cryopexy to the lid margins are [caucasian] patients with normal tear function and localized

trichiasis who are not cosmetically oriented and whose tissue will not shrink. They should not have ocular pemphigoid or reduction of any tear film components.

Trichiasis with Margin Deformity and Marginal Entropion

Increasing degrees of damage to the eyelid margin from inflammatory causes such as Stevens-Johnson syndrome, burns, or postsurgical or traumatic etiologies will not only cause aberrant lash formation and scarring but loss of the architecture of the edge of the eyelid. This margin destruction, when combined with trichiasis, may not respond to cryopexy alone, and reconstruction procedures must be employed to restore the integrity of the eyelid margin.

The technique of tarsal advancement with recession of the lash line and buccal mucous membrane grafting has been used quite successfully over the years (14,16,23,24). A modification of the classic procedure is presented here (Fig. 10). This technique does presume that there is adequate tarsus present to advance. If one is faced with a patient with damaged tarsus to the point that the lid is unstable, then one must employ an eyelid reconstruction procedure to correct the problem.

Epidermalization of the Eyelid Margin

Some patients will manifest scarring and metaplasia of the eyelid margin following traumatic and inflammatory changes that do not produce either abnormal hairs or destruction of margin architecture. These patients will have a metaplasia of the posterior lid margin and palpebral conjunctiva, which produces a roughened surface and will abrade the cornea and produce punctate keratitis and vascularization in the absence of trichiasis (25). This

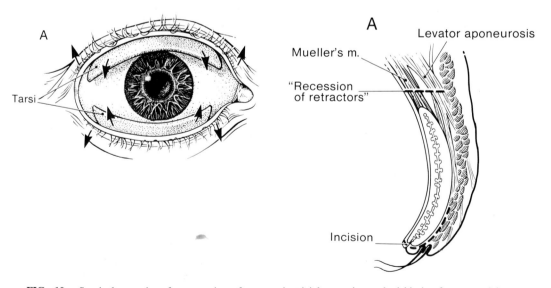

FIG. 10. Surgical procedure for correction of severe cicatricial entropion and trichiasis of upper and lower lids. **A: (Left)** Incisions are made through the eyelid margin, and the tarsoconjunctiva is advanced in the upper and lower lid. It is important to make relaxing incisions at the ends of the tarsoconjunctiva so that the tarsal plate will slide forward. **(Right)** Cross-sectional view showing the initial incision through the entropic lid margin. (From McCord, ref. 1, with permission. © 1985, Lippincott/Harper & Row.)

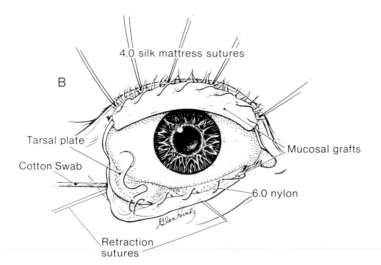

B

4.0 silk mattress sutures

Tarsal plate

Cotton Swab

Mucosal grafts

6.0 nylon

Retraction
sutures

B

4.0 silk mattress
suture

FIG. 10B. **(Top)** Full-thickness buccal mucous membrane graft is sutured to the raw surface of the advanced edge of the tarsoconjunctiva. A 6-0 nylon suture is then introduced from the skin surface and brought in a continuous running manner to close the graft on the anterior and posterior incision. **(Bottom)** Cross-sectional view of the advanced tarsoconjunctival layer. (From McCord, ref. 1, with permission. © 1985, Lippincott/ Harper & Row.)

epidermalization can also manifest itself together with trichiasis and margin destruction in many cases.

The treatment of isolated epidermalization of the margin has been very gratifying. It consists of a technique of abrasion of the margin of the eyelid, with removal of the scar tissue and metaplastic epithelium, and overgrafting of the abraded area with a full-thickness buccal mucous membrane graft (26). This can be used on the margin itself, or can be used for larger areas that include the margin and palpebral conjunctiva. The ability to graft on an intact tarsus is far superior to the excisional methods of repair and those that damage the tarsus or cause it to lose its integrity in some manner, thereby decreasing the

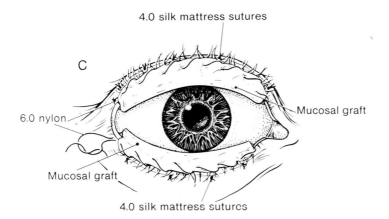

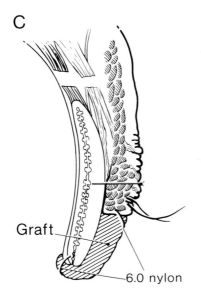

FIG. 10C. (Top) Having been completely sutured around, the graft is then brought back out through the skin in order that it can be tied externally so that the ends of the stitches will not rub against the cornea. It is important to close the eyelid with intermarginal sutures during this period for the graft to take. **(Bottom)** Cross-sectional view of the eyelid showing suturing of the mucous membrane graft into position after the tarsoconjunctival flap has been advanced, following incision through Müller's muscle and the levator aponeurosis.

stability of the eyelid. Figure 11 shows the everted lid of a patient with Stevens-Johnson syndrome with epidermalization of the posterior edge of the eyelid causing cornea vascularization, although very few trichiatic hairs are present.

Surgical Technique of Dermabrasion and Overgrafting of the Eyelid Margin

A full-thickness buccal mucous membrane graft is harvested in the usual manner, as described in Chapter 1 (split-thickness grafts have been found to be inadequate to resurface the margin and palpebral conjunctiva). One must measure the width of the eyelid and the area to be covered before harvesting the graft. One should remember that, after excision of a full-thickness buccal mucous membrane graft from the lip, the graft will contract to a much smaller size and stretching must be used for it to fit the intended recipient site.

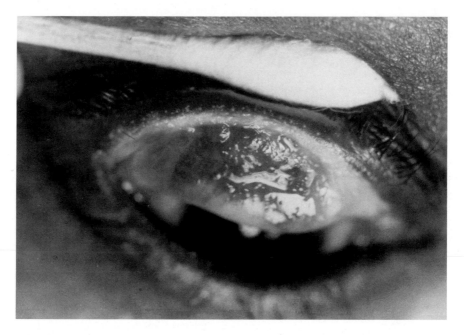

FIG. 11. Patient with Stevens-Johnson syndrome. On lid eversion, the epidermalized, keratinized eyelid margin and tarsoconjunctiva, which abrade the cornea, are visible. There may be a few cilia but mainly there is roughened epithelium. (From McCord, ref. 1, with permission. © 1985, Lippincott/Harper & Row.)

After infiltration of the eyelid with lidocaine (red-label Xylocaine®), the eyelid is everted with traction sutures over a cotton-tipped swab and tensed (Fig. 12A). A 3-mm diamond burr on a microrotary osteotome is used to abrade the entire edge of the eyelid and the palpebral conjuctiva that is epidermalized and scarred. If good vasoconstriction has been obtained, there will be very little oozing in some cases (Fig. 12B). The buccal mucous membrane graft is tailored to fit the defect and the graft is then positioned with a 6-0 nylon running suture. The suture is introduced from the cutaneous surface and sewn in a continuous running manner around the entire graft, and is tied on the external surface of the lid (Fig. 12C).

The lid is then sutured together in a slightly everted position with intramarginal sutures for 1 week (Figs. 12D and 12E). It has been found that almost 100% take of the graft occurs if this eyelid splinting is performed. This graft may take without intramarginal sutures, but in many cases a good bit of shrinkage will occur. Grafts may still have a bluish tinge at the end of 1 week, but generally will "pink up" over the next week.

Improvement noted in patients is largely due to the mechanical effect of the smooth eyelid margin on the cornea. Other possibilities are restoration of the goblet cells or increased corneal oxygenation from healthy mucous membrane opposed to the cornea.

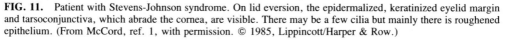

FIG. 12. Technique of tarsal polishing and mucous membrane grafting. **A:** Upper or lower lid is everted and held under tension. **B:** A rotary polishing tip is used to abrade the tarsal conjunctiva. **C:** The graft is sutured in place with the knot exteriorized. (From McCord and Chen, ref. 26, with permission of SLACK Incorporated, Thorofare, New Jersey.)

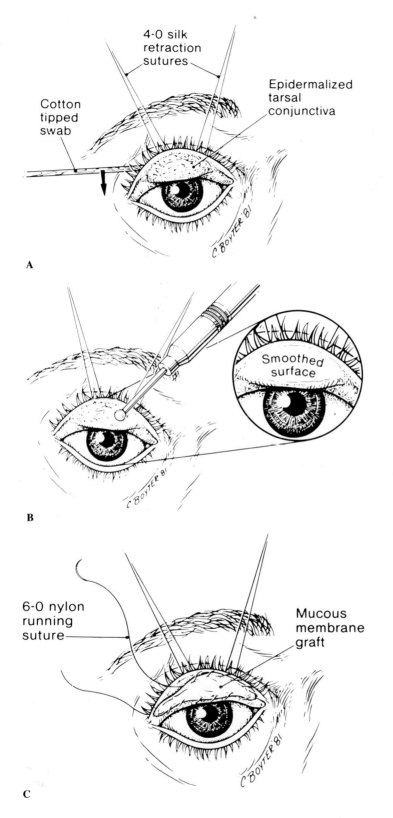

A

B

C

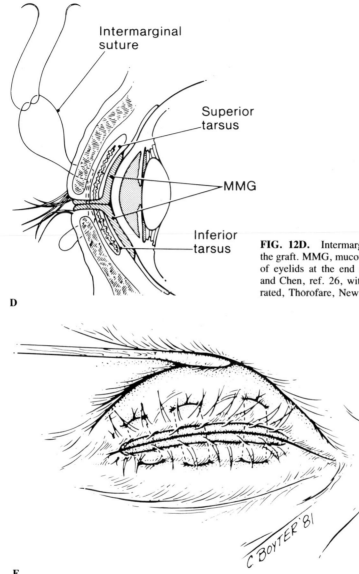

Intermarginal
suture

Superior
tarsus

MMG

Inferior
tarsus

FIG. 12D. Intermarginal sutures are placed to splint the graft. MMG, mucous membrane graft. **E:** Appearance of eyelids at the end of the procedure. (From McCord and Chen, ref. 26, with permission of SLACK Incorporated, Thorofare, New Jersey.)

D

E

ECTROPION

Ectropion of the eyelid is characterized by an outturning of the margin of the eyelid away from the globe and usually a separation of the eyelid from the globe. It can occur as a result of a variety of mechanical forces: laxity of the tarsoligamentous sling, mechanical changes in the tarsus itself, shortening of the musculocutaneous layer of the lid with an outward rotation, and loss of tone of the orbicularis portion of the lid from denervation.

Classifying the types of ectropion is important to assign a specific anatomic cause, which allows a specific anatomic correction of the malposition. The classification of ectropion that has proved to be the most convenient is that of (a) laxity or involutional ectropion,

TABLE 4. *Stages of laxity in involutional ectropion*

Laxity of the ligamentous sling
Usually medially first
Medial ectropion punctal eversion
Tearing
Generalized ectropion
Conjunctival hypertrophy–keratinization

(b) medial ectropion (a subvariant of laxity ectropion), (c) tarsal ectropion, (d) cicatricial ectropion, (e) paralytic ectropion, (f) congenital ectropion, and (g) complex ectropion.

Laxity or Involutional Ectropion

Involutional ectropion [sometimes known] as *senile* ectropion, . . . is caused by laxity of the tarsoligamentous sling. The onset may be gradual, and the laxity may . . . initially [result in] a slight sagging of the lid that can progress to actual eversion of the lid; in most cases this first [begins] medially and [is] subcategorized as *medial ectropion*. As the medial ectropion progresses, there tends to be punctal [eversion. The] tear film cannot enter the punctum [and patients] with adequate tears are intensely symptomatic from epiphora. Patients who have deficient tears do not complain of epiphora but have exposure symptoms, and the exposed conjunctival surface of the lid margin becomes epidermalized, . . . and the punctum itself may be atretic. As the condition progresses further, the lid turns outward more . . . and there is a generalized thickening of the eyelid margin with conjunctival hypertrophy.

Table 4 presents the commonly seen stages in the anatomic progression of laxity in involutional ectropion. As the ectropion progresses, the conjunctiva becomes chronically exposed, producing prominent inflammatory changes within the eyelid tissues. The patient may complain of a red, irritated eye. Inflammatory changes of the eyelid and chronic exposure produce metaplastic changes of the goblet cell, which contains stratified squamous epithelium of the conjunctiva, and keratinization results. The keratinized conjunctiva produces considerable irritation to the globe. If the eyelids are unable to close adequately, the globe exposure produces corneal punctate epithelial breakdown and even corneal ulceration and perforation.

Medial Ectropion

. . . In the early stages of laxity ectropion, the condition may be in a large part helped by a localized medial ectropion procedure [(27). One method of correcting medial ectropion is] the Byron Smith "lazy T" [procedure (Fig. 13) (28)]. There are numerous other procedures for medial ectropion, . . . but generally speaking . . . if there are many procedures for one condition it means that all of them work some of the time and none of them all of the time. Severe cases of medial ectropion cannot be corrected by the "lazy T" procedure, and a more difficult procedure that includes resection of a portion of the canaliculus, reattachment of the medial lid to the posterior reflection of the tendon, and intubation of the lacrimal drainage apparatus can be performed [29].

This technique of lower eyelid and canalicular resection with intubation is described in Chapter 4.

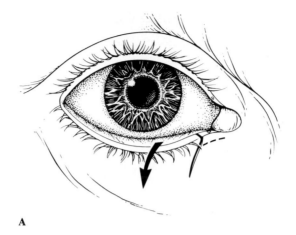

A

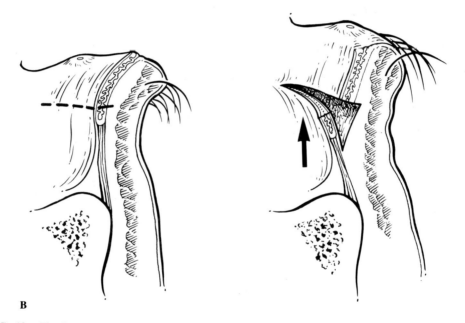

B

FIG. 13. The Byron Smith ''Lazy T'' correction of medial ectropion. **A:** The ''Lazy T'' name is derived from the fact that when the final lid sutures are placed in position they take the configuration of a ''T'' lying on its side. Initially a vertical full-thickness incision is made 2 mm temporal to the punctum of the lower lid in the tarsal plate, followed by an incision horizontally in the posterior lamella. **B:** The medial portion of the bisected lid.

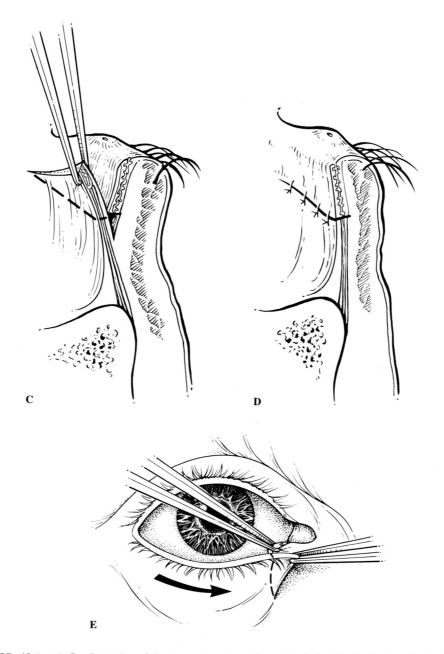

C

D

E

FIG. 13 (cont.) C: Retraction of the tarsoconjunctiva and capsulopalpebral fascia. **D:** Capsulopalpebral fascia and edge of tarsus are resected. **E:** Closure inside the lid with 6-0 Vicryl sutures. **F:** Horizontal tightening: a full-thickness section of eyelid is resected after overlapping the edges to determine the proper tension.

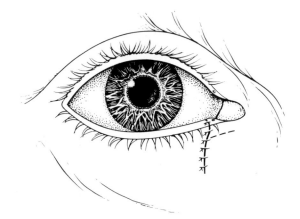

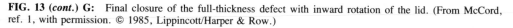

FIG. 13 (*cont.*) G: Final closure of the full-thickness defect with inward rotation of the lid. (From McCord, ref. 1, with permission. © 1985, Lippincott/Harper & Row.)

In cases of laxity ectropion that are more generalized and not localized to the medial canthal area, a horizontal tightening procedure can be performed.

. . . [It is] recognized that in patients with ectropion, the tarsal plate is normal and it is the ligamentous sling at the canthal angles that is abnormal; hence, one should avoid excising healthy tarsal plate whenever possible. Horizontal tightening performed at the lateral canthal angle has become the procedure of choice and has many variations (Fig. 14) [30,31]. Tightening the lid at the lateral canthal tendon will reposition the eyelid margin and, in many cases . . . with medial ectropion, restore the punctum to a reasonably normal position. With [tightening] of the lid, however, the punctum can be displaced temporally. The horizontal tightening for

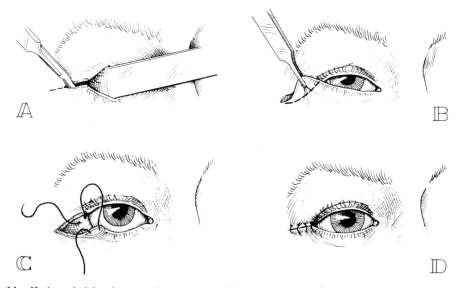

FIG. 14. Horizontal tightening procedure to correct laxity ectropion. **A:** A lateral canthotomy is performed down to the orbital rim periosteum. Malleable retractors are used to protect the eye. The attachments of the inferior crus of the lateral canthal tendon are severed from the orbital rim. **B:** The lower lid is stretched tight to determine the amount of lateral lid to be resected. A 4-0 Prolene vertical mattress suture through tarsus should reattach the lower lid slightly inside orbital rim. **D:** Final closure of musculocutaneous layer with interrupted 6-0 nylon sutures. (From Wesley and Collins, ref. 31, with permission.)

ectropion is performed in a manner similar to the horizontal tightening procedure for [entropion]; however, the placement of the suture that reattaches the tarsus to the orbital rim is different [30]. Tightening of the margin of the eyelid [or superior] tarsal border is important in ectropion [(see Fig. 3E). A more efficient] tightening can be [achieved by] resection of the lid at the lateral canthal tendon and reattachment [to] the periosteum [of] the lateral orbital rim than can be obtained in the mid lid resections. Much less tissue needs to be excised from the lid proper and, in many cases, very little from the tarsus in order to obtain a very dramatic tightening effect. Frequently the lower lid laxity is so severe that a medial ectropion procedure must be combined with the lateral canthal tightening in order to reposition the lid in a more normal position. When combining [a] medial ectropion procedure with the lateral canthal tightening, it

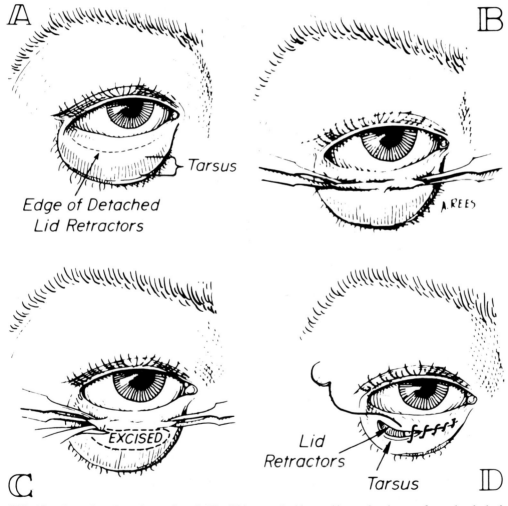

FIG. 15. Correction of tarsal ectropion. **A:** The lid is everted with stretching or detachment of capsulopalpebral fascia to the lower tarsal border. **B:** Bunching the conjunctiva on the inner surface of the lid, judging the amount to be resected. **C:** Incision of conjunctiva beneath the tarsal border, with excision of a segment of conjunctiva and capsulopalpebral fascia. **D:** Closure of the capsulopalpebral fascia, conjunctiva, and lower tarsal border with a continuous suture. (From Wesley, ref. 33, with permission. © 1985, Lippincott/Harper & Row.)

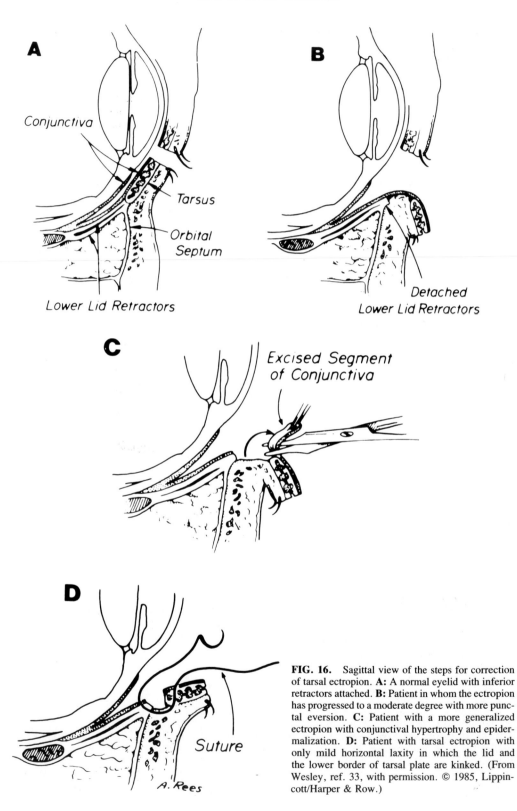

FIG. 16. Sagittal view of the steps for correction of tarsal ectropion. **A:** A normal eyelid with inferior retractors attached. **B:** Patient in whom the ectropion has progressed to a moderate degree with more punctal eversion. **C:** Patient with a more generalized ectropion with conjunctival hypertrophy and epidermalization. **D:** Patient with tarsal ectropion with only mild horizontal laxity in which the lid and the lower border of tarsal plate are kinked. (From Wesley, ref. 33, with permission. © 1985, Lippincott/Harper & Row.)

is best to complete the medial portion of the operation before tightening the lateral canthus so as to not place the medial canthus under [excessive] tension.

Tarsal Ectropion

The term *tarsal ectropion* was originally used . . . to describe an unusual form of ectropion that is not due entirely to horizontal laxity of the tarsoligamentous sling [32]. In these patients the lid is completely everted, with the lower border of the tarsus at the lower limbal margin. . . . There may be some horizontal laxity present. . . . [T]his type of ectropion [has been attributed to dehiscence] or stretching of the capsulopalpebral fascia at the inferior tarsal border in combination with horizontal laxity [32–35]. In some of these patients the laxity may not be striking. Tarsal ectropion may occur in younger people. [Some authors] have advocated a repair of the [lower lid] retractors from an internal approach [33,34]. This repair corrects the lower tarsal eversion; however, it is also recommended that a horizontal tightening procedure be combined with it for correction of the [lid laxity (Figs. 15 and 16)].

Cicatricial Ectropion

Cicatricial ectropion is caused by a shortening of the lid skin or shortening of both skin and muscle as a result of burns, irradiation, inflammatory conditions, or, in many cases, skin removal following blepharoplasty, xanthelasma removal, or skin cancer excision.

Morpheaform basal cell carcinomas may actually present as a cicatricial ectropion in patients with no prior history of eyelid surgery (Fig. 17).

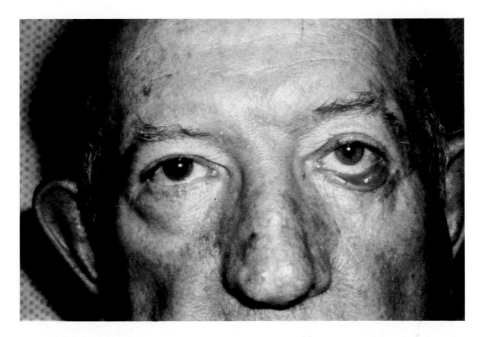

FIG. 17. Clinical photograph of a patient demonstrating a ''spontaneous'' cicatrial ectropion secondary to a morpheaform basal cell carcinoma.

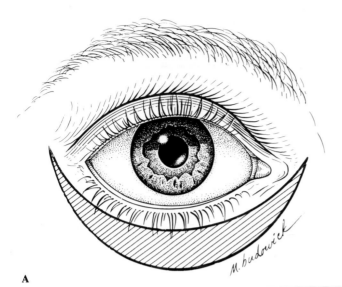

A

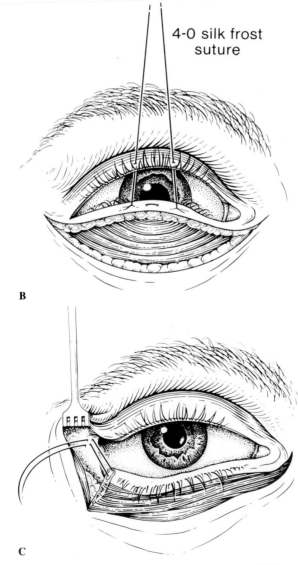

4-0 silk frost
suture

B

C

FIG. 18. Repair of cicatricial ectropion of the lower lid with full-thickness skin graft. **A:** Incision made in the lower lid with skin retraction for placement of a full-thickness skin graft. The incision may be localized if the cicatricial ectropion is localized. If the ectropion is near the canthal angle, the incision must be carried superior to the canthal angles because the graft will straddle the canthal angle. This is because, when contracture occurs, the pull of the graft will be upward, correcting the ectropion, instead of downward, causing recurrence. The incision to create the defect must be placed high as possible under the lashline. **B:** The defect created in the lower skin edge is undermined, allowing the lid to be elevated into position with retraction. **C:** The horizontal tightening procedure should be performed in most cases. Many times simple replacement of skin will not restore the lid to a normal position. A canthotomy and full resection is carried out as described with entropion/ectropion procedures.

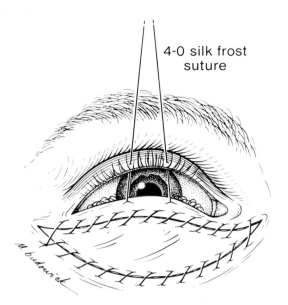

4-0 silk frost suture

FIG. 18 (*cont.*) D: The graft sutured in position. Traction must be placed on the graft with intermarginal sutures or Frost sutures for 1 week so that the graft will heal in the maximally expanded defect.

In most cases the ectropion is caused by the shortage of the skin layer, which must be replaced in order to correct the deformity. [36–39]. [I]n older patients and many times in younger patients, . . . skin [grafting] must be combined with [a] horizontal tightening procedure. Even with skin replacement the antagonizing effect of scarring cannot be completely eliminated, and a borderline laxity of the ligamentous sling may prevent the lid from being [properly repositioned]. The proper steps for application of the skin graft are seen in Fig. 18.

Paralytic Ectropion

Paralytic ectropion is a type of laxity ectropion that results from the denervation of protractor muscles . . . due to a seventh nerve . . . palsy. In many cases it can be aggravated by laxity of the tarsoligamentous sling, a condition that can be striking in older persons but is uncommon in younger people, in whom innervation to the [orbicularis fibers] can often be lost without causing ectropion if there is adequate elasticity of the sling. The treatment of seventh nerve palsy will be [discussed] in another section of this chapter.

Complex Ectropion

Following severe eyelid lacerations, multiple incisions in the eyelid from repeated surgery, or other unusual situations, the anatomic components of the eyelid may be rearranged and many of the elements fused together so that ectropion cannot be blamed entirely on skin muscle shortage, horizontal laxity, or other simple components.

Scarring of the orbital septum and capsulopalpebra fascia is often an important factor in the pathogenesis of complex cicatricial ectropion. These complex cases of ectropion

can be seen following multiple procedures for orbital fractures and certain congenital situations. In many cases, the lower lid malposition can be corrected only with staged procedures of grafting of the external and internal lamella and many times separation of fibrous adhesions from the orbital rim, if they exist.

Congenital Ectropion

Congenital ectropion is a rare condition with multiple causes in which [there] may [be] underlying developmental anomalies. It may be of a temporary nature, or it may require surgical correction [38–40].

FACIAL NERVE PALSY

Facial nerve palsy has many ocular manifestations. There may be merely a cosmetic blemish due to the lack of facial tone on the involved side. In more severe cases, ectropion may manifest itself and the cornea may become involved. Patients with extensive facial nerve paralysis may have intermittent or continuous bouts of exposure keratitis and even progress to corneal ulceration and perforation of the globe. These patients require the attention of the ophthalmologist to manage the ocular sequelae and prevent serious complications.

Etiology

Seventh nerve paralysis may result from injury, tumors, or inflammatory conditions. Facial nerve paralysis from tumors, surgery, or trauma is usually a severe, total paralysis. Functional return is not expected in these patients. Facial nerve paralysis due to parotid tumors is a reflection of the aggressive behavior of the tumor. Eneroth (41) reported 46 patients with facial nerve paralysis due to parotid tumors. All 46 patients died, regardless of the modality of therapy the patient received.

The facial nerve is in close apposition to the auditory nerve. Surgical resection of acoustic neuromas may produce a facial paralysis postoperatively. This paralysis will remain stable with time. Surgical intervention to alleviate exposure keratopathy may be required early in the course of this form of facial paralysis.

Understanding of the anatomy and the course of the facial nerve aids in the comprehension of the signs and symptoms that may occur. The facial nucleus is in the pons. The genu of the facial nerve arches over the abducens nucleus and exits the brainstem. The nerve passes the cerebellopontine angle and enters the internal auditory meatus and a rigid bony canal. This is the longest bony canal in the body. The facial nerve has four anatomic portions prior to exiting from the stylomastoid foramen: the meatal, labyrinthine, tympanic, and mastoid. Involvement of each of these segments will produce specific features. Prior to discussing the specific manifestations of involvement of these areas, it should be noted that the more proximal the involvement of the facial nerve in Bell's palsy, the more profound and permanent the sequelae of involvement. Involvement of taste and salivary flow reflects compression of the mastoid segment. Diminished tear production and disturbances of balance and hearing are associated with involvement of the proximal portion of the fallopian canal, the labyrinthine segment. A diminished stapes reflex is associated with involvement of the tympanic segment.

The recognition of the sites of involvement and electromyographic analysis allow identification of the location of the compression of the facial nerve. If the facial nerve function is markedly diminished and if the tear and/or salivary secretion is reduced, the facial nerve should be explored to prevent irreversible damage (42,43).

Lesions affecting the facial nerve may be central and include other cranial nerves and may occur as a nuclear or intrapontine lesion. Lesions between the pons and the internal auditory meatus (cerebellar pontine angle lesions) are frequently caused by acoustic neuroma, meningioma, basal meningitis, and meningocarcinomatosis. Lower motor neuron damage occurring in the intracanalicular portion of the nerve and causing paralysis of the facial nerve can result from otitis media and chronic mastoiditis, cholesteatoma, middle ear surgery, hemorrhage of the facial nerve, and inflammatory processes such as Guillain-Barré, sarcoidosis, mumps, porphyria, and idiopathic facial palsy (Bell's palsy). As the nerve exists from the stylomastoid foramen, paralysis can be caused by trauma of various kinds, including surgical involvement with tumors, parotid tumors, and neuritis. With one exception, peripheral branches of the facial nerve, if damaged, usually do not cause paralysis because of numerous interconnections; the exception is the temporal branch of the facial nerve to the frontalis muscle, which is vulnerable because of its length.

The etiology of Bell's palsy, or idiopathic facial paralysis, remains obscure. Viral, inflammatory, and immune factors have been implicated as offenders in this disorder. An aggressive approach to Bell's palsy, which has been recently recommended, is to recognize and treat patients with poor prognostic indicators for functional return. Early identification of patients who are likely to proceed to irreversible facial paralysis can be recognized based on clinical features (42,43).

Approximately 70% to 80% of patients with Bell's palsy have a complete or satisfactory return of function (42). Patients who have an incomplete facial paralysis are most likely to have a complete return of function. Approximately 50% of patients who have a complete paralysis at the onset of affliction will have a satisfactory return of function. If the paralysis is incomplete at the time of onset, but progresses to complete, approximately 25% of patients will have a satisfactory return of function (42).

Patients with other neurologic symptoms such as chronic headaches or diminished hearing, or an atypical clinical course, should be evaluated for a structural lesion with a CT scan of the head. The physician must direct special attention to the base of the skull and cerebellopontine angle when requesting the CT scan.

Manifestations of Facial Nerve Paralysis

Facial nerve paralysis produces numerous ocular manifestations (44). The facial nerve supplies the orbicularis oculi muscles, and the loss of tone of this muscle produces a decreased blinking ability. If an increased horizontal laxity of the eyelid exists, ectropion will probably result with the paralysis. If the lid tone is good, ectropion will not result.

Faulty eyelid closure due to orbicularis oculi involvement will produce varying degrees of exposure conjunctivitis and keratitis. In its mildest form, the exposure will be well tolerated. However, depending on the degree of lagophthalmos and underlying integrity of the corneal tear film, varying degrees of corneal breakdown will result. Inferior punctate epithelial staining may progress to corneal ulceration. Clinical and surgical treatments should minimize or control progressive corneal breakdown.

The fifth cranial nerve (trigeminal) may also be involved in facial palsy. May and Hardin (45) reported the polyneuronal nature of Bell's palsy, citing decreased corneal sensation, hearing, and taste discrimination and numbness of the face, shoulder, and neck as evidence. Corneal involvement may be manifested by hypesthesia, thereby aggravating the preexisting condition of lagophthalmos. Neurotropic corneal ulceration may aggravate the exposure difficulties.

Paralysis of the frontalis muscle will produce brow ptosis and a loss of forehead creases (flattening). The brow ptosis and the bulk of the upper lid skin produce a mechanical ptosis on the affected side. Contralateral upper eyelid retraction is frequently observed due to Hering's law of equal innervation.

Epiphora is frequently an annoying sequel of Bell's palsy. This may result from the eversion of the puncta from the lacus lacrimalis (punctal ectropion) or from frank ectropion of the eyelid. Management of these conditions would involve a punctoplasty or ectropion repair, respectively. Epiphora may also result from a nonfunctioning lacrimal pump. The lacrimal pump is postulated by Jones (46,47) and confirmed by manometric studies of Quickert, York, and Dryden (unpublished data). The lacrimal pump involves the orbicularis muscle. The closing of they eyelids increases the volume of the lacrimal sac and creates a negative pressure within the sac. The tears are drawn into the lacrimal sac and then drain into the nose by gravity. The lack of orbicularis function paralyzes the lacrimal pump and causes epiphora.

Surgical Correction

Nonincisional Suture Tarsorrhaphy

Consideration of surgical correction of seventh nerve palsy must include the prognosis for recovery of the facial nerve function without intervention, duration of time since the onset of the facial paralysis, and syndromes of aberrant regeneration that may be present. Patients may suffer facial nerve palsy of a transient nature with the idiopathic inflammation of Bell's palsy or following some surgical trauma to the nerve, from which recovery may be expected within a period of time (6 weeks). If there is exposure of the cornea, it is wise to protect it with a reversible temporary procedure, which may consist simply of an intermarginal 5-0 Prolene suture through the eyelid. The suture can be left for 2 to 3 weeks and replaced if necessary [48]. This is generally tolerated by the patient quite well and avoids unnecessary procedures that may destroy the eyelid margin.

The use of the running serpentine intermarginal suture should be considered for temporizing where the lids need to be closed to protect the globe. The brain-injured individual, temporary seventh nerve palsy, and globe protection prior to having a more definitive procedure are indications. A Prolene 4-0 or 5-0 suture is passed through the lid skin 4 to 5 mm from the eyelid margin near a canthus and tied. The suture then enters the lid skin to exit the lid in the gray line near the canthus. The needle enters the gray line of the opposing lid. A bite is made in the lid prior to exiting the gray line 4 to 5 mm along the lid. The needle then takes a similar bite in the original lid. The process is continued until the entire lid is sutured together in a serpentine manner. The suturing is completed by passing in the lid at the gray line and out the skin 4 to 5 mm above or below the respective lid margin. A bite is made in the skin at that point. The suture is tightened sufficiently to hold the lid margin together. The suture is tied to itself to anchor it in place.

"Reversible" Tarsorrhaphy

There are patients who require a more prolonged closure of the eyelids than can be provided by a nonincisional suture tarsorrhaphy. However, the oculoplastic surgeon should be reluctant to perform the "classic" tarsorrhaphy techniques, which involve either a denuding of the eyelid margin epithelium (49) or actual splitting of the anterior and posterior lamellae (50). These procedures inflict permanent damage to the eyelid margin. Surgical separation of these "permanent" tarsorrhaphy procedures at a later date (as may sometimes be desired) often reveals localized lid notching and intractable trichiasis. This section introduces a surgical tarsorrhaphy that is easy to perform, offers prolonged protection of the globe from exposure, and is readily undone (Fig. 19).

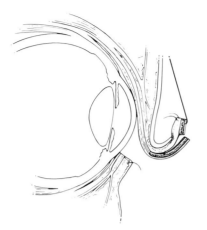

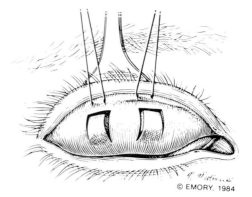

A

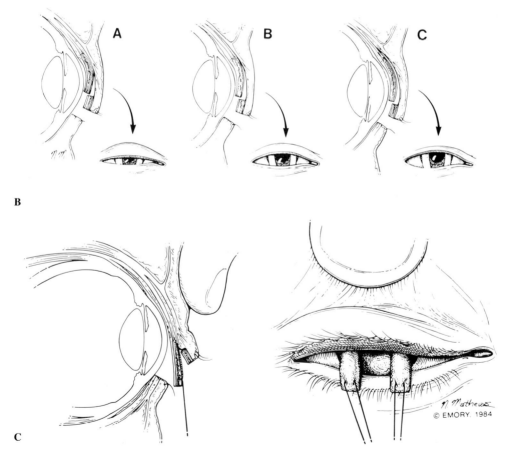

B

C

FIG. 19. Cross-sectional and front views of surgical tarsorrhaphy using upper eyelid tarsoconjunctival strips. **A:** The upper lid is everted and held under tension. Tarsoconjunctival strips, which straddle the pupillary axis, are elevated. **B:** The amount of verticle dissection of the tarsoconjunctival strips will ultimately determine the degree of eyelid closure achieved by the tarsorrhaphy. **A:** Mild. **B:** Moderate. **C:** Maximal. The upper lid tissue strips are mobilized with double-armed 6-0 Prolene mattress sutures. (Courtesy of Donald J. Bergin, M.D.)

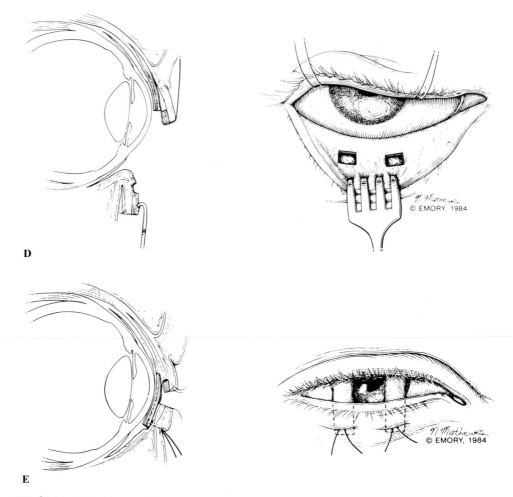

D

E

FIG. 19 (*cont.*) **D:** Divets of lower lid tarsoconjunctiva are excised corresponding to the location of the upper eyelid tissue strips. **E:** The 6-0 Prolene mattress sutures secure the upper lid tarsoconjunctival strips into the lower lid recipient sites. The Prolene sutures are sewn through the lower eyelid and tied externally on the skin. (Courtesy of Donald J. Bergin, M.D.)

For this procedure, the upper and lower lids are infiltrated with lidocaine 2% with epinephrine 1:100,000 and hyaluronidase (Wydase®). The upper lid is everted over a cotton-tipped applicator and held under tension with a 4–0 silk marginal traction suture. A thin strip of tarsoconjunctiva is elevated using a #15 blade. The upper lid margin is spared by at least 4 mm. A single tongue of tissue may be elevated for a lateral tarsorrhaphy or two strips may be used for a combined medial and lateral tarsorrhaphy. The upper lid tarsoconjunctival strips are dissected a variable amount depending on the degree of eyelid closure desired (Fig. 19B). Extensive dissection of the strip above the superior border of the upper lid tarsus will allow for minimal eyelid closure with the tarsorrhaphy. Minimal dissection of the elevated tissue strip will allow for greater narrowing of the palpebral fissure with the tarsorrhaphy.

The #15 blade is used to cut out a divet of tarsoconjunctiva from the lower lid that corresponds to the tongue of tarsoconjunctiva from the upper lid. A double-armed 6–0

Prolene mattress suture is sewn through the upper lid strip of tarsoconjunctiva, into the lower lid recipient bed, and out the skin of the lower eyelid. The suture is tied and cut, and polysporin ophthalmic ointment is applied for the first postoperative week. This tarsorrhaphy may be left in place indefinitely. It is easily undone by simply cutting the tarsoconjunctival strip(s). This is done with a Westcott scissors and topical anesthetic drops.

"Permanent" Tarsorrhaphy

An alternate type of "permanent" tarsorrhaphy can be used when maximum cosmesis of the medial and lateral canthal angles is desired.

Many patients will suffer a more protracted or permanent paralysis of closure with some eyelid malposition.

Historically, medial and lateral canthoplasties have been recommended for the narrowing of the palpebral fissure, but these are seldom used by the authors. These procedures produce a narrowed palpebral fissure, are cosmetically unsatisfactory, and are used only as a last resort. Combining a medial and lateral tarsorrhaphy gives more protection than either alone. The preferred lateral canthoplasty gives a strong bond and acute angle (51). The lateral lid margins are denuded in the areas to be approximated (Fig. 20A). The freshened edges of the lid margin are approximated with a mattress suture that is to brought through the musculocutaneous flap from the lower eyelid (Fig. 20B). A triangle of skin is excised from the upper eyelid to create a bed for the triangle of skin to be rotated in from the lower lid (Fig. 20C).

A medial canthoplasty is performed in the same manner as the lateral canthoplasty. Canalicular probes should remain in place during the procedure to protect the canaliculi, however. Generally, the procedure should be positioned nasally from the puncta.

Paralytic Ectropion (Severe Laxity Ectropion)

The major problems with which one is faced are the ectropion and sagging of the lower lid with resultant corneal exposure or epiphora and the failure of the upper lid to close because of loss of orbicularis tone. . . . [T]he paralytic ectropion that occurs with seventh nerve palsy may be treated simply as an extremely severe laxity ectropion, and an isolated horizontal tightening procedure may be used or combined with the medial ectropion procedure to correct this deformity [see Fig. 14]. In our experience with the horizontal tightening procedure, it has been helpful to perform a wedge resection of the upper lid along with the lower lid tightening at the lateral canthus in order to tighten the tarsoligamentous sling of the upper lid; this combination seems to at least temporarily help upper lid closure [Fig. 21].

Mechanical Prosthetic Devices for Eyelid Closure

Over the years, a variety of mechanical devices have been inserted in paralyzed eyelids in an attempt to achieve movement and eyelid closure. All of these devices attempt to simulate the protractor closure effect of the eyelid muscle and, in some cases, reposition the eyelid. The insertion of magnets in the upper and lower lids to produce closure by magnetic attraction has been described (52). The magnets can be "degaussed" so that the magnetic attraction has the proper degree of force. Lid "loading" with gold weights has been used in the upper lids with varying degrees of success (53,54). However, the gravitational effect only works if the patient is in the upright position and it only moves the upper lid.

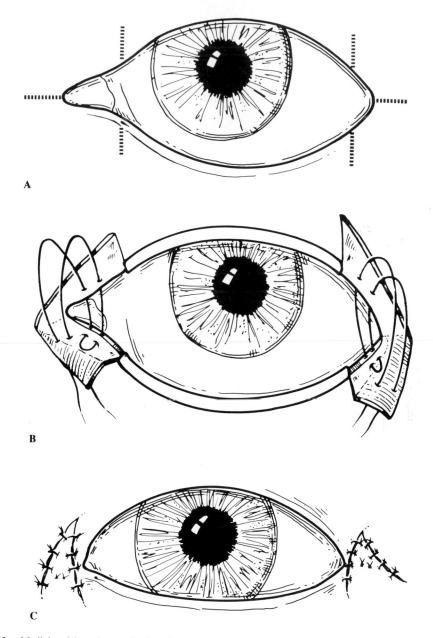

FIG. 20. Medial and lateral tarsorrhaphy of a more permanent nature for chronic seventh nerve palsy. **A:** The lid margin is denuded of its epithelium and the skin is undermined in the areas marked with dashed lines. **B:** Musculocutaneous flaps have been elevated from the lower lid and canthus, and skin and muscle from the upper lid is excised. Closure is performed with a mattress suture spanning from the lower lid margin to the upper lid margin and then out the musculocutaneous flap in the lower lid. **C:** The skin is closed with interrupted sutures.

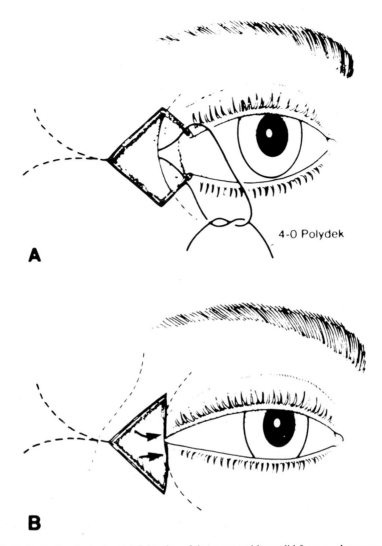

4-0 Polydek

A

B

FIG. 21. Canthal resection for horizontal tightening of the upper and lower lid for seventh nerve palsy. Patients who have poor eyelid closure and some exposure symptoms can be helped to some degree by tightening the upper and lower canthal tendon. **A:** A full-thickness triangular excision extending from the upper lid and the lower lid to the orbital rim. **B:** Attachment of the tendon inside the orbital rim. Approximately 15% to 20% of upper lid tissue has been resected. Skin closure is then accomplished by an advancement flap made temporally, leaving a vertical suture line. This will reposition the lower lid as in an ectropion procedure, cause some narrowing of the fissure, and increase lid closure of the upper lid for a period of time.

Morel et al. (55) introduced a palpebral spring, which mainly affected upper lid closure and has been used on and off for many years; however, in most cases it has not been effective, and most have extruded.

Arion filament

Arion introduced an encircling elastic silicone rod to simulate the squeezing of the protractor muscle (56). Of all the mechanical devices, this seems to be the most effective, although it has its inherent problems of erosion and, in many cases, must be looked upon as a

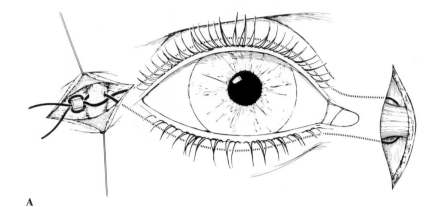

A

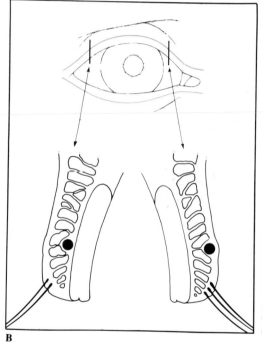

FIG. 22. The Arion sling technique for enhancing eyelid closure. **A:** A silicone rod is passed from the medial palpebral tendon, across the lids to a hole in the lateral orbital rim. **B:** The silicone rod is placed 2 to 3 mm from the eyelid margin. Nasally the rod is subcutaneous; however, laterally the rod is placed beneath the orbicularis muscle. **C:** The silicone rod is tied and looped around a larger silicone sleeve to prevent slippage of the knot.

B

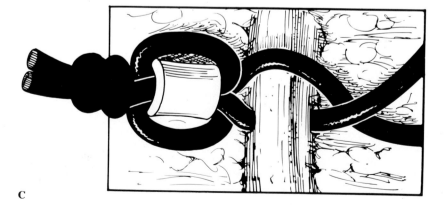

C

temporary procedure. The technique described here is similar to Arion's original technique, but many modifications have been introduced. The most recent modification, which will not be described in detail here, is using the elastic portion of the rod only for the upper lid, with a fascia graft to the lower lids. The fascia will reposition the lower lid while the silicone will affect upper lid closure.

The rationale for the filament is that the elastic silicone is a substitute for the contractility of the orbicularis. The lids and canthi are infiltrated with a local anesthetic. The medial palpebral tendon is exposed with a horizontal incision. The lateral orbital rim is exposed about 3 mm above the lateral palpebral tendon. The 0.8-mm thick silicone rod is passed behind the anterior limb of the medial palpebral tendon. The fil d'Arion introducer is passed through the upper and lower lids from the lateral canthal region. The introducer is passed as close to the lid margin as possible (2–3 mm ideally). In the medial portion of the eyelid, the silicone is placed subcutaneously (Fig. 22A). Nasally and laterally, the silicone is in or under the orbicularis muscle (Fig. 22B). The lateral deep position is necessitated by the origin of the silicone at the orbital rim. The passer is withdrawn with the end of the silicone, which is anchored under the medial palpebral tendon. The silicone ends are drawn across the lids from the medial canthus, first in one lid and then the other. A 1.5-mm hole is then drilled in the lateral orbital rim about 3 mm above the lateral canthal angle. The silicone from the lower eyelid is pulled through the hole created in the lateral orbital wall from the inside to the outside of the orbit. The silicone from the upper arm is brought behind the arm from the lower lid prior to passing anterior to the orbital rim. The two arms of the silicone rod are then secured by passing twice through a larger silicone sleeve (Fig. 22C). The tension is adjusted, preferably in the awake patient. A slight to moderate ptosis should be created because 1 to 2 mm of ptosis is needed in the final result to give adequate protection to the globe. An overcorrection at this stage allows for loosening with time. If the patient is asleep, the pressure achieved with a hanging standard hemostat is a fair approximation of the tension required. After the tension is correct, a square knot is tied in the silicone as additional protection against slippage. The ends are left about 1 cm in length. They are buried under the orbicularis. Closure is made in layers to keep the silicone deep. If adjustments are needed later, these ends may be reexposed, untied, and readjusted. Prophylactic antibiotics should be considered postoperatively to reduce the chance of infection.

Problems encountered with the Arion filament are several. A rod that is not passed through the bone may tear free. Excessive elevation of the rod in the medial area occurs if the rod is too superficial nasally or not well behind the medial limb of the medial palpebral tendon. Infection requires removal and replacement of the silicone rod. Undercorrection is most common and occurs from a reluctance to initially erect enough tension on the silicone rod. Finally, erosion of the silicone through the medial canthal tendon will occur with time in many cases.

Reinnervation

Reanimation of the eyelid itself from reinnervation techniques can be achieved with facial nerve transfer and graft if the facial muscles have not undergone atrophy. If facial nerve transfer or cranial nerve reanastomosis is to be contemplated, it must be performed within a suitable period of time from the onset of the facial nerve palsy, usually within 4 to 6 months, before atrophy of the facial musculature occurs. In cases in which craniofacial anastomosis nerve transfer or nerve grafting cannot be performed, reanimation of the paralyzed face and eyelid muscles can be obtained by temporalis muscle transfer, in which strips of temporalis fascia attached to the temporalis muscle as a circumorbital sling in the upper and lower lid are attached to the medial canthal tendon [57,58]. This is a very successful procedure and has stood the test of time but requires clenching the jaw to effect an eyelid closure. It is beyond the scope of this particular section to discuss surgical techniques of these more complex operations, but the [surgeon] should be aware of the availability of these procedures and should consider the patient on an individual basis to determine whether one of these procedures might be applicable.

Brow Ptosis and Epiphora

Denervation of the brow muscles can cause atonicity of the frontalis muscle and a drooping of the brow or ptosis, which is a significant problem to many patients with seventh nerve palsy. Another side effect of the adynamic eyelids in seventh nerve palsy is deficiency of the lacrimal palpebral pump with resulting epiphora.

Brow ptosis is a problem because of accentuation of dermatochalasis to produce mechanical ptosis or to cover the fissure with redundant skin. Brow ptosis should be measured preoperatively. The brow is moved from its dependent position superiorly to what is considered a normal position to evaluate millimeters of droop. The ellipse of skin to be removed is marked with the inferior border being immediately adjacent to the brow hairs or in a prominent crease to camouflage the incisional scar. The vertical height of the ellipse to be removed should equal the amount of brow ptosis. The skin is removed with care to avoid deep tissues and injury to the supraorbital nerve. Closure is made with a varied running subcutaneous suture and a cutaneous suture. Anchoring to the periosteum is usually advocated but has not been necessary (50) in our experience.

Epiphora may be relieved by managing the exposure or correcting punctal abnormalities. If the lacrimal system is patent to irrigation with an open, well-positioned puncta and is nonfunctioning as confirmed by the Jones I and II tests, a Jones tube may be required to bypass the inadequate pump (see Chapter 14). However, a Jones tube may function poorly with paralyzed lids because of the absence of the palpebral pump for tear elimination.

REFERENCES

1. McCord, C. D., Jr. (1985): Surgery of the eyelids. In: *Clinical Ophthalmology,* edited by T. D. Duane and E. A. Jaeger, Vol. 5, Chpt 5, pp. 1–54. Harper & Row, Philadelphia.
2. Jones, L. T. (1960): The anatomy of the lower eyelid and its relationship to the cause and cure of entropion. *Am. J. Ophthalmol.,* 49:29.
3. Dryden, R. M., Leibsohn, J., and Wobig, J. (1978): Senile entropion: Pathogenesis and treatment. *Arch. Ophthalmol.,* 96:1183.
4. Collin, J. R. O., and Rathbun, J. E. (1978): Involutional entropion. *Arch. Ophthalmol.,* 96:1058.
5. Sisler, H. A. (1973): A biochemical and physiologic approach to corrective surgery for senile entropion. *Ann. Ophthalmol.,* 5:483.
6. Dalgleish, R., and Smith, J. L. S. (1966): Mechanics and histology of senile ectropion. *Br. J. Ophthalmol.,* 50:79.
7. Sisler, H. A., Lebay, G. R., and Finlay, J. R. (1976): Senile ectropion and entropion: A compared and histopathologic study. *Ann. Ophthalmol.,* 8:319.
8. Ziegler, S. L. (1909): Galvano cautery puncture and entropion and ectropion. *JAMA,* 53:183.
9. Quickert, M. H., and Rathbun, E. (1971): Suture repair of entropion. *Arch. Ophthalmol.,* 85:304.
10. Sisler, H. A. (1973): The biomechanical and physiologic approach to corrective surgery for senile entropion. *Ann. Ophthalmol.,* 5:483.
11. Bick, M. W. (1966): Surgical management of orbital tarsal disparity. *Arch. Ophthalmol.,* 75:386.
12. Hornblass, A., Bercovici, S., and Smith, B. (1977): Senile entropion. *Ophthalmic Surg.,* 8:47.
13. Wies, F. A. (1954): Surgical treatment of entropion. *J. Int. Coll. Surg.,* 21:758.
14. Callahan, A: (1976): Correction of entropion from Stevens–Johnson syndrome, use of nasal septum and mucosa for severely cicatrized eyelid entropion. *Arch. Ophthalmol.,* 94:1154.
15. Sheen, J. H. (1974): Supra tarsal fixation in upper lid blepharoplasty. *Plast. Reconstr. Surg.,* 54:424.

16. Tenzel, R. R., Miller, G. R., and Rubnzik, R. (1975): Cicatricial upper lid entropion treated with bank scleral graft. *Arch. Ophthalmol.*, 93:999.

17. Wesley, R. E., McCord, C. D., and Jones, N. A. (1980): Height of the tarsus of the lower eyelid. *Am. J. Ophthalmol.*, 90:102–105.

18. Sullivan, J. H. (1977): The use of cryotherapy for trichiasis. *Trans. Am. Acad. Ophthalmol. Otolaryngolo.*, 83:708–712.

19. Hardy, K., Perry, H., and Kirby, T. (1971): Benign mucous membrane pemphigoid. *Arch. Dermatol.*, 104:467.

20. Fraumfelder, F. T., and Peterson, G. J. (1979): The use of liquid nitrogen cryospray for the treatment of trichiasis. *Opthalmic Surg.*, 10:42–46.

21. Sullivan, J. H., Beard, C., and Bullock, J. D. (1976): Cryosurgery for the treatment of trichiasis. *Am. J. Ophthalmol.*, 82:117–121.

22. Wilkes, T. D. I., and Fraumfelder, F. T. (1979): Principles of cryosurgery. *Opthalmic Surg.*, 10:21–30.

23. Hoschni, R., and Faruk, J. (1974): Repair of trichomatous cicatricial entropion using a mucous membrane graft. *Arch. Ophthalmol.*, 91:49.

24. Leone, C. R. (1974): Mucous membrane grafting for cicatricial entropion. *Ophthalmic Surg.*, 5:24.

25. Maumenee, A. E., (1979): Keratinization of the conjunctiva. *Trans. Am. Ophthalmol. Soc.*, 77:133.

26. McCord, C. D., and Chen, W. P. (1983): Tarsal polishing and mucous membrane grafting for cicatricial entropion, trichiasis and epidermalization. *Ophthalmic Surg.*, 14:1021–1025.

27. Fox, S. A. (1968): A medial ectropion procedure. *Arch. Ophthalmol.*, 80:494.

28. Smith, B. (1976): The "lazy T" correction of ectropion of the lower punctum. *Arch. Ophthalmol.*, 94:1149.

29. McCord, C. D. (1980): Canalicular resection with canaliculostomy. *Ophthalmic Surg.*, 11:440.

30. Bick, M. W. (1966): Surgical management of orbital tarsal disparity. *Arch. Ophthalmol.*, 80:494.

31. Wesley, R. E., and Collins, J. W. (1983): McCord procedure for ectropion repair. *Arch. Otolaryngol.*, 109:319–322.

32. Fox, S. A. (1960): Marginal (tarsal) ectropion. *Arch. Ophthalmol.*, 63:660.

33. Wesley, R. E. (1982): Tarsal ectropion from detachment of the lower eyelid retractors. *Am. J. Ophthalmol.*, 93:491.

34. Putterman, A. M. (1978): Ectropion of the lower eyelid secondary to Mueller's muscle-capsulo palpebral fascia detachment. *Am. J. Ophthalmol.*, 85:814.

35. White, J. W. (1971): Method of correction of tarsal ectropion. *Am. J. Ophthalmol.*, 72:615.

36. Sober, A. J., Grove, A. S., and Muhlbauer, J. E. (1981): Cicatricial ectropion and lacrimal obstruction associated with the sclero dermoid variant of porphyria cutanea tarda. *Am. J. Ophthalmol.*, 91:396.

37. Galentine, P., Sloas, H., Hargatte, N., and Cupples, H. P. (1981): Bilateral cicatricial ectropion following topical administration of 5-fluorouracil. *Ann. Ophthalmol.*, 13:575.

38. Johnson, C. C. and McGowan, B. L. (1969): Persistent congenital ectropion of all four eyelids with megoblepharon. *Am. J. Ophthalmol.*, 67:252.

39. Biglan, A. W., and Burger, G. E. (1980): Congenital horizontal tarsal kink. *Am. J. Ophthalmol.*, 91:552.

40. Gilbert, H. D., Smith, R. E., Barlow, M. H., and Mohr, V. (1973): Congenital upper lid eversion in Down's syndrome. *Am. J. Ophthalmol.*, 75:469.

41. Eneroth, C. M. (1972): Facial nerve paralysis: A criterion of malignancy in parotid tumors. *Arch. Otolaryngol.*, 95:300–304.

42. Jonghees, L. B. W. (1972): On peripheral facial nerve paralysis. *Arch. Otolaryngol.*, 95:313–317.

43. May, M. (1980): Bell's palsy: Diagnosis, prognosis and treatment (update 1980). *Surg. Rounds*, January, pp. 38–60.

44. Jelks, G. W., Smith, B., and Bosniak, S. (1980): The evaluation and management of the eye in facial palsy. *Clin. Plast. Surg.*, 6:397.

45. May, M., Hardin, W. B. (1978): Facial palsy: Interpretation of neurologic findings. *Laryngoscope*, 88:1352–1362.

46. Jones, L. T. (1961): An antomic approach to problems of the eyelids and lacrimal apparatus. *Arch. Opthalmol.*, 66:111–124.

47. Jones, L. T., and Wobig, J. L. (1976): *Surgery of the Eyelids and Lacrimal System*, p. 70. Aesculapus, Birmingham, Alabama.

48. Dryden, R. M., and Adams, J. L. (1985): Temporary nonincisional tarsorrhaphy. *Ophthalmic Plast. Reconstr. Surg.*, 1:119–120.

49. Iliff, C. E., Iliff, W. J., and Iliff, N. T. (1979): *Oculoplastic Surgery*, pp. 162–164. Sanders, Philadephia.

50. Fox, S. A. (1976): *Ophthalmic Plastic Surgery*, 5th ed., pp. 114–115. Grune & Stratton, New York.

51. Beard, C. (1964): Canthoplasty and brow elevation for facial palsy. *Arch. Ophthalmol.*, 71:386.

52. Mühlbauer, W. D. (1978): Palpebral magnets for paretic lagophthalmos. In: *Symposium on the Neurologic Aspects of Plastic Surgery*, edited by S. Fredericks and G. S. Brody. Mosby, St. Louis.

53. Smellie, G. D. (1966): Restoration of the blinking reflex in facial palsy by a simple lid load operation. *Br. J. Plast. Surg.*, 19:279–283.

54. Barclay, T. L., and Roberts, A. C. (1969): Restoration of movement to the upper eyelid in facial palsy. *Br. J. Plast. Surg.*, 22:257.

55. Morel, J., Fatio, D., and Lelardrie, J. P. (1964): Paliative surgical treatment of facial paralysis: The palpebral spring. *Plast. Reconstr. Surg.*, 33:447.
56. Arion, H. G. (1972): Dynamic closure of the lids in paralysis of the orbicularis muscle. *Int. Surg.*, 57:48–50.
57. Masters, F. W., Robinson, D. W., and Simons, N. J. (1965): Temporalis transfer for lagophthalmos due to seventh nerve palsy. *Am. J. Surg.*, 110:607–611.
58. Rubin, L. R. (ed.). (1977): *Reanimation of the Paralyzed Face; New Approaches,* pp. 53–80, 125–131. Mosby, St. Louis.

Oculoplastic Surgery, 2nd edition, edited by
Clinton D. McCord, Jr., and Myron Tanenbaum.
Raven Press, New York © 1987.

Chapter 13

Evaluation and Management of the Ptosis Patient

*Robert R. Waller, **Clinton D. McCord, Jr., and †Myron Tanenbaum

*Department of Ophthalmology, Mayo Clinic, Rochester, Minnesota 55901; and ** Department of*
Ophthalmology, Emory University School of Medicine, Atlanta, Georgia 30308; and † Bascom Palmer
Eye Institute, Department of Ophthalmology, University of Miami School of Medicine,
Miami, Florida 33101

PTOSIS: DEFINITION AND DIFFERENTIAL DIAGNOSIS

Ptosis of the upper lid implies that, in the relaxed position, the upper lid is lower than normal and in most cases obstructs the visual axis. This can occur congenitally or be acquired from a number of causes. However, there are many conditions that simulate ptosis that are not true ptosis. These conditions should be differentiated from true ptosis in order that a proper approach to correction can be undertaken (Table 1).

Contralateral lid retraction from Graves' disease can, in many cases, simulate ptosis in the opposite eyelid. Hypertropia of the eye and a down gaze position will also present as ptosis and may, indeed, have some accompanying ptosis as the eye is rotated downward. Enophthalmos can simulate a true ptosis. As the globe is retracted back, the upper lid will fall over the globe. Conversely, an exophthalmos on the contralateral side can cause an upward alteration in lid position that will produce a relative down position of the side in question. Mechanical pressure on the lid from swelling, edema, tumor, or heavy skin folds can, in many cases, produce a downward position or ptosis of the lid, and it is often difficult to tell whether true ptosis is indeed present in addition to the mechanical pressure. Squeezing or guarding of the eye in the presence of external irritation or photophobia will also simulate ptosis. Retraction of the globe with Duane's syndrome or any other retraction syndromes can cause the eyelid to fall as the globe is retracted.

CONGENITAL PTOSIS

Classification

Beard (1) classifies congenital ptosis into those (a) with normal superior rectus function, (b) with superior rectus weakness, (c) associated with the blepharophimosis syndrome,

TABLE 1. *Causes of pseudoptosis*[a]

Contralateral lid retraction
Hypotropia
Enophthalmos or contralateral exophthalmos
Upper lid pressure (swelling, tumor, or redundant skin)
Guarding
Retraction syndrome

[a] In approximate order of frequency.

and (d) with synkinetic ptosis of the Marcus–Gunn jaw-winking type or ptosis associated with misdirected third nerve palsies. To this classification it might be reasonable to add those patients with apparent congenital ptosis who have aponeurotic defects, as described by Anderson and Dixon (2). There are many ptosis classifications. Beard's classification is simple, practical, and includes most types of congenital ptosis encountered.

Frequency

The frequency of congenital ptosis is difficult to assess. Berke (3) has written that 88% of 200 consecutive cases were congenital, Beard 62% (4), and Fox 90% (5). Of 150 recent consecutive ptosis patients examined at Mayo Clinic, 75 were congenital and 75 acquired.

Pathophysiology

The word "congenital" implies existence from birth. Birth injuries and congenital third nerve paralyses occur at birth but are often considered in the acquired group of disorders, because they are not dystrophic in nature. Congenital ptosis encompasses a group of cases wherein developmental dystrophy exists in the levator muscle without associated innervational abnormalities. There is a lack of peripheral differentiation of the muscle. The levator complex develops at the medial aspect of the superior rectus muscle after the recti and obliques develop. The levator muscle does not reach normal position until the fourth fetal month. Failure or aberration in this late development results in ptosis. Berke and Wadsworth (6) performed muscle biopsies in a series of congenital ptosis cases and found that congenital ptosis of greater than 4.0 mm demonstrated an absence of striated muscle fibers. The histologic picture is somewhat similar to progressive muscular dystrophy, and these authors feel that ptosis is perhaps an isolated form of dystrophy.

Inheritance

Beard stated that, other than isolated family groups, most patients with congenital ptosis have no familial history of a similar condition. Fox reviewed 200 consecutive cases, however, and indicated that 65% of his cases were congenital ptosis present at birth without source of inheritance, and approximately 10% were part of the blepharophimosis syndrome that starts as a mutation and then can be transmitted as a dominant hereditary trait, transmitted equally through both sides.

Associated Ocular Abnormalities

Most patients exhibit no extraocular muscle dysfunction other than the ptosis, but when they do, the muscle involved is usually the ipsilateral superior rectus muscle. This is not innervational but developmental, and is explained by its embryologically close association to the levator muscle.

Marcus-Gunn Jaw-winking Syndrome

The Marcus-Gunn jaw-winking syndrome is the most common congenital synkinetic movement in which ptosis is present. Its incidence is 2% to 6% of congenital ptosis (4) cases [Smith et al. (7) claim a much higher percentage—11%]. The cause is probably the result of abnormal nervous connections in the central nervous system between the levator and the external pterygoid portion of the fifth cranial nerve, which innervates the muscles of mastication (8). Whether this is a supranuclear or intranuclear abnormality is not known. Perhaps it is an atavistic reversion to the association between the mouth and gills. (The gill muscles are associated with the orbicularis and pterygoids.) It is of interest that this phenomenon is sometimes associated with inspiration, and we observe often in children the tendency to open the mouth when opening the eyes, suggesting such an early relationship. Marcus-Gunn jaw-winking ptosis is usually unilateral, often involving the left side. It is rarely associated with other eye or systemic anomalies other than superior rectus weakness. It varies from a minimal to a cosmetically intolerable situation. There is controversy as to whether or not this disorder gets better with age (there are no data to support either side).

Blepharophimosis Syndrome

The blepharophimosis syndrome has classically been described as primarily hereditary with dominant characteristics consisting of a triad of ptosis of the upper lids, telecanthus, and phimosis of the eyelid fissure (9). Other anomalies that co-exist with the syndrome are epicanthal folds, shortage of skin in upper and lower lids, congenital ectropion, and flattening of the glabellar area. This condition is present at birth and in many cases occurs as a sporadic event. The ptosis of the upper lids is usually the first anomaly that is corrected in order to allow adequate visual development. In most cases, the lid is hypoplastic, with poor differentiation of tissue and deficient tarsus, and presents a difficult correction. The frontalis suspension procedure is the most commonly used procedure.

Congenital Anophthalmos

Children who are born with the congenital anophthalmos syndrome have severe anomalies with absence of the eye or a vestigial eye and in many cases hypoplasia of the lids and orbital bones. Ptosis is only a coincidental finding in these children, but must be dealt with at some point in their reconstructive rehabilitation. It also presents a challenge in that there is generally absence of the levator function in the hypoplastic lid.

Co-existent Eyelid Hamartomas

The existence of hamartomatous tissue in the eyelid at birth in children who are diagnosed as having ptosis many times can be unrecognized, but presents a serious problem with correction of the condition. Congenital neurofibromatosis may not be readily apparent in the absence of café-au-lait spots or other stigmata, but can present as a thickened, puffy, S-shaped lid. Lymphangiomas may also be unrecognized initially. Capillary hemangiomas generally are more readily diagnosed because of the surface skin changes. It is important to recognize this tissue in the lid in that it does present an entirely different prognosis for the child in terms of the success of any surgical correction over a long follow-up period.

Co-existent Strabismus and Amblyopia

Neonatal eyelid closure with ptosis has, in the past, been thought to be an entirely benign condition with regard to visual development if the child can "peek under the lid." This has been refuted in that anisometropia or myopia with secondary amblyopia can be induced with lid closure (10–12). True occlusion amblyopia can occur. The mechanisms explaining the higher incidence of ocular abnormalities are occlusion, pressure of the lid on the globe, or coincidental anomalies associated with ptosis itself. This propensity for visual disturbance in children should be recognized in all cases of congenital ptosis.

ACQUIRED PTOSIS

Classification

In contrast to congenital ptosis, the acquired ptoses constitute a heterogeneous group of disorders that are not amenable to simple classification. Beard's classification is perhaps the best and, in the view of many, is the most practical and useful in the clinical setting. He divides the acquired ptoses into four groups: (a) neurogenic, (b) myogenic, (c) traumatic, and (d) mechanical (1).

Neurogenic Ptoses

A host of disease states may afflict the third cranial nerve throughout its course from the nucleus in the floor of the cerebral aqueduct to the muscular portion of the levator complex in the orbit. Beard lists the common causes as vascular lesions, tumors, and neurotoxic and inflammatory states, including diphtheria, poliomyelitis, encephalitis, meningitis, influenza, measles, botulism, syphilis, and heavy metal poisoning. Almost all of these ptoses are not treatable until the underlying process has resolved or stabilized, usually for a period of 9 to 12 months.

Horner's syndrome is the most frequent form of neurogenic ptosis and perhaps the most gratifying to treat. Tumors, aneurysms, injuries, and inflammatory processes are the most frequent causes. Ptosis and headache should alert the ophthalmologist to the association of Horner's syndrome and Horton's headache (histamine cephalgia). Maloney et al. (13) have recently reviewed 450 cases of Horner's syndrome at Mayo Clinic. They provided an in-depth review of causes of Horner's syndrome and reviewed pharmacologic testing for the disorder.

Traumatic ophthalmoplegia with ptosis is common and identifiable usually by history. Beard cautions that paralyses tend to become pareses and advises that patients should be followed for several months prior to surgical intervention (1). Serial photographs, measurements of lid fissure position, and testing such as with the Lancaster red-green screen are invaluable in the selection of the proper time for surgical intervention.

Ophthalmoplegic migraine is extremely rare, at least insofar as the associated ptosis, which is part of an intermittent or permanent third nerve palsy, is concerned. This is a diagnosis of exclusion, and the burden of proof rests with the physician to show that a serious underlying disease process along the pathway of the third nerve does not exist. Walsh and Hoyt (14) have warned that intermittent ptosis with other associated symptoms may be caused by mucocele-pyocele of the sphenoid sinus and may mimic this rare condition.

The ptosis of multiple sclerosis is rarely seen, but this is another cause of neurogenic ptosis. The diagnosis is usually made by associated findings (optic neuritis, internuclear ophthalmoplegia, skew deviation, nystagmus).

Beard lists congenital third nerve palsy as an acquired ptosis, most likely because it can be related to some intrauterine diseases or to birth injury. These children are most difficult to treat, and surgical results in most instances are quite disappointing.

Myogenic (Myopathic) Ptoses

The myogenic (myopathic) acquired ptoses pose a challenge to clinical management. Whereas many patients with myogenic ptosis obtain good results from surgical treatment, some do not because the ptosis can be unstable, slowly progressive, or reversible. While correction of the ptosis at one stage of the disease may be satisfactory, alternative surgical measures may be required at later stages to manage a recurrence of the ocular disability. Associated ocular abnormalities such as poor Bell's phenomenon or weak orbicularis function can make the correction of ptosis difficult or risky. In this group of patients, various approaches must be used to care successfully for the ptosis problem; in some instances surgery perhaps should be avoided altogether.

Senile or involutional ptosis is the most common type of acquired myogenic ptosis. When the condition is mild, the presumed cause is loss of tone and stretching of the levator and Müller's muscle, together with loss of lid support due to enophthalmos resulting from atrophy of orbital fat (1). When the condition is moderate or severe, however, other factors may be present, as suggested by thinning of the upper lid, which allows the color of the underlying iris to be visible through the lid tissues, and the high lid fold, usually in the presence of excellent or good levator excursion. These clinical findings suggest the presence of dehiscence of the levator aponeurosis as first described by Jones et al. (5), the repair of which represents one of the most significant advances in the treatment of ptosis in many years.

Late acquired hereditary ptosis is similar to senile or involutional ptosis but is noted in several members of a family tree. The ptosis is usually symmetric and becomes symptomatic when the patient is in the middle decades of life. Other extraocular muscles are not involved.

Chronic progressive external ophthalmoplegia has been exhaustively reviewed by Walsh and Hoyt (16) in their text. This condition may be a progressive muscular dystrophy that principally affects the extraocular muscles (including the levator muscle), but whether these patients suffer from pure myopathy or associated neurogenic disease is debatable (17,18). Daroff et al. (18) pointed out the difficulties in determining histologically whether partial or total loss of function of extraocular muscles is a result of primary muscle involvement or neural influences. Stephens et al. (19) emphasized that final proof of the myopathic origin of chronic progressive external ophthalmoplegia must be based on more than muscle biopsy data, such as electromyographic findings. Such proof is still lacking. Perhaps neurogenic and myogenic influences both have a role.

Chronic progressive external ophthalmoplegia often begins in childhood or adolescence with a gradually developing ptosis. There is a familial occurrence in 50% of cases (20), with males and females equally affected. The other extraocular muscles soon become affected, but the absence of diplopia is characteristic. Twenty-five percent (17) of these patients have involvement of other muscle groups. Of particular importance is the involvement of the orbicularis oculi, which results in simultaneous inability to open and close the eyelids properly. Oculopharyngeal muscular dystrophy (21) belongs to this same group of diseases, but patients with this disease are slightly older at onset, have more frequent involvement of pharyngeal and facial muscles, and have a higher familial incidence, particularly those of French-Canadian descent.

Patients with chronic progressive external ophthalmoplegia may have other ocular and systemic disturbances (22), particularly retinal pigmentary abnormalities, associated endocrine disorders, and cardiomyopathy (23). These patients suffer progression of their disease without remission or exacerbation. The diagnosis is made primarily on the basis of history, physical findings, and absence of response to edrophonium chloride (Tensilon®) or neostigmine.

Myotonic dystrophy patients usually have mild ptosis. The orbicularis oculi may be weak, and some patients may have myotonia of Bell's phenomenon, which is characterized by maintenance of the elevated position of the eyes after forceful closure of the lids (24). The aphakic patient, particularly if young, who has bilateral (usually symmetric) ptosis and not uncommonly low intraocular pressure, should arouse the suspicion of the presence of myotonic dystrophy (25). Such a patient may have a ptosis problem requiring an approach different from that for the more common type of postsurgical ptosis.

Myasthenia gravis is considered to be myopathic in origin, but the problem is primarily one of an acetylcholine deficiency at the myoneural junction. This is a disease of young women and old men, rarely of children. Ocular symptoms are the initial manifestations in a large majority of patients, and often the presenting symptoms and signs are unilateral or asymmetric ptosis and diplopia, both of which become worse with fatigue. Injection of neostigmine or edrophonium chloride can make the ptosis less noticeable. The presence of Cogan's lid twitch sign can help in the diagnosis (26).

Corticosteroid-induced ptosis occurs in patients on long-term topical corticosteroid therapy, such as for chronic conjunctivitis or uveitis. This is presumed to be of myogenic origin, perhaps a localized form of corticosteroid myopathy.

Beard described several patients who developed ptosis of pregnancy (during or after pregnancy) and several who were heavy users of mascara. Both of these rare ptoses may have some myogenic component.

Graves' disease with ptosis is rare. Usually the disease is quiescent. These patients may have an aponeurotic defect, perhaps resulting from prolonged effects of congestive ophthalmopathy. Because approximately 5% of patients with myasthenia gravis have hyperthyroidism, patients with Graves' disease and ptosis should have an edrophonium chloride test.

Traumatic Ptoses

Damage to the levator complex in acute eyelid trauma can be masked by edema. Allowing the edema to subside for a day or two can facilitate repair. If the patient is cooperative, the levator tissues can be more readily identified using local anesthesia. Horizontal wounds are more prone to levator injury and should be assessed carefully. Proper identification and prompt anastomosis of severed levator tissues can avoid later difficult repairs.

Postenucleation ptosis is rare, fortunately, but can be profound if an injury to the nerve or muscle by the enucleation scissors occurs. Other causes of postenucleation ptosis include dehiscence of the levator aponeurosis, a poorly fitting prosthesis, or adhesions between the muscle stump and the levator. Ptosis following orbital surgery probably results from similar disturbances.

Postsurgical ptosis (following intraocular surgery) is of uncertain etiology, although there is evidence that dehiscence of the levator aponeurosis is sometimes at fault. Some have blamed postsurgical ptosis on the lid speculum or on the improper placement of the superior rectus bridle suture.

Intraorbital foreign bodies or fractures of the orbital roof are additional causes of traumatic ptosis. Orbital hematomas and/or hematic cysts following trauma may also be responsible for ptosis.

Mechanical Ptoses

Beard considers mechanical ptosis to result from increased weight of the eyelid, such as with tumor or from scar tissue interfering with eyelid motility.

The most common eyelid tumors causing ptosis are neurofibroma and hemangioma, but any eyelid tumor can cause ptosis if large enough. Amyloidosis and lymphoma similarly can cause ptosis if present in the upper fornices or on the upper tarsoconjunctiva. Ptosis of the temporal eyelid makes the diagnosis of lacrimal gland tumor suspect.

Blepharochalasis, characterized by repeated attacks of lid edema, may eventually be associated with ptosis, most often as the result of levator aponeurosis dehiscence.

Cicatricial ptosis may result from disease (trachoma, erythema multiforme, ocular pemphigoid) or trauma, either chemical or thermal or surgical, such as for repeated pterygium surgery or following filtration surgery that has been followed by shortening of the upper fornix. It is seen after multiple procedures for retinal detachment, including vitrectomy.

Classification of Acquired Ptosis by Frequency of Cause

Multiple ptosis series, over the years, have shown that the large majority of acquired ptosis patients that present to the surgeon will be either posttraumatic or the involutional myopathic ptosis. Table 2 shows a composite list of the frequencies of the most common types of acquired ptosis as presented to the ophthalmologist. In all series, approximately 40% to 50% are of the involutional myopathic type and 30% are posttraumatic.

EVALUATION AND WORK-UP OF THE PTOSIS PATIENT

The first key element of evaluation and work-up of a ptosis patient consists of determining whether the ptosis is congenital or acquired. The acquired ptosis patient responds differently

TABLE 2. *Causes of acquired ptosis[a]*

Involutional myopathic
Posttrauma—surgical
Chronic progressive external ophthalmoplegia
Mechanical changes with anophthalmos
Third nerve palsy
Horner's syndrome
Myasthenia gravis
Upper lid tumors

[a] In approximate order of frequency.

to levator surgery than the congenital patient, and this determination must be made. If a patient is determined to have an acquired ptosis, the etiology must be determined to rule out any threatening condition that requires further evaluation and possible treatment. The second key element is to determine levator function, since the application of the various corrective surgical procedures depends on the amount of functional strength of the levator muscle. The third key element is the evaluation of eye protective mechanisms to determine whether or not the globe will tolerate the opening of the fissure following the ptosis procedure. Other aspects of the exam are important in the management of the ptosis patient and will be explored in the following section, but these are the three key elements of the ptosis work-up.

Etiology

Major questions to be answered include the presence or absence or family history of ptosis, age of onset of ptosis, whether there has been a history of trauma, medications used by the patient (topical and systemic), whether or not the ptosis worsens with fatigue, and whether or not there are systemic illnesses that might be related to the ptosis.

The most important question requiring an answer preoperatively with regard to etiology may well be related to whether or not the ptosis is congenital or acquired. To answer this question, examine the vertical height of the lid fissures in down gaze. The congenitally ptotic eyelid will not relax just as it does not elevate and, therefore, the lid slit on down gaze will be wider vertically on the ptotic as compared to the nonptotic side. In contrast, when vertical lid slits are measured in acquired ptoses, the lid slit on down gaze will be narrower vertically on the ptotic as compared to the nonptotic side. This is a most important measurement that should be part of every medical record.

Levator Function

One must be absolutely certain of levator function. Ptosis operations can be performed to perfection, but if the amount of levator complex resected is too little or too much, a poor result is inevitable. Levator function is measured in millimeters, measuring the distance from extreme up gaze to extreme down gaze, with the brow firmly splinted by the examiner's thumb so as to eliminate any contribution by the brow to lid elevation. The millimeter rule may be placed vertically at the lateral canthus to accomplish the measurement. Assessment of levator function can be most accurately determined if more than one measurement is taken, perhaps on separate days, and if measurements are taken by separate examiners. If the latter is possible, any disparity in measurements forces closer scrutiny of the problem, which is always to the patient's advantage. Beard (1) stated that levator function can be good (10 mm or more), fair (5–10 mm), or poor (5 mm or less).

Eye Protective Mechanisms

Ptosis procedures, in almost all cases, produce some stiffness of the upper lid and lago-phthalmos, which in some cases can be quite dramatic. If the eye retains its moisture with an adequate tear film and good protective movements, most patients will tolerate this lagophthalmos. Each patient should be examined preoperatively with basic secretion tests and a Schirmer test to determine the adequacy of the tear film. Examination of the motility, including Bell's phenomenon, is important in that severe keratopathy can occur with an eye that cannot move and protect itself. Additional problems such as corneal anesthesia or facial nerve weakness can introduce problems of exposure in patients who ordinarily would tolerate the lagophthalmos. All of these protective mechanisms must be present to use the standard type of corrective procedures safely. In the presence of poor eye protective mechanisms, the patient must be told ahead of time that it may be necessary to reverse the procedure if the cornea will not tolerate the opening of the eyelid.

Amount of Ptosis

Beard (1) wrote that mild ptosis is 2.0 mm or less, moderate ptosis is 3.0 mm, and severe ptosis is 4.0 mm or more. One can assess the amount of ptosis by measuring vertical lids slits with a millimeter rule if lower lid positions are normal and if ptosis is unilateral. On the average, the vertical lid slit normally measures 9 to 10 mm in children and 10 to 11 mm in adults. If for one reason or another vertical lid slits are not useful measurements to take (not all patients can cooperate or ptosis may be bilateral), other measurements are useful to have in mind for assessing the amount of ptosis. The vertical distance between the 12 o'clock and 6 o'clock limbus is approximately 11.0 mm. The normal upper lid covers the upper limbus by approximately 2.0 mm. Having these data in mind can allow the examiner to measure deviations from the norm and estimate the amount of ptosis.

Perhaps the most important assessment of the amount of ptosis can be attained through photographs. Of great assistance to the surgeon is the presence of photographs taped to the X-ray view box in the operating room, showing primary position, up gaze, down gaze, and closure. The subtleties of the amount of ptosis, lid contour, and levator function can be constantly reevaluated as the operation proceeds.

Synkinesis

Is synkinesis present or absent? This should always be determined preoperatively by history or by having the child chew gum or bite down on a tongue blade. More importantly, if the patient has ptosis *and* synkinesis, which of the two concerns the patient and parents more? Is it the ptosis? Is it the bizarre eyelid movement with chewing? Are both equally disturbing? The answers to these questions will have a major impact on the selection of operation for ptosis repair.

Lid Contour

One must document in any ptosis case details of the lid contour:

1. Is the lid crease present or absent? It is often faintly present or absent in severe ptosis with poor levator function.
2. Is the lid crease higher on the ptotic as compared to the nonptotic side? Such a finding is highly suggestive of an aponeurotic disorder, particularly if the ptosis is acquired and levator function is good to excellent.
3. Is the ptosis more severe nasally or temporally? It is not unusual for ptosis to be more significant nasally or temporally, and this is important, particularly in levator resection surgery when one can compensate for asymmetry in ptosis by performing a skewed levator resection.

4. Where is the highest point of the lid arch on the nonptotic side? In most instances the highest point of the normal lid arch is situated just nasal to the pupillary axis in primary position, but this is not always true, and if it is not the case, repair of the ptotic side may need to include suture adjustments to allow lid contour to resemble the nonptotic side.

General Eye Examination

Obviously every patient with ptosis requires the recording of a complete and thorough general eye examination, including a dilated pupil fundus exam. Visual acuity, retinoscopy, and measurement of ocular rotations are of particular interest to the ptosis surgeon.

Measurement of the visual field in ptosis patients has now become standard documentation to represent ptosis surgery as functional in nature. Most insurance companies require a visual field showing the lid in the down position and a visual field with the lid raised. Within the general exam, if it is apparent that there are signs of possible neurologic disease undiagnosed, (e.g., Horner's syndrome), it goes without saying that these must be pursued with a neurologic work-up before any corrective ptosis surgery is undertaken.

Photography

Photographs of the patient before and after the surgery are now considered a standard part of documentation of the patient's condition. Clear photographs are very helpful to the surgeon to demonstrate to patients certain aspects of their ptosis that may be unusual, and aid the surgeon at the time of surgery in adjusting minor contour variations, and postoperatively will be reassuring to patients when they see the improvement in the eyelid position. A standard Polaroid camera with a close-up lens is an adequate instrument for this photographic documentation. A detailed discussion of the use of photography in oculoplastic surgery can be found in Chapter 1.

PROBLEM PATIENTS ENCOUNTERED IN THE CORRECTION OF PTOSIS

Despite an adequate work-up of the ptosis patient ahead of time and the application of an appropriate surgical technique for correction, the ptosis surgeon may encounter other problems that will not only preclude an optimal result but may result in postoperative complications. As the surgeon gains experience with a larger number of ptosis patients, he or she can learn to identify the type of patient that is most likely to present this type of difficulty; these should be classified as "problem patients" (Table 3). A review of a variety of these types of complications will be undertaken here, but this certainly does not imply that these are the only problem cases that may be encountered. It has been previously mentioned that patients with poor eye protective mechanisms should be identified before surgery and warned of the possibility of corneal exposure. This is the most important problem patient to identify because of the possibility of visual damage in these patients.

Many patients encountered will have an unstable upper lid because of deficient tarsus. This presents a problem in correction because the purchase of the eyelid, whether it be from the pull of the levator or the pull of the frontalis suspension, will be uneven and will cause rotation of the lid. These patients are encountered most commonly following surgery in which part of the tarsus has been removed with hamartomatous infiltration of the lid causing it to be much more flexible and unstable, and in many cases of congenital

TABLE 3. *Problems encountered in ptosis surgery patients*

Poor eye protective mechanisms
Deficient tarsus
Paralytic/immobile brow
Eyelid hamartoma
Floppy upper lid
Tarsal shift with involutional ptosis
Co-existent ocular eyelid anomalies
Asymmetric ptosis
Chronic brow elevation
Blepharochalasis syndrome
Canthal dehiscence

anophthalmos and blepharophimosis syndrome with a hypoplastic tarsal plate. Many times, stability to the upper lid can be accomplished with horizontal tightening. In severe cases, grafting of ear cartilage or other stabilizing materials must be performed ahead of time to produce a stable upper lid.

In the presence of a paralytic eyebrow or an eyebrow that has been immobilized from scar tissue, it is extremely difficult to get a full correction utilizing a frontalis suspension. It is universally common to see an undercorrection in these patients, and the patient must be informed of this ahead of time.

The presence of hamartomatous tissue, such as neurofibromas or lymphangiomas, is notoriously difficult in that it tends to recur, causing recurrence of the ptosis, and to produce instability of the tarsus, and may produce severe technical difficulties during surgery. If possible, it may be expeditious to excise all of the hamartomatous tissue from the upper lid and reconstruct it before the ptosis surgery is undertaken.

In older patients and patients who have prosthetic eyes, a very loose and floppy upper lid presents severe difficulties for contour correction and maintenance of eyelid stability when performing ptosis surgery. This is usually more of a problem with the frontalis suspension patient. A horizontal tightening procedure should be performed in conjunction with the levator procedure in patients with floppy or loose upper lids. If one does encounter separation of the eyelid from the globe or notching or contour problems during attempted adjustment at ptosis surgery, one must suspect a floppiness or looseness of the upper lid, and it should be corrected by horizontal tightening.

In many patients with involutional ptosis, a myopathic process in the levator with abiotrophy and dehiscence of the medial horn of the levator and Whitnall's ligament causes outward migration and lateral shift of the tarsal plate (Fig. 1). The peak of the tarsal plate, which is normally centered above the pupil, may be shifted laterally out past the lateral limbus, and if one performs the ptosis surgery at the peak of the tarsus laterally, then one would universally get a temporal overcorrection. This problem must be identified and the contouring sutures must be moved nasally to acquire proper contour of the upper lid.

Congenital cases may have many co-existing problems that must be identified. The co-existing hamartomatous lesions have been mentioned, and the blepharophimosis syndrome has its own additional anomalies and that must be corrected to produce a satisfactory result. It is essential that the ocular function in congenital ptosis be assessed to rule out the high incidence of amblyopia, anisometropia, astigmatism, and strabismus.

Many patients with an asymmetric ptosis will mask the less ptotic eyelid with voluntary effort. Postoperatively, if only the severely ptotic side is corrected, the patient will suddenly

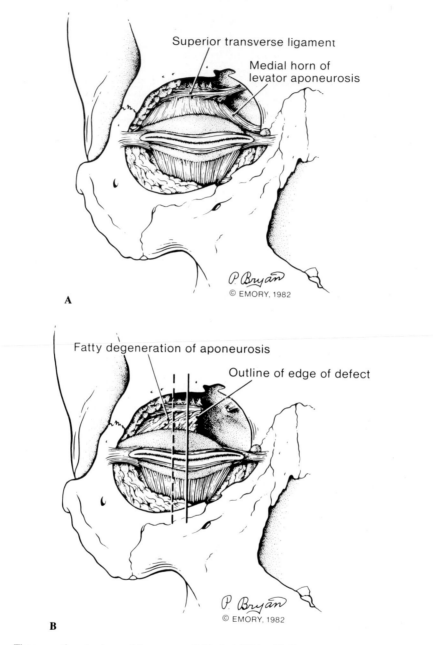

FIG. 1A. The supporting structures of the upper eyelid include Whitnall's ligament (superior transverse ligament) and the medial and lateral expansions (horns) of the levator aponeurosis which, if intact, hold the tarsus in its normal position. **B:** In some cases of involutional blepharoptosis, the medial supporting structures of the upper eyelid are attenuated or missing, leaving a defect that can be seen at surgery. The defect allows the tarsus to shift laterally, shown by the broken line representing the central portion of the laterally displaced tarsal plate. (From Shore and McCord, ref. 28, with permission. © 1984, The Ophthalmic Publishing Company.)

manifest a more severe ptosis in the contralateral side in which the milder ptosis was present. It is very important to recognize this asymmetry and compensatory effort of the patient, point this out to the patient ahead of time, and undertake bilateral surgery to correct it.

The position of the brow in the ptotic eye many times is elevated because of the conscious effort of the patient to open the ptotic eye. Patients with long-standing ptosis may continue to have chronic brow elevation despite a successful correction of the ptosis. This will produce an asymmetrical appearance and a higher lid crease. It must be pointed out to the patients ahead of time that they must learn to relax their brows postoperatively in order to have a symmetrical appearance.

The blepharochalasis syndrome is a rare condition occurring in young people, mainly females, with recurrent idiopathic edema of the eyelid. Recurrent severe swelling of the eyelid results in stretching of the skin and levator aponeurosis, and atrophy of the fat. These patients are correctable but usually require multiple surgical procedures, including blepharoplasty, dermal-fat grafting to correct fat atrophy, and correction of canthal dehiscence that may take place.

Canthal dehiscence can occur in the blepharochalasis syndrome from repeated stretching and can also occur in the involutional patient. It produces a phimotic appearance of the eyelid, and the patients usually complain of a web of skin between the upper and lower lids. In actuality, the upper and lower limb of the canthal tendon has been detached or stretched from the orbital rim, causing this appearance. This canthal dehiscence can mask a true ptosis with a pseudo–upper lid retraction. It is important to point out to the patient that the canthal dehiscence must be corrected if the phimotic appearance of the lid is to be corrected, and that additional surgery may be required to correct the ptosis of the upper lid.

PRINCIPLES OF SURGICAL MANAGEMENT OF PTOSIS

After the surgeon has successfully characterized the ptosis patient, assigned an etiology to the cause, and performed the previously described steps of preoperative evaluation, the decision must then be made on the proper surgical procedure to be used to repair the ptosis. The single most important factor in the choice of surgical procedure is the amount of levator function (Table 4). It is a well-recognized fact that patients who have more levator function have a much better response to levator surgery than those who do not. Another modifying factor in the quantitation of ptosis surgery is the fact that, regardless of levator function, patients with acquired ptosis have a greater response or ''lift'' of the lid to levator surgery than do congenital ptosis patients.

There are three basic procedures to repair ptosis. A frontalis suspension procedure is used in those patients with poor levator function. Resection of the levator may be performed

TABLE 4. *Choice of ptosis procedure with regard to levator function*[a]

Levator function	Procedure
0 to 5 mm (poor)	Frontalis suspension
6 to 10 mm (moderate)	External resection (Berke type)
10+ mm (excellent)	Aponeurotic surgery

[a] Patients with poor eye protective mechanisms must be approached with a reversible procedure, for which the frontalis suspension with the silicone rod offers an excellent alternative.

but will invariably lead to undercorrection. The second generic procedure is the levator resection procedure (as popularized by Berke), in which extensive dissection of the levator aponeurosis and Müller's muscle is carried out. This is applied to those patients with moderate levator function. The third basic procedure is that of aponeurotic surgery or surgery on the anterior portion of the levator muscle as it inserts in the lid. This can take the form of aponeurotic repair or anterior aponeurotic resection. This procedure lends itself well to those patients with excellent to normal levator function and requires a minimum amount of dissection.

Other procedures have been prescribed for patients in this specific category of excellent levator function, such as the Fasanella-Servat procedure and the external tarsal aponeurectomy. Both of these procedures involve excision of the tarsal plate and, although effective, are falling into a less desirable category because they must be viewed as nonanatomic procedures that require excision of the tarsus, which introduces possible instability to the eyelid.

The cutoff points in amount of levator function that are used to group patients into the poor, moderate, and good categories remains rather arbitrary among ptosis surgeons. In general, patients with 4 to 5 mm of levator function or less must be considered to have poor levator function, those with between 5 and 10 mm to have moderate levator function, and those with above 10 to 11 mm to have good levator function.

One factor that may override levator function as a consideration in selection of the type of procedure appropriate for a specific ptosis patient is the presence of eye protective mechanisms. In patients with poor Bell's phenomenon or dry eyes from any cause, one must consider only a ptosis procedure that can be reversed easily and preferably one that can be adjusted downward in the office. Exposure following ptosis surgery is one of the most dreadful complications that one can encounter and is visually threatening. The patient who has this risk potential should be treated very cautiously with any ptosis procedure.

A procedure that is useful in third nerve palsy, myasthenia gravis, and chronic external ophthalmoplasia is the frontalis suspension procedure with silicone rod implants, which can be adjusted postoperatively in the office if necessary. This will be described, and is recommended because of its safety.

The following sections will describe the various methods of ptosis repair, including: frontalis suspension with the use of autogenous fascia lata, frontalis suspension with the use of the silicone rod, external resection of levator with dissection (Berke-style external levator resection), and methods of anterior aponeurotic surgery. The Fasanella-Servat procedure will also be described because it is still quite a useful procedure in experienced hands. Because of the problems mentioned (excision of tarsus and the nonanatomic nature of the procedure), it is to be emphasized that this procedure should be used only by the experienced surgeon because of potential serious complications in certain groups of patients. The Fasanella-Servat procedure has been largely replaced by the newer, more anatomic, aponeurotic approach to ptosis surgery in patients with excellent levator function. The method of levator excision for the correction of patients with Marcus-Gunn jaw-winking ptosis will also be discussed.

SURGICAL METHODS OF REPAIR

Ptosis Surgery on Patients with Excellent Levator Function

The patients in this category, by and large, are the involutional patients, most of whom have an aponeurotic defect. Three repair techniques will be described: the levator aponeurosis repair under local anesthesia with adjustment of the lid position with voluntary opening of the patient's eyes, aponeurotic resection and repair and adjustment by gapping of the eyelids without voluntary patient eye opening, and the Fasanella-Servat procedure.

Levator Aponeurosis Repair

Classic signs suggesting the presence of an aponeurotic defect causing ptoses include (a) significant ptosis (commonly, but not always, as much as 3–4 mm), (b) good to excellent levator function, (c) a high lid fold, and (d) thinning of the upper eyelid tissues. Figures 2A through 2E show photographs of such a patient. Note the significant ptosis with the high lid fold in Fig. 2A. Levator excursion is excellent, as shown in Figs. 2B and 2C. (Note also in Fig. 2C that the palpebral fissure is more narrow in down gaze on the ptotic side, a hallmark of acquired ptosis.) Closure is normal, as shown in Fig. 2D, and one can observe, as in Fig. 2E, the color of the underlying iris because of marked thinning of the upper eyelid tissues.

A simplified schematic of upper eyelid anatomy in sagittal section is depicted in Fig. 3A. Three of the major attachments of the levator complex are demonstrated, including Müller's muscle, which inserts into the upper tarsal border, the anterior tarsal attachments of the aponeurosis that insert primarily onto the lower one-third of anterior tarsus, and the aponeurotic bands that penetrate the orbicularis muscle and insert into the skin, creating the lid crease. In the involutional ptosis patient, lid crease attachments remain intact (Fig. 3B); however, the anterior tarsal attachments are defective and, with stretching or disinsertion,

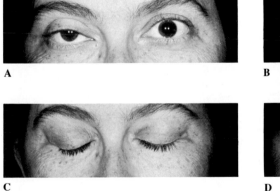

A

B

C

D

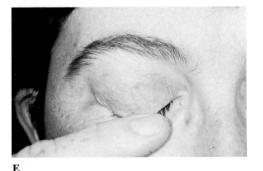

E

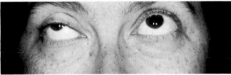

FIG. 2. **A:** Ptosis with a high lid fold. **B and C:** Levator excursion. **D:** Closure is normal. **E:** One can observe the underlying iris because of marked thinning of the upper eyelid tissues.

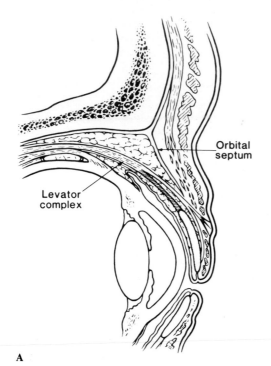

Orbital
septum

Levator
complex

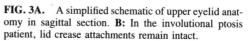

FIG. 3A. A simplified schematic of upper eyelid anatomy in sagittal section. **B:** In the involutional ptosis patient, lid crease attachments remain intact.

A

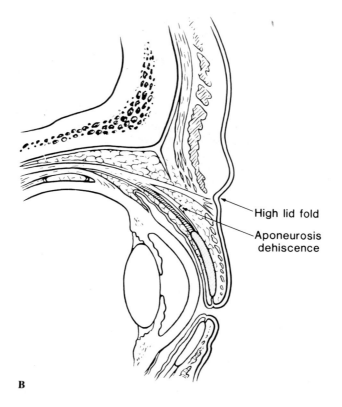

High lid fold

Aponeurosis
dehiscence

B

ptosis occurs. The preservation of lid crease attachments allows creation of the high lid crease and explains the usual finding of good to excellent lid excursion, often in the presence of significant ptosis.

Indications

One can reasonably argue that most, if not all, involutional ptosis cases are caused primarily by abnormalities in the distal aponeurosis, which lends itself readily to repair by the technique to be described. Most ptosis surgeons approach the involutional ptosis patient solely by aponeurosis repair.

At least some post-ophthalmic-surgery ptosis patients have ptosis because of aponeurotic defects, and they should be repaired by a direct approach to the distal aponeurosis. This is true also for the blepharochalasis patients, many of whom may be in the younger age groups.

A history of trauma, often associated with prolonged lid edema, should alert the surgeon to search for signs of aponeurosis disinsertions, as should the history of insect bites, especially bee stings. Finally, Anderson and Gordy have called to our attention that a small but significant number of patients with congenital ptosis may have aponeurotic defects requiring repair as described below (27).

Surgical technique, pitfalls

Local anesthesia is desirable, because aponeurosis repair under general anesthesia for most surgeons can be a formidable task. One-half to 0.75 ml of a short-acting infiltrative anesthetic placed along the site of the intended lid crease, just beneath the skin, is usually all that is necessary.

A lid crease incision is made at the desired level, usually near the upper border of the tarsal plate (Fig. 4A). Avoid the pitfall of marking the lid crease incision too high; this is easy to do when the pathophysiology is such that a high lid crease exists preoperatively. Gentle separation of the orbicularis muscle horizontally will expose the orbital septum, which can then be horizontally incised, exposing preaponeurotic fat.

At this point in the procedure, it is wise to gently retract skin, muscle, orbital septum, and orbital fat at the superior edge of the wound. More importantly, the scissors should be discarded and surgical dissection should be blunt, preferably with cotton-tipped applicators, to avoid the pitfall of inadvertent injury to the aponeurosis. Blunt retraction of preaponeurotic fat will allow the distal aponeurosis to become identified (Fig. 4B).

We employ three 5–0 Prolene sutures to perform the repair (Fig. 4C), placing a double-armed suture into the nasal, central, and temporal-most edge of the aponeurosis. Shown in Fig. 4D, the 5–0 Prolene sutures are used to secure the levator aponeurosis to the anterior surface of the tarsus. Incorporating these sutures into the skin of the wound edges (Fig. 4E) allows for the preservation of the lid fold along with ptosis repair and usually precludes the need to place additional skin sutures, unless blepharoplasty has been performed concomitantly.

Complications

Failure to place one's sutures precisely in the distal defective aponeurosis is a potential complication. Proper identification of the aponeurosis is confirmed once the initial sutures are secured by having the patient look up and down with maximum effort. When performed under local anesthesia, the glistening aponeurosis will move with lid excursion and be readily identified, so that this improper identification of tissue planes may be avoided.

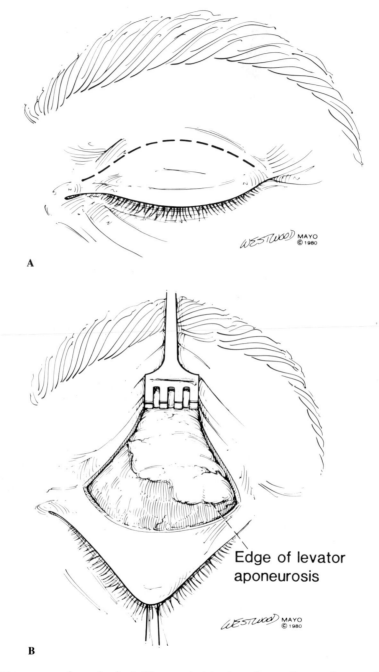

FIG. 4. Levator aponeurosis repair. **A:** A lid crease incision is made, usually near the upper border of the tarsal plate. **B:** Blunt retraction of preaponeurotic fat will allow the distal aponeurosis to become identified.

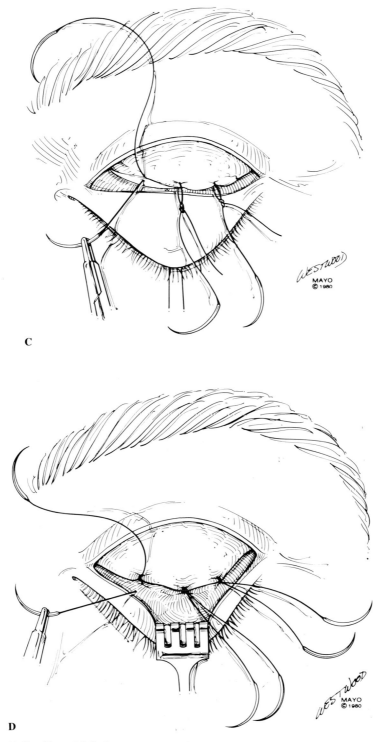

FIG. 4 (*cont.*) **C:** Three 5-0 Prolene sutures are used to perform the repair. **D:** The aponeurosis is sutured to the anterior surface of the tarsus.

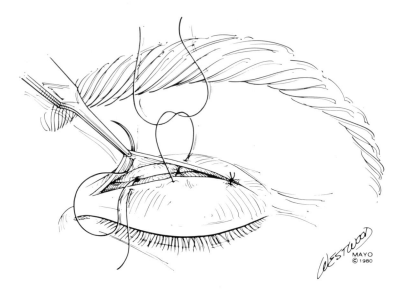

FIG. 4 (*cont.*) **E:**   The double-armed suture is incorporated into the skin of the wound edges.

Overcorrection and undercorrection can occur and can be corrected quickly, one or more days postoperatively, by adjusting the sutures. We prefer generally to place our sutures at the time of operation so that the lid arch falls at or near the upper limbus, that is, slightly higher (0.5 mm) than the anticipated final position of the lid, which is in contrast to the general philosophy for repair of acquired ptoses. If the lid position is too high postoperatively, it is usually easier to remove a suture to allow the lid to fall than it is to readjust sutures to compensate for undercorrection.

Lid arch peaking or obliquity is usually noted at the operating table and should be corrected when recognized. In our experience arch asymmetry results from sutures that are tied too tightly or are placed too far down on the anterior tarsal surface. Perhaps the most exciting feature in performing this procedure is the usual absence of lid arch deformities. Aponeurosis repair, if correctly performed, provides the most natural lid arch of any ptosis operation thus far devised.

Preoperative bilateral aponeurosis disinsertions are shown in Fig. 5A. Postoperative appearance 3 months following aponeurosis repair is depicted in Fig. 5B.

Levator Aponeurosis Surgery by the Gapping Method without Patient Cooperation

An alternative method of aponeurosis surgery is sometimes needed that does not involve patient cooperation. This occasion arises when the aponeurosis surgery must be done under general anesthesia, or if the patient is uncooperative under local anesthesia as far as gaze and eye opening, or if the local anesthetic infiltrated affects movement of the levator and the patient is unable to cooperate because of levator anesthesia.

The exposure of the aponeurosis is similar, as described in the previous procedure, but is reillustrated for the reader's convenience (Fig. 6). A lid crease incision is made through the musculocutaneous layer with dissection into the orbital septum and the pretarsal area, as shown in Fig. 6A. The levator aponeurosis is then opened while the lid is under tension, preferably using the cutting needle Bovie. In some patients, the aponeurosis may be extremely

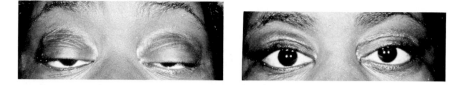

FIG. 5. **(Left)** Preoperative bilateral aponeurosis. **(Right)** Postoperative appearance 3 months following aponeurosis repair. (Courtesy of John D. Bullock, M.D., Dayton, Ohio.)

rarified because of the pathologic state of the aponeurosis. Figure 6B shows the incision made through the aponeurosis exposing the superior vascular arcade found just above the tarsal plate, which is very tortuous and lies in the superficial portion of Müller's muscle. With the aponeurosis procedure, it is not necessary to involve Müller's muscle or the superior arcade, and good dissection can be performed sparing those structures and reducing the amount of bleeding during the procedure. After the levator is dissected free from Müller's muscle and separated superiorly so that a suture can be passed underneath, a 6–0 silk suture with a small cutting needle is then introduced one-half thickness into the tarsal plate at the juncture of the lower two-thirds and upper one-third of the tarsus. This can be a double-armed suture that which is brought out through the levator aponeurosis or the muscular portion of the levator, as shown in Fig. 6C. This suture is the central lifting suture and it should be placed at the exact vertical plane of the pupil. This becomes extremely important in dealing with involutional patients who have, in many cases, a lateral displacement of the tarsal plate.

Figure 1A shows the normal anatomic structures, as one perceives them to be present in patients for ptosis surgery, and Fig. 1B shows a common occurrence in the involutional patients who have loss of integrity of the medial horn of the levator because of degeneration in the aponeurosis and levator, which allows the tarsal plate to shift laterally. If one uses the central position of the tarsus to introduce the central suture, then the entire ptosis procedure will be performed lateral to the pupillary plane and a so-called *temporal flare* will be encountered postoperatively (28). In many cases, the central lifting suture in the involutional patient will be, in effect, placed in the nasal portion of the tarsus. To quantitate the ptosis correction in these patients by the gapping method, a formula has been developed that has a good degree of predictability correlating the gapping of the eyelid at the surgical table with the postoperative position of the eyelid. Figure 6D shows the calipers being used to measure the gapping of the eyelid. In general, the patients with acquired ptosis are gapped on the operating table 1 mm more than the amount of ptosis one wishes to correct. In congenital cases, the amount of gapping is 3 mm more than the amount of ptosis that one wishes to correct. This means that in a patient with acquired ptosis of 3 mm the eyelids will be gapped 5 mm on the operating room table, and in a patient with congenital ptosis of 3 mm the eyelids will be gapped 7 mm on the operating room table. It is to be emphasized that there are other variables involved, that all formulas are simply a starting point, and that each ptosis surgeon must adapt these formulas to his or her own specific technique.

After the gapping has been obtained with the central lifting suture, additional nasal and temporal sutures to ensure proper contour are then placed, as shown in Fig. 6E. It is to be emphasized that three sutures must be used because the additional two sutures must act as suspenders to maintain the lid contour when orbicularis tone returns. The surgeon

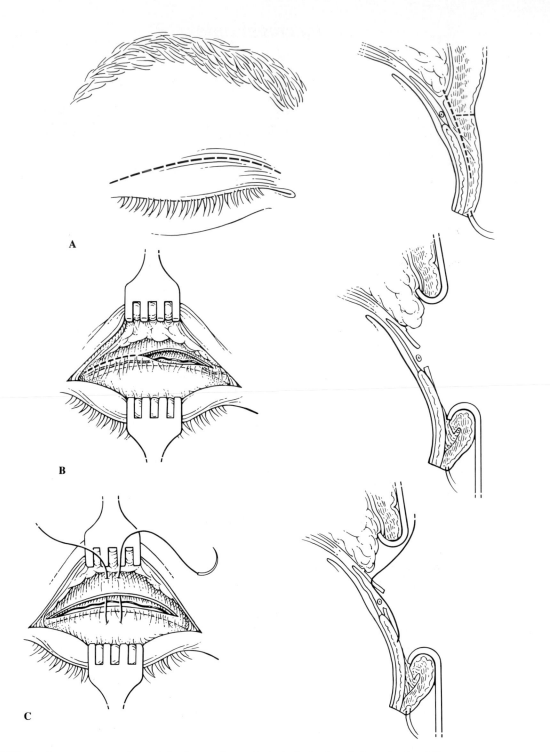

FIG. 6. Levator aponeurosis repair by the gapping method. **A:** In the frontal view, the *dotted line* represents the incision line across the upper lid crease. The cross-sectional view indicates that the dissection is carried into the orbital septum and the pretarsal tissues. **B:** Following the incision and dissection as indicated in Fig. 6A, retraction exposes the anterior surface of the tarsus and the levator aponeurosis. The frontal view indicates the incision line along which the levator aponeurosis is disinserted from the tarsus. The superior marginal vascular arcade is visualized underneath the levator. **C:** A central lifting suture in the pupillary plane is used to anastomose the tarsus to the levator aponeurosis or the levator muscle.

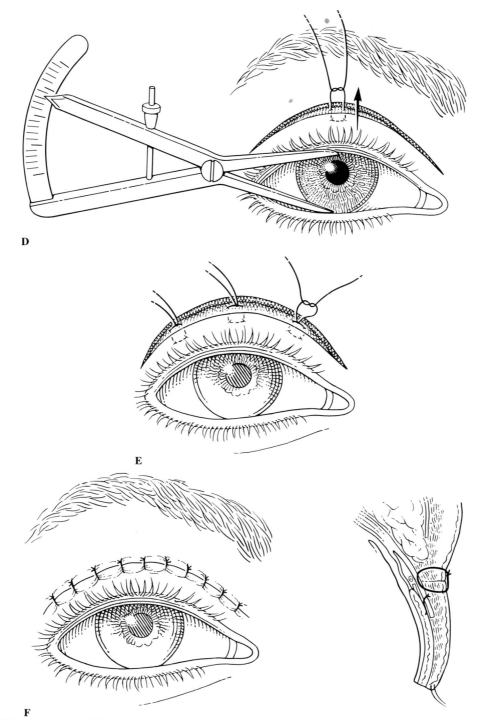

FIG. 6 (cont.) D: With the central lifting suture secured, a caliper is used to measure the eyelid gapping, as described in the text. **E:** The placement of medial and lateral tarsus–to–levator sutures maintains an even lid contour. **F:** Everting sutures are used for final musculocutaneous closure. The cross-sectional view demonstrates the lid crease formation via supratarsal fixation of the musculocutaneous edge to the levator.

must be forewarned in the patients with lateral tarsal shift that the temporal suture must
be tied in a conservative manner to avoid the "temporal flare." Figure 6F shows final lid
closure with attachment of the musculocutaneous edges to the levator aponeurosis at the
superior tarsal border.

Fasanella-Servat Procedure (Tarsomyectomy)

The Fasanella-Servat procedure is commonly termed a conjunctival approach levator
resection, but in reality very little tissue is removed except for the upper tarsus, supratarsal
conjunctiva, and some of Müller's muscle (29). Histologic studies of the specimens demonstrate that levator aponeurosis is rarely present (30).

Indications

Tarsomyectomy should usually be chosen in those situations where there is mild to
moderate ptosis, with good to excellent levator function. Whereas most patients with involutional ptosis are better treated by aponeurosis repair, tarsomyectomy can be employed in
those situations where there is 2.0 mm or less of ptosis. Late-acquired hereditary ptosis is
usually accompanied by good to excellent levator function, and at some point in the management of this problem tarsomyectomy may be useful. Management of Horner's syndrome
may include tarsomyectomy as an alternative to the performance of Müller's muscle resection.
Ptosis is usually mild, and levator function excellent. Some patients with myopathic ptosis
(chronic progressive external ophthalmoplegia, myotonic dystrophy, myasthenia gravis,
steroid-induced ptosis, and the ptosis of pregnancy) respond to tarsomyectomy (31). When
levator function is less than good, this procedure is occasionally useful in the myopathic
group of patients when one is attempting to elevate the eyelid for functional rather than
cosmetic purposes.

Surgical technique, pitfalls

Local anesthesia may be used, infiltrating along the upper border of the tarsus sbuconjucti-
vally with the lid everted (Fig. 7A). When everting the lid, do so gently and do not push
the skin and orbicularis into the crease, for it is possible, especially on reoperations, to
include these tissues in the clamp and excise a full-thickness defect into the lid. Gentle
massage of the eyelid held over a Desmarres retractor after infiltration will help to distribute
the anesthetic evenly and will help to minimize distortion of the soft tissues (Fig. 7B).

We prefer to use curved hemostats to perform the operation, because their placement
can compensate readily for the variable sizes of the tarsus in any given patient. Figure 7C
demonstrates the *wrong* way to place the clamps. Placing the hemostats in such a manner
allows for excessive tarsal excision centrally and thus causes peaking of the lid arch with
an undesirable cosmetic result. Figure 7D demonstrates the *correct* way to place the clamps.
The points of the clamps should meet at a level that is approximately above the pupil or
at the position where the highest point of the lid arch is desired: The points of the clamps
should also be directed slightly toward the patient's feet. Consequently, a lesser amount
of tarsus is resected centrally, peaking of the lid arch is minimized, and the arch has a
more natural appearance.

We prefer to use a 6–0 plain double-armed suture; this suture is placed from the temporal
to the nasal aspect of the lid in serpiginous fashion, 1.5 mm beneath the clamps (Figs.
7E and 7F). The clamps are then removed, and the tissues in the clamp are excised,
generally within the bed of the crush marks left by the clamp (Figs. 7G and 7H).

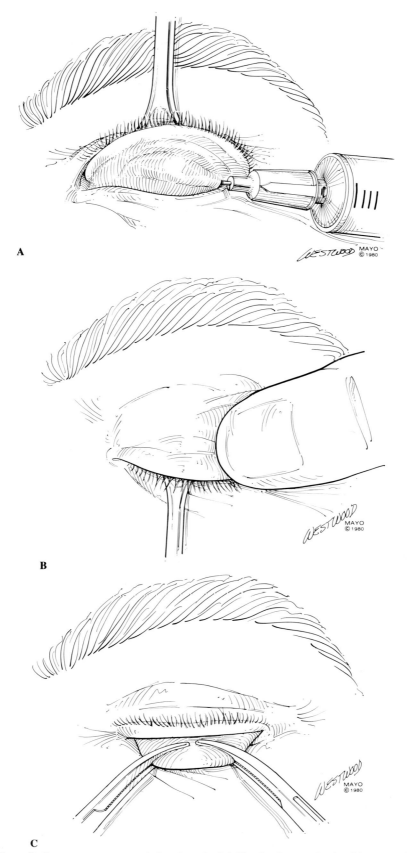

FIG. 7. Fasanella-Servat tarsomyectomy. **A:** Local anesthesia infiltrating the upper border of the tarsus subconjunctivally with the lid everted. **B:** Gentle massage of the eyelid to help distribute the anesthetic evenly. **C:** The *wrong* way to place the clamps. **D:** The *correct* way to place the clamps.

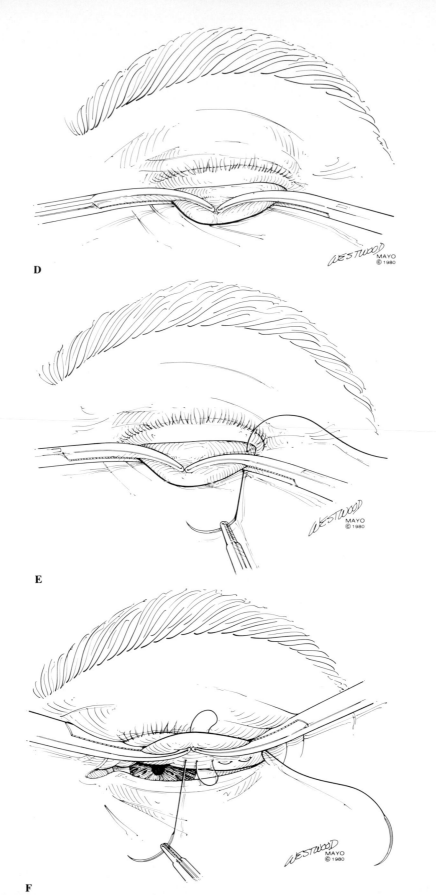

D

E

F

FIGS. 7E and F. A 6-0 plain double-armed suture is placed from the temporal to the nasal aspect of the lid in serpiginous fashion, 1.5 mm beneath the clamps.

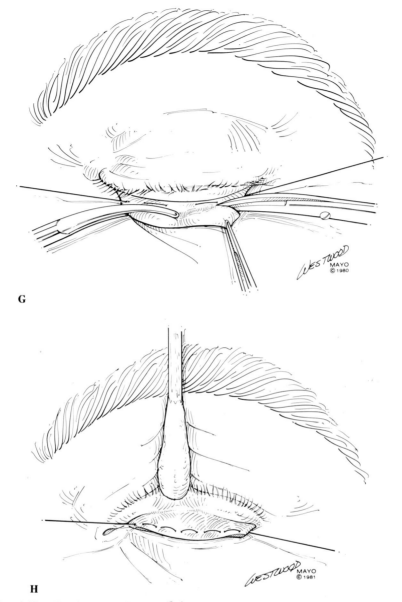

G

H

FIGS. 7G and H. The clamps are removed, and the tissues that were in the clamp are excised, generally within the bed of the crush marks left by the clamp.

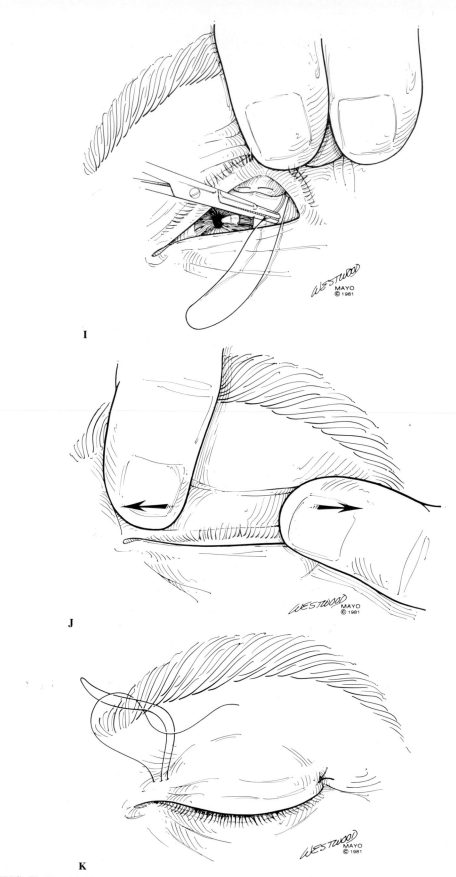

I

J

K

FIGS. 7I, 7J, and 7K. Each end of the double-armed suture is passed through the full thickness of the eyelid, into the lid fold, and tied into the skin after gentle massage to distribute equally the tension in the suture line.

Each end of the double-armed suture is then passed through the full thickness of the eyelid nasally and temporally (as suggested by Bullock), into the lid fold, and tied into the skin after gentle massage to distribute equally the tension in the suture line. The procedure is then complete (Figs. 7I, 7J, and 7K).

Complications

The most common complication of tarsomyectomy relates to the faulty placement of the clamps. This takes some practice to do correctly. If the clamps are not placed properly and the lid arch is "peaked" postoperatively, it is best to do nothing for a few days. In 3 to 4 days, one can snip the suture at the site of the peak and gently stretch the lid to smooth out the irregularity. Slight peaking can exist because of sutures that are too tight. Massage at the operating table can minimize peaking at times (see Fig. 7J). If the clamps are placed more temporally then they should be or if more tarsus is resected temporally than nasally (which generally is the reverse of what it should be), then one gets a disturbing "temporal flare" that can only be corrected by levator tenotomy.

The next most frequent complication is cutting the suture, either with a scissors or with the edge of the cutting needle. One cannot tie the suture together and leave a knot on the conjunctival surface. Simply rethread another double-armed suture and proceed as previously planned.

Postoperative keratitis is a disturbing problem, but usually is self-limited and subsides in 24 to 48 hr. This usually causes nothing but some mild discomfort to the patient and embarrassment to the surgeon. The use of 6–0 plain catgut, placed as described above, minimizes suture irritation, which presumably causes the keratitis.

Suture granuloma is rare, as is postoperative hemorrhage, but the latter can occur several days after surgery, usually during sleep. Because of this possibility, we recommend that a metal shield be worn for 14 days postoperatively during the sleeping hours.

Precautions

Beware of performing tarsomyectomy when other lid pathology is present. Examine the undersurface of each eyelid before scheduling ptosis repair. One may find some surprises (granuloma, lymphoma, amyloid) that may alter one's approach.

Beware of performing tarsomyectomy unilaterally when the patient has bilateral ptosis. Make certain that the matter of unilateral versus bilateral ptosis is settled before the operative procedure is initiated.

Beware of keratitis sicca. Some ophthalmologists are critical of this procedure in such cases because normal eyelid tissues are excised. Performing this operation can place the patient with keratitis sicca at higher risk and therefore it should be used with caution. All tarsomyectomy patients should be evaluated preoperatively for tear deficiency.

Beware of excising more than 3 mm of tarsus. This procedure is difficult to quantify (as are all ptosis procedures). Small resections yield minimal results, large resections yield greater results, and only the experience of the individual surgeon will aid in quantifying the procedure. As a guide, however, a 3.0-mm resection should be considered as the upper level of maximum tarsomyectomy.

Preoperative left upper lid ptosis (Horner's syndrome) is depicted in Fig. 8A, and postoperative results after tarsomyectomy in Fig. 8B. Preoperative left upper lid ptosis, left lower lid ectropion, and a poorly fitting prosthesis are shown in Fig. 9A, and postoperative results after left upper lid tarsomyectomy, left lower lid ectropion repair are shown in Fig. 9B.

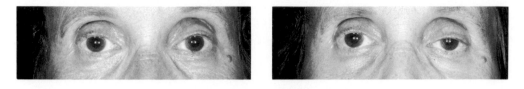

FIG. 8 **(Left)** Preoperative left upper lid ptosis. **(Right)** Postoperative repair by tarsomyectomy.

External Levator Resection

External levator resection as advocated by Leahy (32), and Johnson (33), and Berke (34) has stood the test of time as a sound surgical approach for a variety of ptosis problems. However, failure to pay meticulous attention to detail can yield a poor postoperative result. There are 10 major steps in this procedure. Pitfalls to avoid will be highlighted as each step is reviewed.

Indications

The first step has to do with patient selection and preoperative evaluation. External levator resection is ideally suited for most patients with moderate or severe congenital ptosis. It may be useful in the treatment of mild congenital ptosis or in the treatment of acquired ptosis, but one should consider alternatives for these problems, because there are other approaches that may be desirable.

Again, be certain of levator function. Many resections have been performed to perfection, only to have a disappointing result because of failure to assess properly levator function. Evaluating levator function is no different from evaluating strabismus. One is on more solid ground if the patient is studied more than once, and the data checked and rechecked, thus avoiding the major pitfall of faulty assessment of levator function.

Is there more ptosis temporally than nasally? Notation of this fact preoperatively allows the surgeon to slant or skew the resection so that asymmetry may be avoided.

Take photographs. They are another source of information, and they are helpful in minimizing postoperative misunderstandings.

Surgical Technique, Pitfalls

The second step relates to the lid crease incision (Fig. 10A). Ordinarily the lid crease incision is 25 mm long, at the level of the upper tarsal edge, curvilinear, and slightly closer to the lash line at the nasal and temporal ends of the lid. It is wise to visualize the

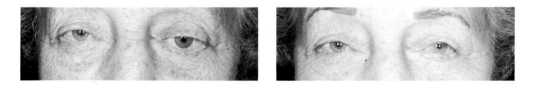

FIG. 9 **(Left)** Preoperative left upper lid ptosis. **(Right)** Postoperative repair by left upper lid tarsomyectomy, and repair of left lower lid ectropion.

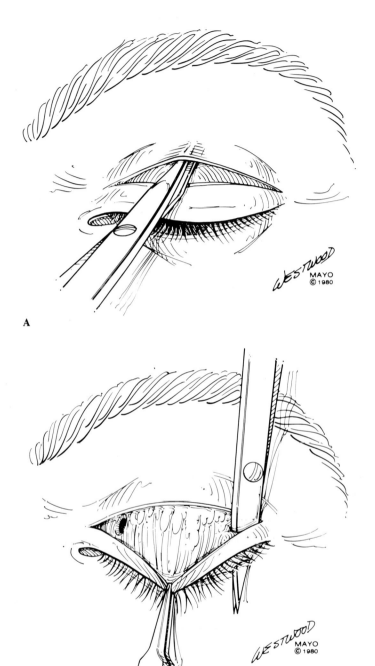

FIG. 10. External levator resection. **A:** Lid crease incision. **B:** The anterior tarsal surface exposed.

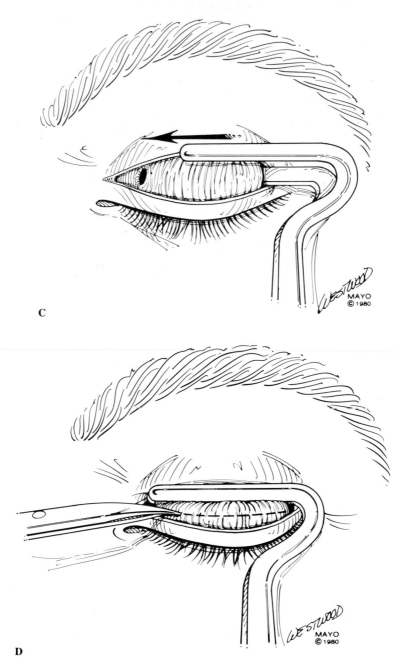

C

D

FIG. 10 (*cont.*) **C:** Isolating the levator complex and conjunctiva by punching through the nasal- and temporal-most ends of the skin incision. **D:** The ptosis clamp is applied at or near the upper edge of the tarsus.

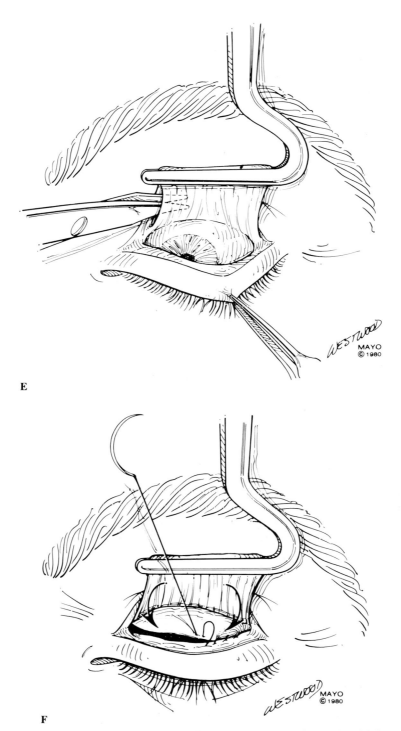

E

F

FIG. 10 (*cont.*) E: Dissection of the conjunctiva. **F:** Conjunctival closure is complete; Muller's muscle, the levator aponeurosis, and the orbital septum are contained in the ptosis clamp.

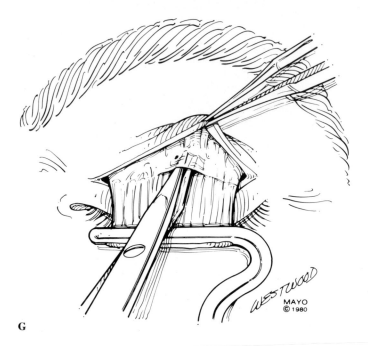

G

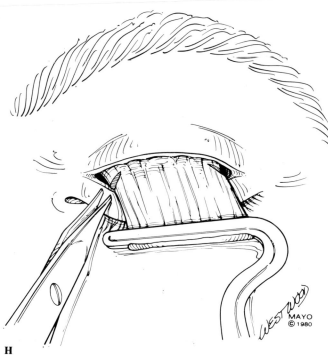

H

FIG. 10 (*cont.*) G: Orbital dissection of the levator complex. **H:** The orbital septum has been partially incised vertically, exposing preaponeurotic fat.

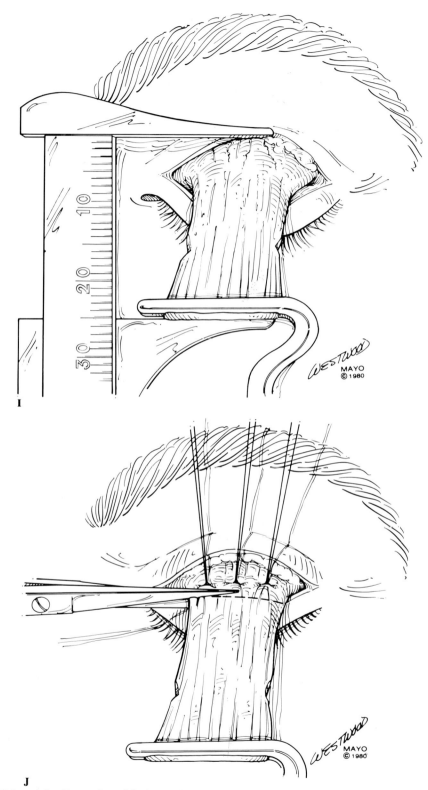

FIG. 10 *(cont.)* **I:** Transection of the levator horns. **J:** Additional attachments of the orbital septum are freed, and the levator complex comes easily into view. Resection is accomplished by straight scissors after three double-armed 5-0 catgut mattress sutures are placed just above the resection line.

359

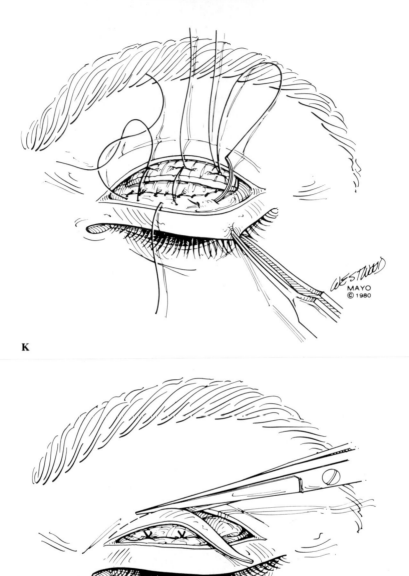

K

L

FIG. 10 (cont.) K: The resection of the levator complex is complete; tarsal sutures are placed. **L:** After resection is complete, skin excision is performed.

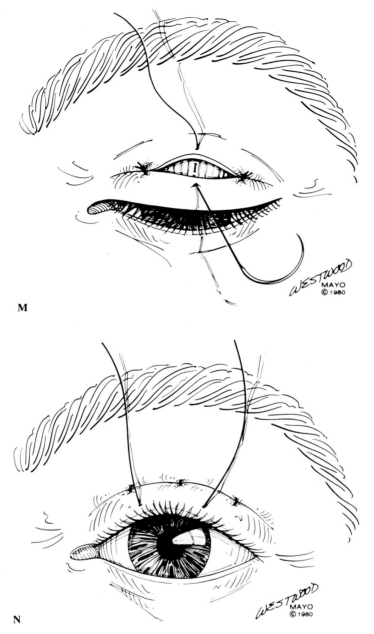

M

N

FIG. 10 (cont.) M: The placement of the tarsal sutures. **N:** The re-creation of the lid fold.

site of the intended lid crease incision in the office with the patient awake and seated, comparing the ptotic with the nonptotic side. An undercorrected lid arch may be salvaged by a perfectly placed lid crease. A perfectly corrected ptosis may be compromised by a lid crease that is too high or too low.

In the third step we expose the anterior tarsal surface (Fig. 10B). Skin and orbicularis muscle should be reflected from the anterior tarsal surface to allow for proper insertion of sutures later in the procedure. If this is done early, bleeding will subside and visualization for suture placement will not be compromised. Avoid the pitfall of too vigorous dissection toward the lash line, because trauma to the lash roots can result in loss of cilia.

In the fourth step it is very important to secure the distal levator complex early before extensive dissection takes place; this prevents wasted time searching for tissue planes, risking increased bleeding and potential levator injury. Isolating the levator complex and conjunctiva can be achieved quickly by punching through these structures at the nasal- and temporal-most ends of the skin incision (Fig. 10B). The "punch-through" maneuver should be done with the globe in full view.

Nasally, one should be superior to the canaliculus. Temporally, one should be inferior to the lacrimal gland ductules. The ptosis clamp (Fig. 10C, and 10D) should be applied at or near the upper edge of the tarsus. In detaching the levator complex, one should avoid excising excess tarsal plate, because excision is not necessary; it may make suture placement more difficult, and if too much tarsus is removed ectropion can result.

The fifth step is dissection of the conjunctiva (Fig. 10E). Loope magnification and/or saline injection to "balloon up" the conjunctiva is optional in removing conjunctiva from Müller's muscle. Blunt scissors minimize the risk of conjunctival laceration. Dissection should avoid the fornix attachments of the conjunctiva to prevent later conjunctival prolapse. Resuturing conjunctiva to the upper border of the tarsus can be accomplished with 6–0 catgut, which should be placed to avoid exposure to the globe. In Fig. 10F conjunctival closure is complete; Müller's muscle, levator aponeurosis, and orbital septum are contained in the ptosis clamp.

In the sixth step orbital dissection of the levator complex is initiated (Fig. 10G). Proper dissection depends upon identification of the orbital septum—the first goal is to separate the orbital septum from the anterior levator surface. A gentle ballottement of the orbital contents by using a cotton-tipped applicator against the lower lid will usually cause orbital fat to bulge forward behind the orbital septum. The most valuable sign to the surgeon performing levator resection is identification of preaponeurotic fat; upon finding the fat, he or she knows that the levator complex is just beneath to be quickly isolated and identified.

In the seventh step (Fig. 10H) we transect the levator horns. Severing of the horns should be done to avoid the trochlea nasally and the orbital lobe of the lacrimal gland temporally. Slightly curved scissors directed away from these structures will allow these pitfalls to be avoided. Once the levator horns are severed, additional attachments of the orbital septum may be freed, after which the levator complex should come easily into view (Fig. 10I).

There are two major approaches in quantitating the amount of levator to be resected in the external levator resection. A common method, one that is favored by Beard (1), is measuring the amount of levator that is "cut out." If this is the method to be used, one should proceed with the operation as described, measuring the amount of levator to be resected according to Table 5.

An alternate method, and one commonly used, is that described by Berke (34) in which one does not actually measure the amount of levator resected, but measures the amount

TABLE 5. *Choice of operation for congenital ptosis*

Amount of ptosis	Levator contraction amplitude	Levator resection
Normal (no ptosis)	Excellent (15 mm)	—
Mild (1–2 mm)	Good (8 mm or more)	10 to 12 mm
Moderate (3 mm)	Fair (5–7 mm)	18 mm
Severe (4 mm)	Poor (less than 4 mm)	24 mm
Severe (4 mm or more)	None (0 mm)	Frontalis sling

From Illif et al. (35) with permission.

of gapping or separation of the upper and lower eyelids on the operating room table, which is then correlated with the postoperative lid position. Berke, with a series of hundreds of patients, was able to make this correlation and has developed a table of the expected lift or fall of the lid postoperatively, according to how much levator function the patient has preoperatively. One advantage to this technique is that it does neutralize many surgical variables, such as how much the levator is stretched when measuring and how extensive a dissection is carried out. Table 6 illustrates the amount of gapping of the eyelid or the position of the upper lid in relationship to the upper limbus with the expected postoperative result. It has been adapted for use in patients who have levator function of from 5 to 10 mm. It is to be emphasized that no "formula" is perfect, and any formula is a starting point for the ptosis surgeon to make his or her own judgment. Only with experience can each individual ptosis surgeon adapt the formula to his or her specific techniques to gain predictable results.

The eighth step is the resection (Fig. 10J). If one has chosen to resect an amount of the levator complex based on preoperative measurements, the precise amount to be resected should be measured twice to make certain that suture placements are accurate; it is desirable to "measure the measuring device" once to twice to make certain that the instrument is not improperly set. Resection (Fig. 10J) can then be accomplished by straight scissors after three double-armed 5–0 catgut mattress sutures are placed just above the resection line.

The ninth step is placement of tarsal sutures (Fig. 10K). The three 5–0 chromic sutures should be placed anteriorly, usually within the lower third of the tarsus. Avoid placing them through full-thickness tarsus, because this can expose the globe to suture abrasion. Sutures should be tied first with a surgeon's knot. Any slippage at this point will promote undercorrection; after the knot is completely tied, careful inspection to look for slippage will avoid this pitfall. Suture should not incorporate orbital septum, because this will

TABLE 6. *Adaptation of berke's table for placement of ptotic lid for various amounts of levator action of congenital monocular ptosis when normal lid covers cornea 2 to 3 millimeters and the external approach is used*

Amount of levator action	Ptotic lid should cover cornea	Expected "lift"	Postoperative "fall"	Expected overcorrection
4 to 5 mm	1 to 2 mm	0 mm	0 to 1 mm	0 to 1 mm
6 to 7 mm	2 to 3 mm	0 to 1 mm	0 mm	0 to 1 mm
8 to 9 mm	3 to 4 mm	2 to 3 mm	0 mm	0 to 1 mm

Based on data in Berke (34).

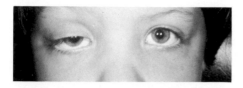
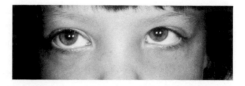

FIG. 11. Moderately severe congenital ptosis. Patient looking straight ahead, preoperatively **(left)** and postoperatively **(right)**.

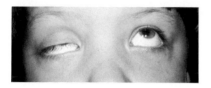
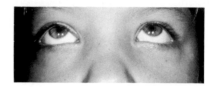

FIG. 11B. Patient looking up, preoperatively **(left)** and postoperatively **(right)**.

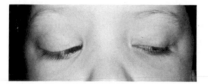
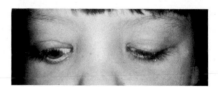

FIG. 11C. Patient looking down, preoperatively **(left)** and postoperatively **(right)**.

promote lagophthalmos. Pay particular attention to the temporal suture. Lid arch deformities are often the result of temporal sag, and this can be avoided.

The tenth step is re-creation of the lid crease (Figs. 10L–10N). In most levator resections, it is important to perform a small skin excision in order to avoid redundant skin in the newly elevated lid (Fig. 10L). It is critical to include in the skin closure sutures that will allow incorporation of the advanced levator complex into the closure. The blepharoplasty is usually small but should not be forgotten. Three 5–0 chromic catgut sutures are placed first through skin, then through advanced levator, then through skin (Fig. 10M). The closure is then completed. Additional skin sutures are optional. A Frost suture is placed to protect the eye for 24 hr (Fig. 10N).

The patient in Fig. 11 had moderately severe congenital ptosis. A 24-mm external levator resection was performed. Preoperative photos are on the left and 6 months postoperative photos are on the right.

Levator Excision for Correction of the Marcus-Gunn Jaw-winking Syndrome

The presence of jaw winking in children introduces a second anomaly in addition to the ptosis that may need correction. The general approach to these two problems, jaw winking and ptosis, depends on the severity of the wink or the excursion of the lid as the jaw is moved from side to side. If the wink excursion is very small, one should simply ignore the wink and proceed with the indicated ptosis surgery. If the excursion of the wink is large, then one must eliminate the wink before performing ptosis surgery because levator surgery may amplify the wink itself and aggravate the anomalous lid movement.

To inactivate the wink, it has been recommended, in the past, to inactivate the levator with excision; historically the excisions have been performed as an anterior levator resection followed by frontalis suspension. It has also been the habit to divide the procedure into two stages because if the frontalis suspension is inserted at the same time as the levator incision, there has been some recurrence of winking because of fibrous adhesions of the levator stump. There has also been a tendency for undercorrection in the lids in which the levator has been excised, leading Beard (1) to propose a bilateral levator excision with frontalis suspension.

The technique of levator excision proposed by Dillman and Anderson (36) and others, has provided the best approach to this problem in that the levator is excised behind Whitnall's ligament in the thin orbital portion, leaving the anterior levator, Whitnall's ligament, horns, and support structures intact. Upon excising levators in this manner, it has been noted that the undercorrection with subsequent frontalis suspension seen previously is no longer present.

Surgical Technique

A lid crease incision and dissection through the orbital septum, exposing the levator, is performed as described in the previous section. A retractor is used at Whitnall's ligament (small rake or skin hook) to retract the orbital portion of the levator anteriorly. A muscle hook is then inserted under the ribbon-like levator to isolate it from the surrounding tissue. At this point, forceps are introduced to grasp the superior rectus and make sure that it has not been also hooked in conjunction with the levator, since they travel together very closely. Once this has been ascertained, the hemostat is applied to the levator, just behind Whitnall's ligament and approximately 1 cm further in the orbit, and the segment of levator between the two clamps is excised and cauterized. An alternative is not to excise the levator but to incise it and suture the segment of the orbital portion to the orbital roof so that the levator pull is transmitted to the roof. This method also leaves the anterior portion of the levator attached.

Either method preserves the anterior support of the levator and prevents the undercorrection previously seen. The second stage of this procedure is to then repair the ptosis by frontalis muscle suspension (see following section).

Frontalis Muscle Suspension Procedures

Indications

The most common indication for frontalis suspension is the presence of bilateral severe congenital ptosis with very poor or no levator function (Fig. 12). Many (but not all) children with belpharophimosis syndrome (Fig. 13) also require frontalis suspension, because the ptosis is often severe and cannot be repaired by levator resection. In addition, children with synkinetic ptosis (Marcus-Gunn syndrome) pose special problems, as discussed in the previous section.

Levator resections for severe unilateral ptosis (Fig. 14) result in a high percentage of undercorrections, but asymmetry in blinking and vertical lid fissures, especially in down gaze, are also major problems. Levator resection in the synkinetic ptoses can not only exaggerate the synkinesis but also cause asymmetry. For these reasons, bilateral brow suspension procedures have been advocated for the above unilateral ptosis problems, especially by Beard (1), who feels that better symmetry is achieved with bilateral surgery (37). In the case of synkinetic ptosis, levator excision of the abnormal side is performed prior to bilateral brow suspension if the synkinesis is a significant cosmetic liability. Beard also advocates excision of the levator aponeurosis on the normal side because he has

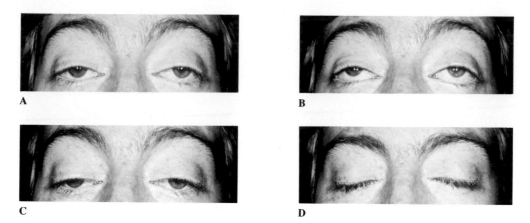

FIG. 12. The presence of bilateral severe congenital ptosis with very poor or nil levator function. **A:** Patient looking ahead. **B:** Patient looking up. **C:** Patient looking down. **D:** Patient with eyes closed.

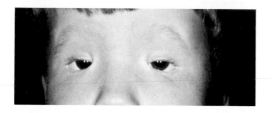

FIG. 13. Child with blepharophimosis.

found that even better symmetry is achieved when both the normal and abnormal levator complexes are excised.

In past years many substances, including a variety of synthetic suture materials, preserved eye bank sclera, and preserved fascia lata, have been employed to perform the brow suspension procedure. Surgical techniques employing orbicularis or skin flaps within the ptotic lid have been advocated. However, the most commonly used material in brow suspension at present may well be autogenous fascia lata (38). Certainly many would argue that this is the best substance for elevating the severely ptotic eyelid and perhaps provides the most

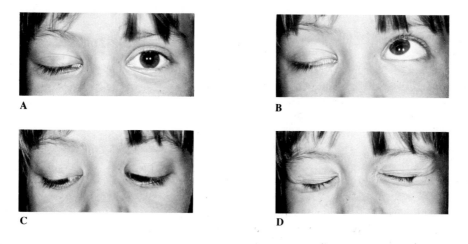

FIG. 14. Levator resections for severe unilateral ptosis result in a high percentage of undercorrections. **A:** Patient looking forward. **B:** Patient looking up. **C:** Patient looking down. **D:** Patient with eyes closed.

long-lasting results. Preserved fascia lata relieves the surgeon of the burden of obtaining the autogenous material and is the favorite of many. Finally, Supramid suture material has remained useful, although the complication rate (infection, extrusion, etc.) is high (15–20%).

Technique of Frontalis Suspension with Autogenous Fascia Lata

Fascia lata can be obtained from the patient in a manner described in Chapter 1. The fascia is generally divided into strips approximately 3 mm in width for easy manipulation. With the Crawford (39) method of placement of the fascia, six markings are made on each eyelid. In the supralash area three marks are made; one at the central pupillary area and one at each limbal area, with methylene blue; corresponding marks are made with methylene blue in the central brow area and in the suprabrow area (Fig. 15A). These areas are infiltrated with lidocaine (red-label Xylocaine® and incisions are made through the musculocutaneous layers. The classic mechanism of passage of the fascia is then accomplished with the use of the Wright fascia needle, depicted in Fig. 15A.

It is important to protect the globe in the passage of the fascia needle from the brow incisions down into the lid. The fascia is threaded through the eyelet of the Wright fascia needle and then retracted into the brow area. Care must be taken in the horizontal passage between the incisions in the supracilliary area not to penetrate the tarsal plate. The fascia should find a resting place between the musculocutaneous layer and the tarsus. Little dissection should be carried out so that the fascia will be anchored into position with passage.

The final positioning of the fascia takes the form of two triangles, as shown in Fig. 15B. Adequate dissection should be made in these brow incisions to allow a single square knot to be made with the thin fascial strip and then buried beneath the skin area in the brow tissue. The pathway of the fascia strips from the supracilliary incisions to the brow should be in the submuscular plane and should not penetrate the orbital septum, or it will cause additional lagophthalmos. In the brow area, there is a plane of fatty tissue that is present between the skin and the frontalis muscle, and dissection must be carried through that in order for the knotted fascia to find a resting place on the frontalis muscle. The knot is reinforced with a nonabsorbable suture. One arm of each of the fascial bands is then brought out through the third central brow incision as part of the classic Crawford method (39). It is important that all of the knotted fascia in the brow be buried deep beneath the skin to avoid granuloma formation.

Adjustment of the upper lid position before securing the knot must be made and, in general, placement of the lid elevation on the operating table should be slightly higher than one wishes it to be postoperatively. In adjusting patients with frontalis suspension, care must be taken that all traction on the forehead, including drapes, be relieved to eliminate any false elevation of the brow. Once the desired elevation and contour have been obtained by adjusting the knots in the brow, a permanent suture is placed into the knot, securing it. Skin closure should take place in layers in the forehead area, again to avoid granuloma formation. Preoperative and postoperative photos of the Crawford method are shown in Fig. 16.

Frontalis Suspension Ptosis Repair using Fascia Lata, with Direct Tarsal Suturing and Lid Crease Formation

The classic Crawford-style method of frontalis suspension with fascia lata has stood the test of time and works very well in a majority of cases. As the surgeon gains more experience

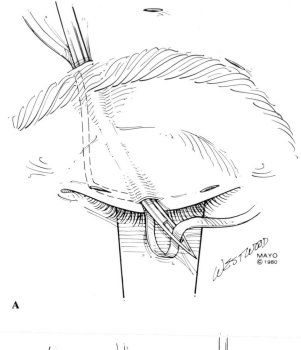

A

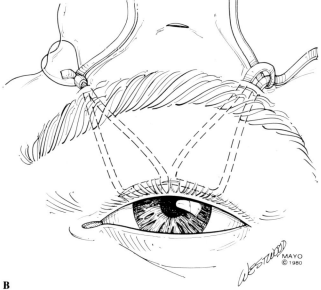

B

FIG. 15A. The Crawford method uses two strips of fascia and requires three lid incisions in the brow and lid. **B:** Passage of the fascia is in the form of two triangles.

with ptosis patients requiring frontalis suspension, he or she will encounter some postoperative problems that can be prevented by additional modifications and techniques.

The most common postoperative problems found in patients who have undergone frontalis suspension in the lid itself are loss of lid crease and postoperative entropion of the upper lid, due to slippage of the frontalis suspensory material. This alternate technique is offered

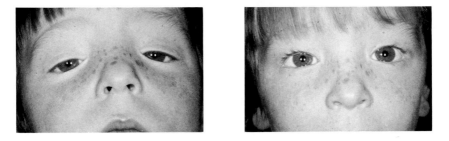

FIG. 16. (Left) Patient with bilateral ptosis preoperatively. (Right) Patient following Crawford method to achieve postoperative frontalis suspension.

as a method to gain the superb correction that the Crawford procedure yields but also, with additional steps, to prevent certain complications that can occur.

Incisions are outlined with methylene blue (Fig. 17A) in the lid crease area and the suprabrow area. Incisions are made through the marked areas, through the musculocutaneous layer in the upper lid, with dissection down to the tarsal plate exposing the tarsal plate, and through the thick brow skin down through the subbrow fatty pad to the frontalis muscle. The fascia strips obtained are then threaded through the eyelid crease incision with a general half-circle closure cutting needle. The advantage of using this needle is that it is less bulky than the Wright fascia needle and that it allows one to direct the point of the needle away from the eye instead of toward the eye. The fascia strips are threaded through the lid crease incision and through both brow incisions (Fig. 17B). Fixation to the tarsal plate of the fascia strip is then accomplished by suturing a horizontal segment of both strips of fascia across the tarsal plate, just above the cilia; 6–0 silk has served well for this, although any nonabsorbable suture can be used.

After adequate fixation to the tarsal plate has been obtained in this manner (Fig. 17C), the lifting power and contour can then be tested by pulling on the fascia strips, which exit the brow incision (Fig. 17D). At this point, if it is determined that there is some difficulty with contour or elevation, one simply can open the lid crease incision and rearrange the fixating sutures to the tarsal plate until the desired contour and lifting power have been obtained.

Following this, the lid crease incision can be closed with sutures, attaching the musculocutaneous edges to the upper tarsal border. It is imperative that the skin between the lashes and the lid crease be tense to avoid an entropion and to ensure good lid crease formation. In any case, skin sutures, in an interrupted manner, are sufficient for this. In problem cases, or cases in which one is unsure about the ability to form the lid crease (reoperated cases or cases with deficient tarsus) one should use through-and-through mattress sutures to accomplish the tensing of the skin and the crease formation. These sutures are best made using double-armed 4–0 silk (Fig. 18). It is important to recognize that the suture placement beginning on the internal surface of the lid must be above the tarsal plate so that, when tied, the suture will nestle within the mucosal conjunctival fold and not abrade the cornea. If the sutures are placed directly through the tarsal plate, this will result in corneal abrasion. These sutures are quite excellent in producing a lid crease incision, having been described in the past by Pang (40). They have served as an excellent supplement to the frontalis suspension procedure, ensure lid crease formation, and avoid complications with entropion. Three sutures are generally enough, but more can be used if necessary. The brow incision is then closed, as previously described.

Frontalis Suspension Using the Silicone Rod

Silicone rod frontalis suspension is recommended in patients with poor eye protective mechanisms because of its ease of reversibility or adjustment in the office setting. Lagophthalmos from any ptosis procedure can produce severe exposure keratopathy in patients with

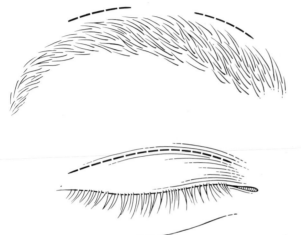

A

FIG. 17. Frontalis suspension repair. **A:** The dotted lines indicate the lid crease and suprabrow incisions used for frontalis suspension ptosis repair with direct suturing of the suspension material to the tarsus, and lid crease formation. **B:** On a semicircular needle, the fascia strips are threaded in the submuscular plane from the lid incision up to and out of the brow incisions.

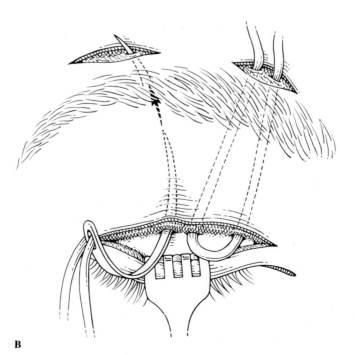

B

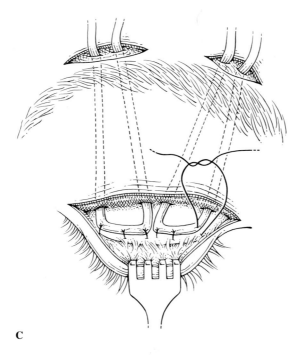

C

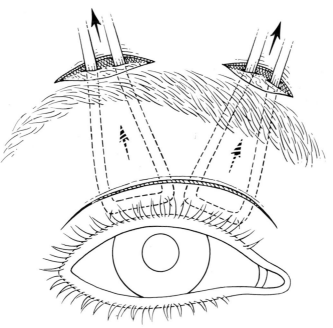

D

FIG. 17 (*cont.*) **C:** The fascia strips are directly sewn to the tarsus at a level just above the cilia. **D:** The fascia strips are pulled through the brow incisions to raise the upper lid to the correct level; at this point, the fascia is secured to frontalis muscle with 4-0 nonabsorbable sutures. Lid crease formation and final closure are as described in the text.

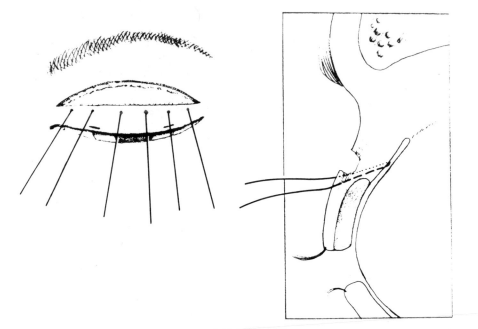

FIG. 18. **(Left)** Frontal view shows three sets of double-armed 4-0 silk Pang sutures used for upper lid crease formation. **(Right)** Cross-sectional view shows the full-thickness mattress sutures that enter the conjunctiva above the superior tarsal border and exit the musculocutaneous edge overlying the anterior tarsal surface.

poor eye movement or extremely dry eyes. Patients who have weakness of eyelid closure from denervation or corneal anesthesia are also at risk for exposure keratopathy following ptosis surgery. Table 7 lists the types of patients at risk for exposure following ptosis procedure. It is to be emphasized that the 1-mm Dow Corning solid silicone rod is the silicone device to be used. Various retinal bands have been used in the past and cannot be configured to the eyelids successfully.

If one wishes to ensure the formation of a lid crease to prevent lash ptosis or correct a preexisting entropion, the through-and-through lid mattress sutures, (Pang sutures) can be used as shown in Fig. 18 to supplement placement of the silicone rod.

TABLE 7. *Conditions associated with poor eye-protective*
mechanisms

1. Neuroparalytic keratitis.
2. Third cranial nerve palsy.
3. Chronic progressive external ophthalmoplegia.
4. Myasthenia gravis.
5. Orbital fibrosis syndromes.
6. Seventh cranial nerve paresis associated with ptosis.
7. Severe keratoconjunctivitis sicca.
8. Double elevator palsy with ptosis.

From McCord and Shore (41) with permission.

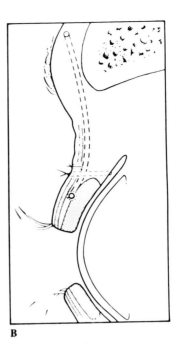

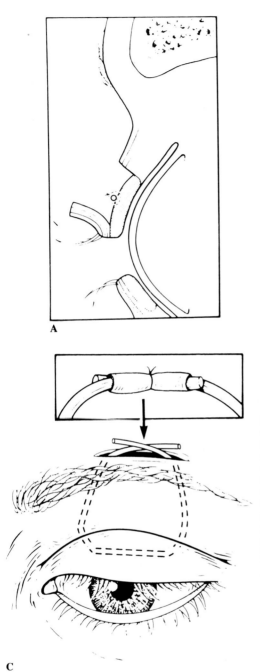

FIG. 19. Method of tarsal fixation and lid crease formation. **A:** The rod is sutured to the tarsus with interrupted 7-0 silk prior to passing the rod through the suprabrown incision. **B:** The lid crease is formed by closing the musculocutaneous layer with a running 5-0 prolene subcuticular suture and three double-armed 4-0 silk Pang sutures. **C:** Technique of suprabrow fixation. When passing the rods through the upper eyelid, the medial arm must be directed toward the glabella for 1.5 cm prior to turning cephalad and bringing the rod out through the brow. The ends of the rod are passed through a Watzke sleeve (*inset*) and secured with one 4-0 Prolene suture that, in turn, is fixated to the underlying frontalis muscle. (From McCord and Shore, ref. 41, with permission.)

Surgical Technique[1]

The surgery can be done under local or general anesthesia. The brow and upper eyelid are injected with red-labeled Xylocaine and Wydase. A 2 cm supra-brow incision is made centered over the pupil. The frontalis muscle is exposed and the superior wound edge undermined for 1 to 2 mm for later fixation of the rod to the frontalis muscle. The proposed lid crease is marked, and a skin-muscle incision made to widely expose the tarsus [Figs. 19A and 19B]. The silicone rod is sutured to the tarsus 2 mm below the superior tarsal border with 2 or 3 interrupted sutures of 7–0 silk [42]. . . . The medial and lateral sutures are centered over the medial and lateral limbus respectively. The position of these sutures can be changed later if necessary to make fine adjustments in lid contour. A general closure needle is then used to pass the rods through the eyelid. The needle is passed in the plane of the levator aponeurosis, through the pre-aponeurotic fat, exiting the brow in the center of the supra-brow incision, 4 to 5 mm apart. The arcus marginalis and frontalis muscle should not be engaged because this inhibits postoperative mobility of the eyelid. When passing the medial rod, the needle should first be angled towards the glabella for [a] distance of 1.5 cm before turning cephalad towards the center of the brow [Fig. 19C]. This gives the correct vector forces on the tarsus and prevents bunching, tarsal buckling, and contour deformities from horizontal forces on the tarsus as the rod is tightened, elevating the lid. The ends of the rod are now passed through a Watzke sleeve and pulled tight to adjust the eyelid to its upper height. The ends of the rod are trimmed long for later loosening if this becomes necessary. Do not overcorrect lid height by more than 1 mm. One, 4–0 Polydek suture is tied around the Watzke sleeve, which in turn, is sutured to the frontalis muscle. Bites deep in the Galea should be avoided except in patients with facial nerve paresis who have no frontalis motility. The supra-brow incision is closed in two layers. It is important to avoid superficial placement of the silicone to avoid granuloma formation. The eyelid wound is closed with a 5–0 subcuticular suture. The eyelid crease is formed with three double-armed 4–0 silk sutures [40]. . . . A [F]rost suture is not required. Ocular lubricants and ice provide comfort and decrease postoperative lid edema. If there is excess skin in the upper lid, a small strip of skin and [orbicularis] may be excised prior to closing the wound, but one should be conservative when excising skin.

One can adjust the eyelid position in the office if necessary. Infiltrate the brow with red labeled Xylocaine. A 1.5 cm incision is made through the previous scar in the brow and the Watzke sleeve is exposed. The Polydek suture is removed and the rods tightened or loosened to adjust the lid to the desired position. The sleeve is again secured to the frontalis muscle as previously described and the wound closed in two layers.

REFERENCES

1. Beard, C. (1976): *Ptosis,* 2nd ed. Mosby, St. Louis.
2. Anderson, R. L., and Dixon, R. S. (1979): Aponeurotic ptosis surgery. *Arch. Ophthalmol.,* 97:1123–1128.
3. Berke, R. N. (1964): Blepharoptosis. In: *Ophthalmic Plastic Surgery,* 2nd ed., edited by W. L. Hughes. American Academy of Ophthalmology, Rochester, Minnesota.
4. Beard, C. (1966): The surgical treatment of blepharoptosis: A quantitative approach. *Trans. Am. Ophthalmol. Soc.,* 64:401–487.
5. Fox, S. A. (1958): *Ophthalmic Plastic Surgery,* 3rd ed. Grune & Stratton, New York.
6. Berke, R. N., and Wadsworth, J. A. C. (1955): Histology of the levator muscle in congenital and acquired ptosis. *Arch. Ophthalmol.,* 53:413–428.
7. Smith, B., McCord, C. D., and Baylis, H. I. (1969): Surgical treatment of blepharoptosis. *Am. J. Ophthalmol.,* 68:92–99.
8. Sano, K. (1959): Trigemino-oculomotor synkinesis. *Neuralgia,* 1:29–51.
9. Kohn, R., and Romano, P. E. (1971): Blepharoptosis, blepharophimosis, epicanthus inversus, and tenecanthus—A syndrome with no name. *Am. J. Ophthalmol.,* 72:625.
10. Merriam, W. W., Ellis, F. D., and Helveston, E. H. (1980): Congenital blepharoptosis, anisometropia, and amblyopia. *Am. J. Ophthalmol.,* 89:401–407.

---

[1] Modified from McCord and Shore, ref. 41, with permission.

11. Hoyt, C. S., Stone, R. D., Fromer, C., and Billson, F. A. (1981): Monocular axial myopia associated with neonatal eyelid closure in human infants. *Am. J. Ophthalmol.*, 91:197–200.

12. Anderson, R. L., and Baumgartner, A. (1980): Amblyopia in ptosis. *Arch, Ophthalmol.*, 98:1068–1069.

13. Maloney, W. F., Younge, B. R., and Moyer, N. J. (1980): Evaluation of the causes and accuracy of pharmacologic localization in Horner's syndrome. *Am. J. Ophthalmol.*, 90:394–402.

14. Walsh, F. B., and Hoyt, W. L. (1969): *Clinical neuro-ophthalmology*, 3rd ed. Williams & Wilkins, Baltimore.

15. Jones, L. T., Quickert, M. H., and Wobig, J. L. (1975): The cure of ptosis by aponeurotic repair. *Arch. Ophthalmol.*, 93:629–634.

16. Walsh, F. B., and Hoyt, W. F. (1969): Progressive muscular dystrophy principally affecting extraocular muscles: Chronic progressive external ophthalmoplegia. In: *Clinical Neuro-Ophthalmology*, 3rd edited by F. B. Walsh and W. F. Hoyt. Williams & Wilkins, Baltimore.

17. Kiloh, L. G., and Nevin, S. (1951): Progressive dystrophy of the external ocular muscles (ocular myopathy). *Brain*, 74:115–143.

18. Daroff, R. B., Solitare, G. B., Pincus, J. H., et al. (1966): Spongiforme encephalopathy with chronic progressive external ophthalmoplegia: Central ophthalmoplegia mimicking ocular myopathy. *Neurology*, 16:161–169.

19. Stephens, J., Hoover, M. L., and Denst, J. (1958): On familial ataxia, neural amyotrophy, and their association with progressive external ophthalmoplegia. *Brain*, 81:556–566.

20. Moses, L., and Heller, G. L. (1965): Ocular myopathy. *Am. J. Ophthalmol.*, 59:1051–1057.

21. Victor, M., Hayes, R., and Adams, R. D. (1962): Oculopharyngeal muscular dystrophy: A familial disease of late life characterized by dysphagia and progressive ptosis of the eyelids. *N. Engl. J. Med.*, 267:1267–1272.

22. Drachman, D. A. (1968): Ophthalmoplegia plus: The neurodegenerative disorders associated with progressive external ophthalmoplegia. *Arch. Neurol.*, 18:654–674.

23. Kearns, T. P. (1965): External ophthalmoplegia, pigmentary degeneration of the retina and cardiomyopathy: A newly recognized syndrome. *Trans. Am. Ophthalmol. Soc.*, 63:559–625.

24. Dyken, P. R. (1966): Extraocular myotonia in families with dystrophia myotonica. *Neurology*, 16:738–740.

25. Burian, H. M., and Burns, C. A. (1967): Ocular changes in myotonic dystrophy. *Am. J. Ophthalmol.*, 63:22–34.

26. Cogan, D. G. (1965): Myasthenia gravis: A review of the disease and a description of lid twitch as a characteristic sign. *Arch. Ophthalmol.*, 74:217–221.

27. Anderson, R. L., and Gordy, D. D. (1979): Aponeurotic defects in congenital ptosis. *Ophthalmology*, 86;1493–1499.

28. Shore, J. W., and McCord, C. D. (1984): Anatomic changes in involutional blepharoptosis. *Am. J. Ophthalmol.*, 98:211–27.

29. Fasanella, R. M., and Servat, J. (1961): Levator resection for minimal ptosis: Another simplified operation. *Arch. Ophthalmol.*, 65:493–496.

30. Putterman, A. M., and Urist, M. J. (1975): Müller's muscle-conjunctiva resection. *Arch. Ophthalmol.*, 93:619–623.

31. Waller, R. R. (1975): Management of myogenic (myopathic) ptosis. *Trans. Am. Acad. Ophthalmol. Otolaryngol.*, 79:697–702.

32. Leahey, B. D. (1953): Simplified ptosis surgery: Resection of the levator palpebrae by the external route. *Arch. Ophthalmol.*, 50:588–596.

33. Johnson, C. C. (1954): Blepharoptosis: A general consideration of surgical methods, with results in 162 operations. *Am. J. Ophthalmol.*, 38:129–162.

34. Berke, R. N. (1959): Results of resection of the levator muscle through a skin incision in congenital ptosis. *Arch. Ophthalmol.*, 61:177–201.

35. Iliff, C. E., Iliff, W. J., and Iliff, N. T. (1979): *Oculoplastic Surgery*. Saunders, Philadelphia.

36. Dillman, D. R., and Anderson, R. L. (1984): Levator myectomy in synkinetic ptosis. *Arch. Ophthalmol.*, 102:422–423.

37. Callahan, A. (1972): Correction of unilateral blepharoptosis with bilateral eyelid suspension. *Am. J. Ophthalmol.*, 74:321–326.

38. Crawford, J. S. (1968): Fascia lata: Its nature and fate after implantation and its use in ophthalmic surgery. *Trans. Am. Ophthalmol. Soc.*, 66:673–745.

39. Crawford, J. S. (1956): Repair of ptosis using frontalis muscle and fascia lata. *Trans. Am. Acad. Ophthalmol. Otolaryngol.*, 60:672–678.

40. Pang, H. G. (1961): Surgical formation of upper lid fold. *Arch. Ophthalmol.*, 65:783–784.

41. McCord, C. D., and Shore, J. W. (1982): Silicone rod frontalis suspension. *Adv. Ophthalm. Plast. Reconstr. Surg.*, 1:213–219.

42. Leone, C. R., Jr., Shore, J. W., and Van Gemert, J. V. (1981): Silicone rod frontalis sling for the correction of blepharoptosis. *Ophthalmic Surg.*, 12:881–887.

Oculoplastic Surgery, 2nd edition, edited by
Clinton D. McCord, Jr., and Myron Tanenbaum.
Raven Press, New York © 1987.

Chapter 14

Lacrimal Drainage System Disorders: Diagnosis and Treatment

*Robert B. Wilkins, **Craig E. Berris, †Robert M. Dryden,
‡Marcos T. Doxanas, and §Clinton D. McCord, Jr.

*Department of Ophthalmology, University of Texas Medical School, Houston, Texas 77025;
**Department of Ophthalmology, University of California Medical School, Davis, California 95616;
†Department of Ophthalmology, University of Arizona Medical School, Tucson, Arizona 85721;
‡Department of Ophthalmic Plastic Surgery, Greater Baltimore Medical Center, Baltimore, Maryland
21204; and §Department of Ophthalmology, Emory University School of Medicine,
Atlanta, Georgia 30308*

Patients with lacrimal drainage insufficiency usually present to the ophthalmologist with the complaint of tearing. The tearing may be unilateral or bilateral, constant or intermittent. The tears may blur the vision, interfere with contact lens wear, or overflow onto the cheek. Occasionally there is a buildup of mucopurulent material in the nasolacrimal sac above an obstruction. Patients will then complain of "mattering" of the eyes, especially in the morning. They may learn on their own to push on the area of the sac to express this material. If the area of the common canaliculus also becomes temporarily obstructed from secondary inflammation, an acute distension may develop. The infected, distended nasolacrimal sac will form a red, tender mass below the medial canthus. The offending organism is usually streptococcus, but pneumococcal organisms may also be present (1). Treatment for acute dacryocystitis consists of warm compresses, nasal spray decongestants, and topical and systemic antibiotics. If the patient is in significant pain, it may be necessary to incise and drain a markedly distended nasolacrimal sac. Even if the dacryocystitis clears, the patient may have recurrent attacks until the underlying obstruction of the nasolacrimal duct is relieved by a dacryocystorhinostomy.

There are other etiologies for tearing besides lacrimal drainage insufficiency. Organizing the causes of tearing into a system will help one understand the work-up of the tearing patient and the rationale of therapy.

It is helpful to differentiate between lacrimation, which is an overproduction of tears, and epiphora, which is a decreased ability to manage the outflow of tears through the nasolacrimal system. Lacrimation results from stimulation of the lacrimal gland by any of a variety of means:

1. Supranuclear. Stimulation of the lacrimal nucleus in the pons by emotion, psychological problems, or central nervous system disorders can lead to lacrimation.
2. Reflex lacrimation. Stimulation to the ophthalmic division of the fifth nerve, which supplies sensation to the eye, in turn stimulates the lacrimal nucleus to increase nerve impulses via the seventh nerve to the main lacrimal gland. The result is increased tear production. This reflex arc may be stimulated by pain or irritation from iritis, glaucoma, diseases of the cornea or conjunctiva, foreign bodies, contact lenses, or other causes. A type of reflex tearing called pseudoepiphora requires special attention, because it may mislead the casual examiner. In pseudoepiphora, the basic tear secretors in the glands of Krause and Wolfring are not producing a sufficient quantity of tears to keep the cornea moist. This dryness stimulates the reflex arc between the fifth and seventh nerves, causing the main lacrimal gland to produce a gush of tears. The lacrimal drainage system, which could handle a normal flow of tears, cannot manage this sporadic, sudden volume of tears, and overflow tearing occurs. If the cornea is kept moist with artificial tears, this reflex arc is not stimulated, and the patient will be relieved of this pseudo-epiphora. Other reflex arcs for lacrimation include retinal stimulation from bright lights, yawning, and laughing.
3. Infranuclear factors. Tumors of the cerebellopontine angle can cause irritation of the nervus intermedius and result in excessive lacrimation. After Bell's palsy, a patient may have misdirection of regenerating salivary axons in the peripheral portion of the seventh nerve. These fibers grow out of the nerve innervating the lacrimal gland, producing a gustatory-lacrimal reflex, or "crocodile tears," when the patient eats or thinks of food.
4. Direct stimulation of the gland. An inflammatory process or tumor of the lacrimal gland may cause either an increase or a decrease of tear production. Parasympathomimetic drugs such as Mecolyl®, which mimic the neurotransmitter of the seventh nerve, or cholinesterase inhibitors such as physostigmine or some pesticides, which block its breakdown, can cause lacrimation.

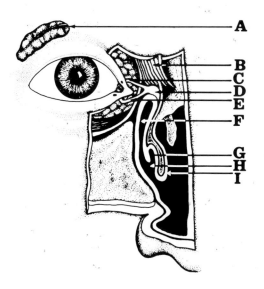

FIG. 1.   Lacrimal system anatomy. A, lacrimal gland; B, reflected medial canthal tendon; C, punctum; D, common internal punctum; E, canaliculus; F, lacrimal sac; G, valve of Hasner; H, inferior meatus; I, inferior turbinate.

Epiphora can be caused by problems anywhere along the nasolacrimal passage from the eye to the nose (Fig. 1).

1. Punctal. There may be a congenital absence of the puncta, keeping the tears from entering the nasolacrimal system. This may consist of just a membrane occluding the opening or total absence of the punctum and canaliculus. The punctum may be everted, because of an ectropion, and not be in contact with the tear lake due to eyelid malposition.

2. Canalicular. There may be stenosis of the punctum or canaliculus from viral infections or drugs, such as idoxuridine and phospholine iodide (2). The canaliculus may become occluded from dacryoliths from *Actinomyces* or mycotic infections. Also, there may be scarring from previous injuries or lacerations.

3. Nasolacrimal sac. The sac may be obstructed by stones, tumor, or inflammation (3–5).

4. Lacrimal pump. The tear pumping action of the orbicularis muscle during blinking may be absent, because of a facial paralysis. This can happen with a Bell's palsy or after surgery to the cerebellopontine angle.

   Abnormal stiffness of the eyelid resulting from burns, scleroderma or other cicatrizing processes can interfere with the lacrimal pump mechanism. Figure 2 shows the insertion of the orbicularis fibers anterior and posterior to the lacrimal drainage apparatus encompassing it in such a way as to exert a squeezing effect when the muscle contracts. Figure 3 shows, with opening of the eyelids, the negative pressure created in the ampulla of the canalicular system drawing tear film into the canalicular system; with closure, the tears are then expelled into the lacrimal sac, which is expanded by contracture of the outlet muscle. This lacrimal pump mechanism is critical to the elimination of tears (6).

5. The nasolacrimal duct. The duct can be stenosed from inflammation or scarred from injuries or surgery (7). In a child, the duct may have an imperforate membrane.

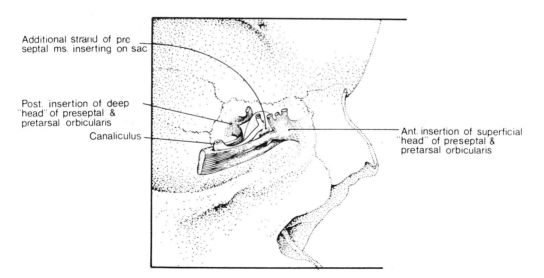

FIG. 2. Diagram of the tendon insertions of the eyelid muscles on and around the lacrimal sac and canaliculus. (Adapted from Jones, L. T. An anatomic approach to problems of the eyelids and lacrimal apparatus. *Arch. Ophthalmol.*, 66:111 124, 1961.) (From McCord, ref. 26, with permission. © 1985, Lippincott/Harper & Row.)

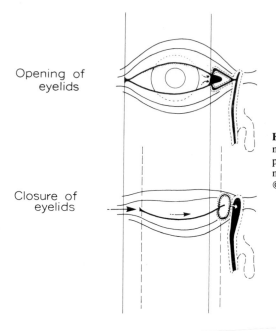

Opening of
eyelids

Closure of
eyelids

FIG. 3. The lacrimal pump. Mechanics of eyelid movement during a blink showing the actions of the palpebral pump, ampulla-canalicular system, and lacrimal sac pump. (From McCord, ref. 26, with permission. © 1985, Lippincott/Harper & Row.)

6. Valve of Hasner. The distal opening of the nasolacrimal duct may be imperforate or be obstructed by the inferior turbinate impinging on it (1,8).

DIAGNOSTIC WORK-UP

The evaluation of the tearing patient should begin with a good history. This may help determine whether the patient's complaints are from lacrimation or from epiphora. The patient may describe associated symptoms such as itching and burning (as with allergies) or pain and photophobia (as with an iritis). The patient with lacrimal drainage insufficiency may give a history of recurrent dacryocystitis, or may relate having injured or had surgery to the eyes or nose. There have been reported cases of lacrimal duct obstruction secondary to rhinostomies (7) and migrating implants after orbital surgery (9). In addition to a thorough eye history, obtain a general review of systems to determine if other conditions may be contributing to the patient's tearing. The patient may state that he or she has had a Bell's palsy in the past and now has tearing, most marked when eating or thinking of food.

Before going to more elaborate diagnostic tests, examine the patient grossly, and at the slit lamp. Check the area of the nasolacrimal sac for any redness, mass, or fistula. If there is an obstruction below the level of the nasolacrimal sac and the sac is distended, one frequently can express mucopurulent material back through the puncta. Palpate under the superior orbital rim for signs of lacrimal gland enlargement. The patient may demonstrate orbicularis weakness by decreased muscle strength on forced lid closure, or lagophthalmos. Look for an ectropion causing punctal eversion or an entropion or trichiasis that may cause irritation and reflex lacrimation. Also note if the puncta are patent. A careful slit-lamp examination may uncover diseases of the conjunctiva, cornea, or anterior chamber that may cause reflex lacrimation.

Quantitation of Tear Production

Rough quantitation of tear production has been aided by the introduction of the Schirmer test strips. These filter paper strips, 5 mm wide and 35 mm long, can be obtained from SMP Division of Cooper Laboratories, Inc. Fold the strip at the notched indentation and drape the short end over the lower lid margin. Jones and Wobig have found that it is not important where on the lid the strip is placed (10). Wetting of the strip is measured after a period of time. Jones and Wobig have found that the amount of wetting after 1 min multiplied by 3 is approximately the same as after the traditional 5-min period. Wetting between 10 and 30 mm is considered normal. One should not automatically conclude, however, that over 30 mm of wetting represents an abnormal production of tears.

The results of this test (Schirmer #1) are compared to the basic secretion test. This second test eliminates the reflex tearing from the main lacrimal gland caused by irritation from the filter paper strips. In this test, the conjunctiva is anesthetized with a topical anesthetic as well as a 5% solution of cocaine applied with a saturated cotton-tipped applicator. If the patient feels the filter paper, the result of the basic secretion test may be invalid. Dry the conjunctiva with a cotton-tipped applicator prior to placing the strip. Also subdue the room lighting to avoid any photopic contribution to tear production. Wetting of the filter paper strips of less than 10 mm in 5 min (or 3 mm in 1 min) indicates a deficient basic secretion of tears. This would mean the patient's tearing is probably reflex lacrimation creating pseudoepiphora (especially if other tests demonstrate a patent nasolacrimal system).

The Schirmer #2 test is sometimes confused with the basic secretion test. The Schirmer #2 is used when the Schirmer #1 and the basic secretion test indicate no reflex secretion from the main lacrimal gland. This could be caused by either primary disease of the gland or a fatigue block, in which the reflex arc between the nerve fibers of the fifth nerve innervating the eye and the seventh nerve is not functioning. Fatigue block is tested by stimulating the posterior nasal mucosa with a cotton-tipped applicator while performing the Schirmer test for 2 min. With fatigue block, the strip will be completely wet. Jones and Wobig (10) believe fatigue block is usually transient, with recovery possible. If there is no increased tearing with stimulation of the nasal mucosa, then the problem is most likely in the gland itself.

Patency of the Nasolacrimal System

The patency of the nasolacrimal system can be evaluated by employing the primary and secondary dye tests described by Jones and Wobig (10). The primary test consists of instilling fluorescein dye (2%) in the conjunctival sac and, after 5 min, attempting to retrieve the dye in the nose with a cotton-tipped wire applicator (Figs. 4–7). The retrieval of dye is probably the most difficult problem for the general practitioner of ophthalmology, who performs this procedure only occasionally. Attention to details is important to avoid false-negative results, which could lead patients to unnecessary surgery. The opening of the nasolacrimal duct, the valve of Hasner, lies anteriorly beneath the inferior turbinate (see Fig. 1). A cotton-tipped applicator soaked in 5% cocaine is placed under the inferior turbinate under direct visualization to shrink the nasal mucosa and obtain anesthesia. The shrunken mucosa aids the visualization and placement of the cotton-tipped wire applicator. The applicator should be curved slightly to slide up under the inferior turbinate. A wire is used because the inferior turbinate is closely approximated to the wall of the nose and a

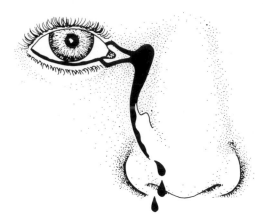

FIG. 4. Positive Jones 1 test (primary dye test). Fluorescein dye (2%) has been retrieved from beneath the inferior turbinate 5 min after its instillation in the cul-de-sac of the eye. Interpretation: lacrimal drainage system is normal.

normal cotton-tipped applicator cannot enter this passageway. The successful placement of the wire applicator requires a nasal speculum and a head light. An indirect ophthalmoscope makes a convenient light source. Occasionally, the inferior turbinate will be impacted against the wall of the nose and may need to be fractured away in order to retrieve dye.

If no dye is retrieved with the wire applicator, the patient is instructed to occlude the opposite nostril and to blow into a tissue, which is then checked for dye. Occasionally, dye may be retrieved by irrigating a stream of saline under the inferior turbinate and catching the dye in a white porcelain basin. Other authors have described alternate techniques for performing this test. One asked patients to bow their heads after instillation of dye in the conjunctival sac and the placement of cotton applicators in the nose (11). The head position allows the dye to run forward and be retrieved by the cotton-tipped applicators, rather than running backward into the throat. This may avoid the need for instrumentation with the wire applicator. In a unilateral test, one may also check the pharynx with a fluorescent light for the appearance of dye (12).

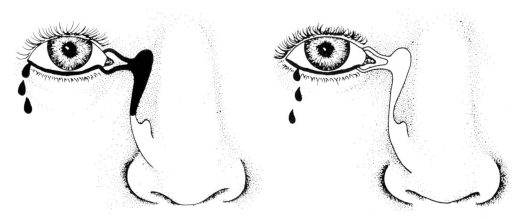

FIG. 5. Negative Jones 1 test (primary dye test). **(Left)** It can be seen in the drawing that the dye has entered the sac but has not passed the nasolacrimal duct. **(Right)** It can be seen from the illustration that dye has not entered the sac, and the obstruction is somewhere proximal to the sac. In neither case, of course, can these determinations be made clinically; further testing (a secondary dye test) must be done.

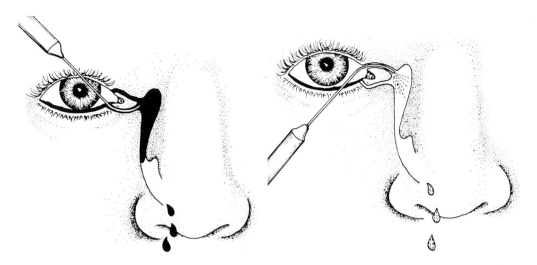

FIG. 6. Jones 2 test (secondary dye test). **(Left)** Positive test. The dye had entered the sac in the primary dye test, but, of course did not go past the nasolacrimal duct and therefore resulted in a negative primary dye test. On irrigation, however, dye flows out of the nose, indicating a partial obstruction of the nasolacrimal duct. DCR is the treatment of choice. **(Right)** Negative test. Dye did not enter the sac in the primary dye test, and when irrigation occurred with clear fluid in the secondary dye test, only clear fluid came out of the nose. This indicates that no dye entered the sac, and the obstruction lies somewhere in the puncta or canaliculi. DCR would be of no benefit to this patient.

The rate of disappearance of the fluorescein dye from the conjunctival sac has been used by some as an indirect estimate of the patency of the drainage system. The amount of dye remaining after 5 min is graded from 0 to 4^+. A 0 to 1^+ would indicate little remaining dye and, therefore, a drainage system that is working. Hornblass has recommended a subjective test employing a drop of 2% saccharin instilled in the anesthetized eye (13). After a period of time, the patient is asked if he or she can taste the saccharin. In a negative test, a drop is placed on the tongue to determine if the patient can actually taste saccharin. This test has not become widespread, partly because of its subjectivity and also because of the inability to test both sides at the same time.

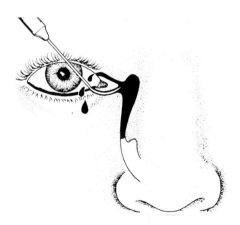

FIG. 7. Irrigation in the lower canaliculus results in reflux from the upper canaliculus, indicating total obstruction of the nasolacrimal duct. DCR is the treatment of choice.

If the Jones primary dye test is negative (no demonstration of dye in the nose), one can assume there is a blockage in the system, either actual obstruction or a functional block. One can differentiate these, as well as estimate the level of blockage, by the Jones secondary dye test. First, the remaining dye in the conjunctival sac is irrigated from the eye. The punctum is anesthetized with a cotton-tipped applicator soaked in cocaine and then dilated with a punctal dilator. An irrigation cannula, attached to a 3-ml syringe, is inserted through the inferior punctum and canaliculus. The irrigant employed is normal saline or any sterile irrigant solution. The patient is instructed to tip his or her head over a white porcelain basin so that any dye irrigated through the system will be retrieved. There are four possible results of this irrigation:

1. The irrigation of fluid through the system with the appearance of dye in the basin and no reflux of irrigant indicates a partial stenosis or a functional blockage. A functional blockage is an indication for a dacryocystorhinostomy (DCR), even though the patient irrigates through freely. With a medial ectropion, one may not recover dye in the primary dye test and yet irrigate fluid through the nasolacrimal duct easily. These patients require repair of this ectropion and not a DCR.
2. If the irrigant comes through clear, this indicates no dye reached the nasolacrimal sac, because of either a stenosis of the punctum or canaliculus or an abnormality of the opening of the common canaliculus into the sac (value of Rosenmüller). The irrigation cannula was able to cross this barrier and irrigate solution through the system. Depending on the findings at surgery, these patients may require a resection of the valve of Rosenmüller with silicone tubing, or a Jones tube.
3. If there is reflux of fluid from the opposite punctum with none entering the nose, there is probably an obstruction at or below the level of the nasolacrimal sac. These patients are candidates for DCR.
4. If there is a reflux around the irrigating cannula, with no fluid refluxing through the opposite punctum or entering the nose, there is a blockage in the inferior or common canaliculus. If attempts at irrigation through the upper canaliculus are also unsuccessful, these patients are candidates for a Jones tube procedure (a conjunctivodacryocystorhinostomy). If the lower canaliculus is obstructed, yet one can irrigate through the upper canaliculus, the patient's complaint of tearing should be reevaluated. The upper canaliculus can provide adequate drainage for the normal eye without the contribution of the inferior canaliculus. The patient may have tearing, in spite of a patent upper canaliculus, if a medial ectropion does not allow the formation of a tear lake from which the upper punctum may draw fluid.

Dye tests should not be done initially in cases of acute dacryocystitis. The infection alone is an indication of an obstruction of the nasolacrimal system, and forcing fluid into an inflamed, distended sac could produce more harm than information. We do not routinely employ special tests such as dacryocystography and dacryoscintigraphy (14). Other authors have described their usefulness in suspected lacrimal sac tumors, but we have not found them valuable in the everyday work-up of the patient (15).

CONGENITAL DACRYOSTENOSIS

The lacrimal drainage apparatus is embryologically derived from a pouch of epithelial cells at the nasal end of the lower eyelid, and extensions progress nasally to form the nasolacrimal duct and temporally to form the canaliculi and puncta. Should development of either of these extensions be interrupted, an obstruction will be present at birth. About 30% of normal infants will show an obstruction of the nasolacrimal duct at birth, and a much higher percentage of premature infants will. Development will generally continue, and these obstructions will open spontaneously in the first 3 to 4 weeks after birth. Some do not open, however, and such infants will present with tearing and purulent exudate. Many will have been treated with antibiotic drops for conjunctivitis and, while they are on the drops, the conjunctivitis will resolve; however, tearing will persist, and when the drops are stopped the exudate will recur.

Definitive treatment should begin with massage of the canthal region in an attempt to perforate the persistent membranes blocking the nasolacrimal duct (16). Massage alone will effect a greater than 90% success rate within the first 12 months of life (17–19). If the symptoms persist, or a lacrimal system infection develops, the patient is a candidate for a nasolacrimal duct probing.

Technique for Probing Congenital Dacryostenosis

In the hospital, under general anesthesia, the lacrimal system is irrigated on both sides. The obstructed side should, of course, demonstrate regurgitation from the lower punctum when the upper is irrigated, and vice versa. A purulent exudate will usually accompany the refluxed irrigation solution. In order to shrink the mucosa, the inferior meatus is packed with ½-inch gauze packing that has been soaked with a solution of equal parts of 0.25% phenylephrine hydrochloride (Neo-Synephrine®) and 4% cocaine. After 5 min the pack is removed and the initial probing is done. Probing is carried out through the upper and lower puncta using a 00 Bowman probe (Fig. 8A). Great care must be taken not to create a false passage. One should keep in mind the anatomy of the area.

The probe should enter the lower punctum and pass initially downward about 2 mm, then gently turn toward the nose. The lower lid should be retracted temporally in order to straighten the canaliculus and not accordion loose tissue in front of the probe, contributing to a false passage (Fig. 8B). When the probe meets a soft bony resistance, it is in the sac and against the lateral wall of the nose. The probe is then raised vertically and gently passed downward. Several very gentle probes downward with the probe in the direction of the molar tooth area of the same side will result in the probe slipping into the nasolacrimal duct and then into the nose. A gentle pop will sometimes be felt. When the probe is removed, it should have traversed a distance of about 20 mm. A repeat probing is then done with a size 0 probe. The probe is left in place and, with a nasal speculum and a head light, the probe should be visualized. If the probe cannot be seen, it should be located with a small curved hemostat. This is done by gently probing and feeling in the nose until the probe is felt and can be moved about with intranasal manipulation. The probe may be located quite posteriorly, may be hidden by a large turbinate, or may actually be submucosal. When the probe is located, an effort is made to grasp it with the hemostat and gently manipulate it back and forth in an attempt to slightly enlarge the nasolacrimal duct opening into the nose.

After these manipulations are completed, with direct visualization and illumination, a Freer periosteal elevator is placed beneath the inferior turbinate, and the turbinate is cracked in an upward rotation toward the nasal septum (sometimes called an infracturing; Fig. 8C). A definite cracking of bone is only occasionally heard, but one should definitely get the feel and visualization of a larger space being created in the inferior meatus.

One should be able to irrigate fluid through the system into the nose after these manipula-

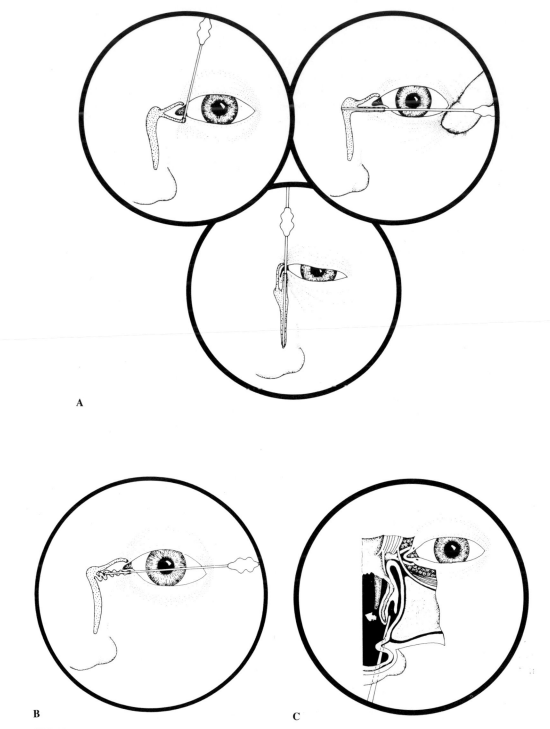

FIG. 8. Technique for probing in congenital dacryostenosis. **A:** Probing in infants. **(Top left)** Initial vertical probing, 2 mm. **(Top right)** Horizontal probing. Note lateral tension on lower lid. **(Bottom)** Final vertical probe through nasolacrimal duct. **B:** ''Accordioning,'' which can lead to false passage. This can be avoided with lateral tension on lower lid. **C:** Infracturing of turbinate. Freer elevator cracks turbinate toward nasal septum.

tions. Irrigation can then be carried out in the lower canaliculus with saline stained with fluorescein. A suction catheter is then introduced into the intranasal cavity and as one irrigates the stained fluid can be withdrawn from the nose, indicating successful probing.

Children who have had a technically adequate probing and fracture of the inferior turbinate, and still have continued epiphora, are candidates for intubation with silicone tubes. It is obvious that a prerequisite for implantation of the silicone tubes is the ability to probe into the nose. If one has encountered an inability to pass the probe into the nose then one cannot pass the tubing, and the DCR is indicated in these children.

Technique of Silicone Intubation

The passage of lacrimal probes that are swedged onto the silicone tubing is performed in a similar manner, as previously described. Successive generations of probes with swedged-

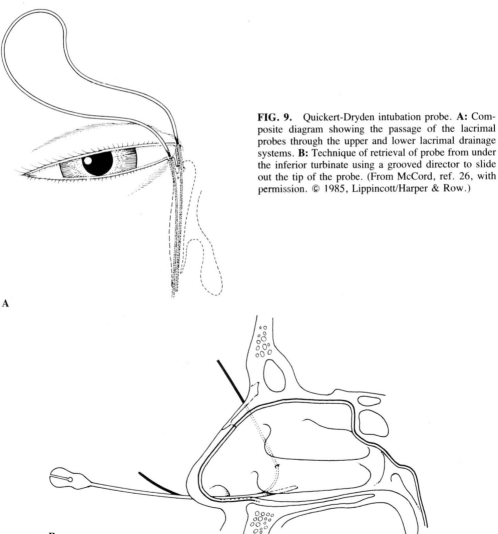

FIG. 9. Quickert-Dryden intubation probe. **A:** Composite diagram showing the passage of the lacrimal probes through the upper and lower lacrimal drainage systems. **B:** Technique of retrieval of probe from under the inferior turbinate using a grooved director to slide out the tip of the probe. (From McCord, ref. 26, with permission. © 1985, Lippincott/Harper & Row.)

A

B

on silicone have found their way into the ophthalmic surgeon's hands. The initial Quickert-Dryden (20) probes were of silver and their removal from the inferior turbinate was accomplished by directing them into a grooved director for subsequent extraction (Fig. 9). The silicone had to be glued on by the surgeon, and many times pulled off of the probe with passage. Also, the extraction from the nose was extremely tedious.

This probe was subsequently replaced with the stainless steel probes, which had the silicone commercially attached to the probe. There was less problem with the silicone pulling off. However, extraction from the nose was extremely difficult with the grooved director and required the use of a grasping hemostat (Fig. 10). The stiffness of the probes and the difficulty of inserting the hemostat lead to the development of the third-generation intubation set designed by Crawford (available from Jed Med) (21). The advantage of this probe is that it has a small soldered olive tip. Once the probe is introduced into the nose, an extracting hook is introduced under the inferior turbinate, grasping the probe above the olive tip; the probe can then be withdrawn very easily from under the inferior turbinate. Shore and McCord (22) modified the extracting hook with a simple bend so that one can actually visualize the tip of the probe under the inferior turbinate, which simplifies the ease of extraction (Fig. 11). In children, the intubation must be performed under a general anesthetic and the inferior turbinate must be thoroughly vasoconstricted with either 4% cocaine or a mixture of oxymetazoline hydrochloride (Afrin®) and 0.25% phenylephrine hydrochloride. In adults, the procedure can be performed under local anesthesia with a nasocilliary block and a packing of the inferior turbinate with 4% cocaine.

After the tubing has been threaded through the upper and lower canaliculi, the probe is excised from the end of the silicone tubes, which have exited the external nostril. The silicone tubing is then tied. Our technique for securing the tubes is to introduce the first half of a square knot and tighten the knot until the eyelids close. One must then manually open the eyelids to produce enough slack in the silicone tubing so that the eyelids can open. The second half of the square knot is then introduced and tied under the inferior turbinate (Fig. 12). It has been our experience that a single square knot is quite sufficient to keep the tubing anchored in the nose, and allows for ease of extraction later. If the

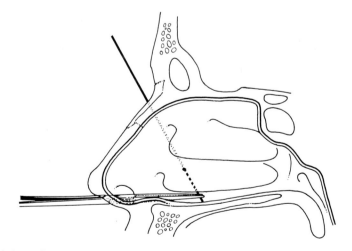

FIG. 10. Technique of retrival of a Quickert-Dryden lacrimal probe by grasping the tip of the probe with a straight hemostat. (From McCord, ref. 26, with permission. © 1985, Lippincott/Harper & Row.)

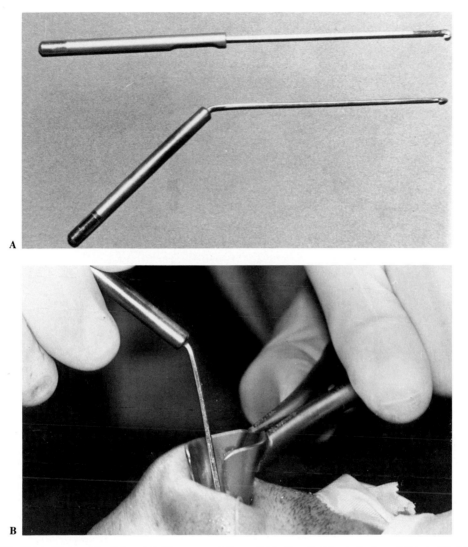

FIG. 11A. Photograph of the straight, commercially available Crawford hook (*top*), and the modified hook with a 45° bend (*bottom*). (From Shore and McCord, ref. 22, with permission. © 1982, Ophthalmic Publishing Company.) **B:** Photograph demonstrating the use of the modified (bent) Crawford hook for retrieval of a lacrimal probe. The bend in the hook allows for use of the hook without obstructing the surgeon's view of the intranasal space.

single square knot is used, removal of the tubing can be accomplished by pulling the knot up through the nasolacrimal duct and into the tear sac and then rotating the knot out through the upper punctum. This can be done in children if there is no eyelid squeezing and in adults with topical anesthesia. An alternative is to extract the knot and ends from the nose. However, in many cases, particularly if the tubing has been in place for many months, the identification of the tubing may be very difficult. If one does extract the tubing from the nose, it is obvious that the loop between the upper and lower canaliculi must be cut before pulling the tubes out of the nose.

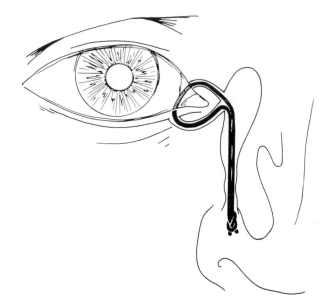

FIG. 12. Technique for securing silicone tube by tying the ends tightly with a square knot.

There are some special manipulations that must be used for the passage of the Crawford tube that are different from that of the standard lacrimal probe. In all patients, it is our practice to make the initial passage with the standard 00 probe to determine the trajectory of the nasolacrimal duct. In adults with prominent foreheads, it is oftentimes necessary to bend the probe so that the tip of the probe curves forward, in order that it may find its way down the angled nasolacrimal duct (Fig. 13). The proper curve of the Crawford probe can be determined from the curve needed in the preliminary Bowman probing. The Crawford probe is much more flexible than the silver Bowman probe, and it is helpful to grasp the probe with a needle holder just as it enters the punctum, immediately after it has been rotated to the vertical position. This allows one to have the proper purchase to push the tube down the nasolacrimal duct, which in many cases is a more anterior direction than the distal part of the curved probe may take.

The nasolacrimal duct normally exists under the inferior turbinate in the vault of the meatus at the juncture of the anterior one-fourth and posterior three-fourths of the turbinate. There are anatomic variations of which one should be aware in which the meatus can open further down on the lateral wall and nearer the floor. This can introduce difficulties in extracting the probe in some cases (Fig. 14).

Most individuals tolerate the silicone tubing extremely well. An occasional patient will complain that his or her eye is irritated and even red. Additionally, sensation of the tube may be associated with adduction.

Most patients with the tube in place will not tear after mucosal swelling has resolved. Tearing 2 to 3 weeks following intubation does not signify poor prognosis. Tearing several months following intubation generally does indicate a poor prognosis for functional patency after tube removal. Remarkably, some individuals with total blockage do not complain of tearing after removal of the tube. Additionally, a flaccid pumping system would also cause tearing when the tubing is removed even if the system is patent to irrigation.

Occasionally the tubes themselves appear to irritate the canaliculus and promote localized

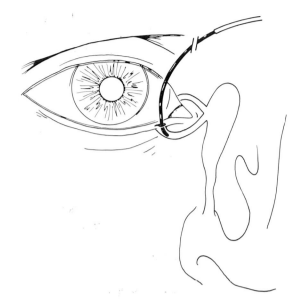

FIG. 13. Tip of Crawford probe placed into punctum showing the curve in the probe necessary to intubate the lacrimal system.

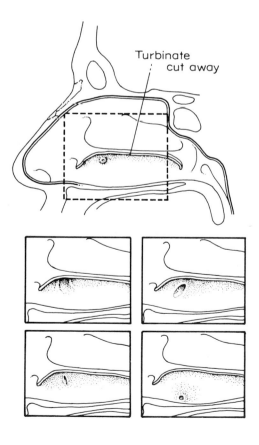

FIG. 14. Variations in the positions and shapes of the distal opening of the nasolacrimal duct under the inferior turbinate. (Adapted from Shaffer, J. P.: Am. J. Anatomy 13:185, 1912.) (From McCord, ref. 26, with permission. © 1985, Lippincott/Harper & Row.)

infection. Usually, however, topical antibiotics will control such difficulties. A crack in the silicone will occasionally facilitate infection in association with the accumulation of material in the tube. A broken tube must be replaced. An individual sometimes develops granulation tissue. If this granulation is unsightly, inflamed, or bleeding, cauterization or removal of the tissue may be needed.

Certain preventable problems are associated with loop tension or length. A tight silicone tube can cause a "cheese-wiring" effect on the canaliculi with the silicone loop moving nasally in the canaliculi. If cheese-wiring occurs, the tube should be removed. The failure to secure the tubing in the nose may be associated with a large loop of silicone appearing between the puncta. The initial repositioning should be attempted by feeding the arms of the silicone back into the canaliculi. The knot may be pulled into the nasolacrimal duct. An attempt to retrieve the knot can be made by passing a probe down the nasolacrimal duct. If pushing the knot into the inferior meatus is unsuccessful, the tube may be removed directly through the canaliculus with gentle but persistent tension.

Other Conditions

Another anomaly more rarely seen is the developmental failure of the puncta. Patients with this condition have no tear drainage, and therefore increased tearing; but because there is no exudate and no hyperemic, tender dacryocystitis with this maldevelopment, it is usually not noticed until early childhood. This is a slit-lamp diagnosis. Either the puncta will be totally absent or a fine transparent membrane will be seen covering the opening. These patients, depending on their age, can be treated either in the office with local anesthesia or as hospital outpatients. Magnification is required, and a #11 Bard-Parker blade is gently thrust into the punctal area as seen through the microscope in an attempt to open the punctum. This will either be a very easy task, or be impossible if the distal canaliculus is also absent. When unsuccessful, a Jones tube procedure must be done, preferably at the same surgery. If successful, however, a one-snip is done on the puncta, and then followed by dilations in the office, when possible, every other day for a week. This has been enough, in our experience, to treat punctal stenosis successfully. There are those, however, who will place silicone tubes through the openings for several days. We have not found this necessary. Some of these punctal stenosis patients will also have nasolacrimal duct obstruction, which, of course, is not diagnosed until the puncta are open. These patients will require in most instances a punctal opening plus a DCR. Some will get by with punctal opening and nasolacrimal duct probing, and this procedure should be tried, although success is rare.

A very rare condition, referred to by Jones and Wobig (10) is amniocentele (dacryocystocele). This presents in infants as a bluish mass in the lacrimal sac area that is usually nontender but visible and palpable. The mass is the result of a nasolacrimal duct obstruction combined with an obstruction in the area of the common internal punctum. A probing of the system may result in the complete resolution of the problem, although all patients should be followed after probing because the fluid may reaccumulate (23–25).

LACERATIONS OF THE CANALICULUS[1]

Acute lacerations to the canaliculi may occur following sharp penetrating wounds or as a result of shearing or ripping wounds of the eyelid with hooklike devices or teeth.

---

[1] Extracted portions of this chapter are reprinted from McCord, ref. 26, with permission. © 1985, Lippincott/Harper & Row.

Always repair upper as well as lower canalicular lacerations. Repair may be delayed for as long as 48 hours with the use of ice compresses [(27). Delayed repair of canalicular lacerations (i.e., weeks to months following injury) is more difficult and much less likely to be successful (28)]. Injection of hyaluronidase (Wydase) will . . . reduce the amount of swelling at the time of the repair if needed. For ease of examination, general anesthesia should be used, if possible. Injection of the area with a local anesthetic often distorts tissue. . . . [Magnification] is often necessary to find the severed ends of the canaliculus.

Internal splinting of the canaliculi is mandatory to repair the laceration, and the splinting material should be soft and pliable [(29) (Fig. 15)]. End-to-end anastomosis of the canaliculi is ideal with 7–0 to 8–0 sutures, however, it may be difficult to suture the edges for 360° . . . [Many m]aterials . . . have been used for intracanalicular splinting:

1. Large caliber sutures such as 3–0 gut may be brought out through the tear sac.
2. A 1-mm silicone rod may be "dead-ended" through the canaliculus into the sac and sutured to the punctum.
3. Metal rods and polyethylene tubes have been used with varying success. Rigid materials are best avoided in the canaliculus, which is under constant motion with each blink.
4. Silicone tubing wedged onto lacrimal probes [(Crawford probes) (21)] can be threaded through the upper and lower canalicular system to the sac and nasolacrimal duct and tied under the inferior turbinate. This is the procedure of choice, particularly in double canalicular lacerations or in those which extend through the canaliculus and into the sac.

The identification of the proximal cut end of the canaliculus (canaliculi) is perhaps the most trying experience in canalicular repair. If the laceration is distal and swelling is minimal there is generally no problem with identification since the canalicular diameter is fairly large, 1.0 to 1.5 mm. If the laceration is close to or into the lacrimal sac and swelling is present, identification is difficult because the tissues are distorted and the membranous conduit is compressed. Allowing tissue swelling to subside with time and with the application of ice compresses and the injection of Wydase solution and massage may restore normal contour and alignments so that the opening of the membranous conduit laceration may be identified. If the opening cannot be identified, then irrigation of the opposite canaliculus with air and flooding the field with water is helpful in detecting where bubbles occur under the water [30]. Milk used as an injected material can be irritating. The injection of methylene blue is not advised as it may totally obscure the field after its injection in the canaliculus. The pigtail probe has been shown to be of little help and perhaps dangerous and should be avoided [31].

DACRYOCYSTORHINOSTOMY

Anatomy of the Lacrimal Sac Pertinent to Dacryocystorhinostomy

The lacrimal sac rests in the bony lacrimal fossa within the nasal frontal process of the maxilla at the anterior portion of the orbit. From the inferior portion of the sac, the nasolacrimal canal extends in the medial wall of the antrum through the bony canal to exit under the inferior turbinate (Fig. 16). If the lacrimal sac is viewed looking at the lateral wall of the nose, it is normally positioned just anterior to the middle turbinate, and it is in this area where the rhinostomy will enter into the nose (Fig. 17). Many variations can occur in this portion of the nose. Figure 18 shows the usual relationship seen together with other anatomic variations that may be commonly encountered.

Technique for Dacryocystorhinostomy

Administration of either a local or a general anesthetic with packing of the inferior meatus, using half-and-half 4% cocaine and 0.25% phenylephrine hydrochloride for hemostasis, is the first step. When a local anesthetic is used, one performs general infiltration of

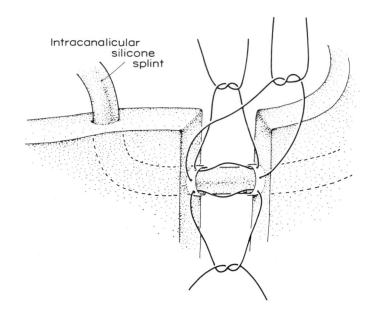

Intracanalicular
silicone
splint

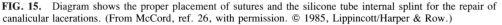

FIG. 15. Diagram shows the proper placement of sutures and the silicone tube internal splint for the repair of canalicular lacerations. (From McCord, ref. 26, with permission. © 1985, Lippincott/Harper & Row.)

the incision site, including the area of the medial canthus and the distribution of the infra-trochlear nerve. The skin is then marked with a straight line that is about 3 to 4 cm in length and runs tangent to the inferior nasal border of the orbital rim (Fig. 19A). This incision should be 11 mm from the medial canthus and should have its highest point on the skin immediately inferior to the medial canthal tendon area. This location should then

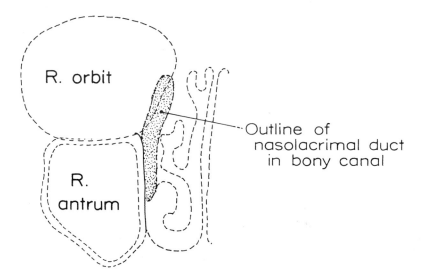

R. orbit

R.
antrum

Outline of
nasolacrimal duct
in bony canal

FIG. 16. Frontal view of the nasolacrimal duct demonstrating its course in relation to the orbit, maxillary sinus, and nasal turbinates. (From McCord, ref. 26, with permission. © 1985, Lippincott/Harper & Row.)

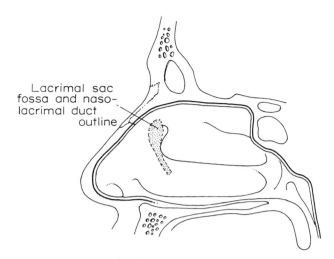

FIG. 17. Outline of the lacrimal sac fossa and nasolacrimal duct in its course under the inferior turbinate, as viewed from inside the nose looking at the lateral wall of the nose. (From McCord, ref. 26, with permission. © 1985, Lippincott/Harper & Row.)

place the incision above the large angular vessels. After the mark is made, an injection of 1 to 2 ml lidocaine (Xylocaine®) with epinephrine is used in the area for hemostasis.

An incision is made through the skin only using a #15 Bard-Parker blade. The incision is then carried down to the periosteum with gentle blunt dissection (Fig. 19B), taking care to cauterize the vessels meticulously as one proceeds. The large angular vessels can be avoided in the dissection by carefully retracting them out of the field.

The periosteum is next incised with the Bard-Parker blade, and a Freer periosteal elevator is used to expose the raw bone down to the anterior lacrimal crest. Elevation of the periosteum is continued into the lacrimal fossa, retracting the lacrimal sac out of the fossa, away from the bone (Fig. 19C).

The next step is to break through the bone in the fossa to expose the nasal mucosa. This is done after the nasal pack is removed and is achieved in a variety of ways by different individuals. Some actually punch through the thin bone with a curved hemostat,

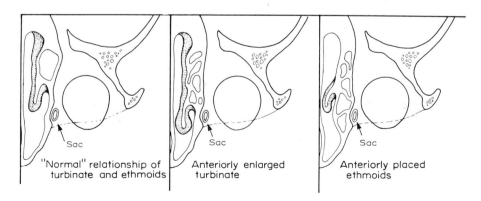

FIG. 18. Axial view diagrams showing the relationship of the lacrimal sac fossa, the ethmoidal air cells, and the tip of middle turbinate, and the anatomic variations that the surgeon may encounter. (From McCord, ref. 26, with permission. © 1985, Lippincott/Harper & Row.)

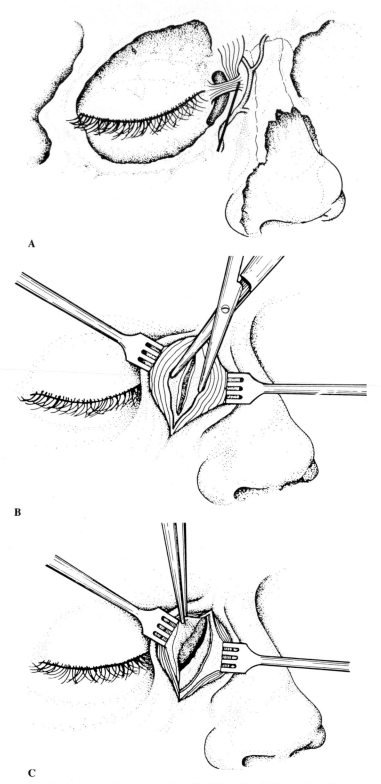

FIG. 19. Dacryocystorhinostomy technique. **A:** Site of incision. Careful blunt dissection is necessary to avoid the angular vessel. **B:** Blunt dissection down to periosteum, with sharp dissection through periosteum. **C:** Lacrimal sac is pulled out of lacrimal fossa.

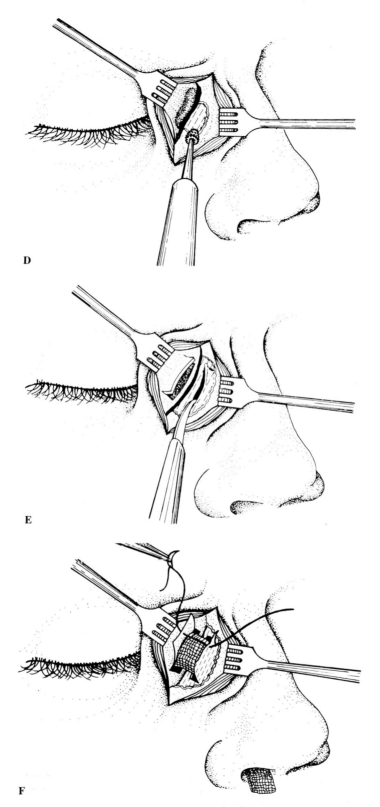

FIG. 19 (cont.) D: Burr on air drill is used to create bony opening. **E:** Incisions into lacrimal sac and nasal mucosa to create flaps. **F:** Suturing of lacrimal and mucosal flaps.

others use a trephine attachment on a Stryker saw, and still others, including these authors, prefer to use an air drill with a burr attachment to grind through at and posterior to the anterior lacrimal crest (Fig. 19D). A hole large enough to allow the jaw of a small Kerrison punch is made, attempting not to break through the nasal mucosa. The bone is then removed, taking out the anterior lacrimal crest, the nasal wall of the nasolacrimal duct, and most of the nasal wall to the lacrimal fossa, including the bone beneath the medial canthal tendon. This will involve the removal of the frontal process of the maxilla and the lacrimal bone. Inadequate bone removal is a common and serious error that can lead to reobstruction.

After the bone is removed, a 0 or 00 probe is placed in the lower punctum and canaliculus and the sac is tented into the wound. With a #12 Bard-Parker blade, an incision is made into the sac from the upper part of the fundus of the sac and down toward the nasolacrimal duct opening (Fig. 19E). This incision is placed so as to create a flap of sac wall that can be pulled anteriorly toward the wound opening, thereby creating a large opening in the sac facing the nasal mucosa. The sac wall below this flap is excised. One must remember in incising the sac wall that there are actually two layers of tissue in the wall; that is, the wall of the sac itself and the adherent periosteum must both be cut through. Irrigation with a lacrimal cannula and a syringe is then carried out through the puncta and canalicular system.

If the fluid flows easily into the wound, one can be comfortable that the obstruction was indeed in the nasolacrimal duct and the common internal punctum is open and clear. However, if the fluid does not enter the wound but continues to regurgitate through the opposite punctum, attention must be turned to the common internal punctum, which may be occluded by overlooked adjacent bone or soft tissue flaps of sac wall. These need to be clear, and if the obstruction persists, the opening of the common internal punctum within the sac itself must be excised. This is done by tenting the internal punctal area into the wound with a probe and grasping the peak of the tent and snipping it off with a Westcott scissors. The fluid should then flow easily.

We then deal with the nasal mucosa. A curved hemostat is placed in the nose and the mucosa is tented into the wound. A #12 Bard-Parker blade is used to cut an identical incision opposite the one previously cut in the lacrimal sac. An anterior flap is created, the posterior mucosa is exposed, and the bony window is excised. When we pull both flaps (lacrimal sac and nasal mucosa) up into the wound, there will exist two openings facing each other—the open lacrimal sac and the adjacent nasal cavity at the level of the middle meatus (see Fig. 19E).

A probe is again placed through the canalicular system into the wound, one end of an 8-inch piece of umbilical tape thoroughly impregnated with antibiotic steroid ointment is placed up in the area of the common internal punctum (the area where the probe enters), and the probe is removed. The tape is then packed up into this area, and the opposite end is grasped, pulled out of the nose, and cut within the nose so that it can be easily grasped and removed later. The two flaps (lacrimal sac and nasal mucosa) are then sutured together over the gauze using a 4–0 chromic suture on a half-circle needle (Fig. 19F). Meticulous suturing of the anterior flaps and posterior flaps of the lacrimal sac and nasal mucosa is important in maintaining a patent rhinostomy, a principle of the DCR. The wound is closed using deep absorbable sutures and interrupted or running skin sutures of choice.

Some recommend that a Quickert silicone tube be left in place for several weeks when extensive manipulation is carried out in the area of the common internal punctum. We highly recommend this, and also use a 1-mm silicone rod in traumatic cases with a great deal of scar tissue and in children under 7 or 8 years of age, because of their tremendous capacity for healing and sealing off the surgical fistula created. We often place postoperative DCR patients on prophylactic antibiotics and use, in place of saline, a dilute solution of polymyxin B–neomycin-gramicidin (Neosporin®) for irrigation during the case. This is important because of nasal contamination and the frequency of purulence in the infected lacrimal sac contaminating the wound.

Occasionally casts forming in the lacrimal sac and nasolacrimal duct will be present. These can either be removed with forceps or irrigated out of the sac.

Patients leave the hospital the day after surgery and will rarely, if ever, experience any pain. When bilateral stenosis is present, both sides can be operated at the same surgical session.

It will sometimes be necessary to shrink the nose down to find the pack, and occasionally vigorous bleeding can occur when the pack is removed. In about 6 cases of approximately 250, we have had to get ENT consultation to control the persistent ooze of blood. This usually results from the pack drying, sticking to mucosal vessels, and rupturing the vessels when it is removed.

Patients will generally get very little scarring, but the wound will become elevated and hard as the scar matures. The complete healing to the final scar takes about 3 months, and the patient should be told to expect this. Some patients will react to the absorbable subcutaneous sutures and begin to form pustules and spit the sutures out. This occurs about 2 to 5 weeks postoperatively. We treat them with local incision and drainage, systemic antibiotics, and heat compresses. A properly done DCR should yield a success rate in the high 90th percentile (32,33).

Iliff recommends a somewhat different technique, in that he omits the umbilical tape and instead uses a piece of rubber or silicone French catheter to bridge the gap between the sac and the nasal mucosa. Since it is sutured with chromic, it can be pulled out in 10 days to 2 weeks.

We have attempted in the text of our DCR description to point out common errors and pitfalls that could lead to surgical failure. In spite of careful adherence to these techniques, an occasional recurrence results. If a DCR is not successful, passage of a Quickert tube can be made, and if one still has no success, a repeat DCR must be done, attempting with this second procedure to discover the reason for failure. Everything should be exaggerated on the repeat DCR (larger bony window, longer duration of umbilical packing, Quickert silicone tubing); however, the most common causes of DCR failure are fibrous overgrowth of the rhinostomy and common canalicular obstruction (32).

JONES TUBES

Closure of the . . . canaliculus may follow repeated probing, occur post dacryocystorhinostomy, and follow inflammation such as herpes simplex and other inflammatory agents, [trauma, surgery, and irradiation]. A bypass procedure for tear elimination is indicated when the lacrimal canaliculi have been destroyed or the remnants of canaliculi cannot be anastomosed satisfactorily with [the] intranasal cavity to establish tear drainage. It is also indicated in some cases in which the eyelids are totally paralyzed or tethered by scar tissue so that the pumping action of the canaliculus is absent [10]. A small Pyrex glass tube is placed to drain the tears from the lacrimal lake into the nose, and its mechanism is [largely] that of gravity drainage, although some lid movements must be present to move the tears into the lake area. Materials other than glass have been used as the bypass conduit, however, these are not as effective because they are hydrophobic and repel a smooth flow of tears. Since no canalicular system has ever been successfully reconstructed even on a short-term basis with skin grafts, mucous membrane grafts or vein grafts, this is the only available procedure. Fortunately, it is usually successful.

The Jones tube is not indicated for a focal block such as occurs with internal common punctum obstruction. These cases are helped with internal punctoplasty and intubation with silicone at the time of DCR. Similarly, an isolated canalicular obstruction can usually be resected and reconstructed over silicone tubing.

It is most important to have a full set of Pyrex glass tubes available with collar sizes of 3, 3.5, and 4 mm. Tubes are available with and without holes in the collar. The nasal end should be flared slightly. The tubes we prefer are manufactured by Gunther Weiss.[2] A useful method of storing the tubes and keeping a current inventory is to have the autoclavable Jones tube steel box (Gunther Weiss).

A conjunctivodacryocystorhinostomy is a specialized DCR performed in conjunction with placing a Jones tube (34). A Jones tube may also be placed after a DCR if the bony ostium is correctly positioned. After completing the DCR, as described previously, attention is directed toward placement of the Jones tube. This is done before closure of the anterior flaps in the DCR procedure. A linear slit is made in the caruncle so the tube will be well situated in the nasal end of the palpebral fissure. No carunclar tissue is removed. A 15-gauge needle is passed into the nose through the canalicular slit (Fig. 20A). The direction is anterior and inferior. The tip of the needle is visualized anterior to the tip of the middle turbinate. The intranasal septum must be sufficiently away from the lateral wall of the nose for adequate space. The middle turbinate tip should be trimmed or excised as needed. The passageway from the medial canthus to the nose is enlarged with a knife or scissors (Fig. 20B). A Quickert-Dryden lacrimal intubating 00 probe is placed through the needle lumen into the nose (Fig. 20C). As the needle is withdrawn from the nose, the distance from the caruncle to the nose should be measured. With the tip of the needle in the midaspect of the nostril, the hemostat is placed on the needle next to the caruncle. The marked needle length indicates the distance into the nose and the length of the Jones tube needed. A Quickert-Dryden probe remains in the nose as the needle is withdrawn. The new passageway should be in soft tissues so that the Jones tube has a soft tissue suspension. The Quickert-Dryden probe is used as a guide for passing the glass Jones tube directly into the nose (Fig. 20D). A suture is placed through the hole in the collar to fixate the tube to adjacent tissues. Another method for placing the tube is to use the glaucoma trephine over a solid guide. The glaucoma trephine cuts the hole into the nose. The probe is then pushed into the nose with care.

The length of the tube should be such as to extend well into the nose without touching the septum (Fig. 20E). The collar size should be initially 3.5 to 4.0 mm. As the tube becomes well seated, it is not unusual to need a shorter length or smaller collar size. Straight tubes are preferred by the authors. A spectrum of tube sizes should be available in Pyrex glass. The plastic tubes are never placed initially or late.

Postoperatively, the patient should be on topical antibiotics. The patient should also be encouraged to aspirate water or saline through the tube daily on a long-term basis to prevent protein buildup.

Tubes are an excellent bypass appliance. However, the surgeon must be willing to follow the tubes for a long term. Changing the tube length or collar size is expected in the postoperative period. Decreased tissue swelling may cause the need for a shorter tube. A large collar may be irritating. Expected maintenance also includes cleansing with alcohol annually or biannually. Tube placement or cleansing is facilitated by passing a Quickert-

---

[2] 14380 N.W. Science Park Dr., Portland, Oregon 97229.

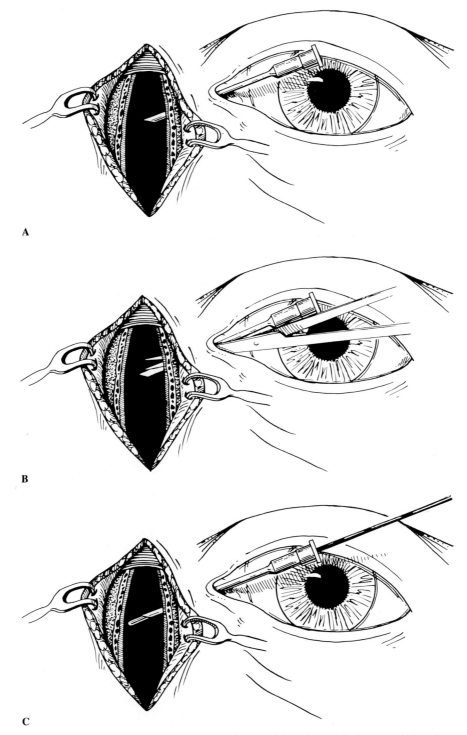

FIG. 20. Jones tube placement. **A:** A 15-gauge needle passed through a slit in the caruncle into the nose. **B:** A sharp scissors is used to enlarge the path into the nose along the 15-guage needle. **C:** A Quickert-Dryden probe (00) is passed into the nose through the lumen of the needle.

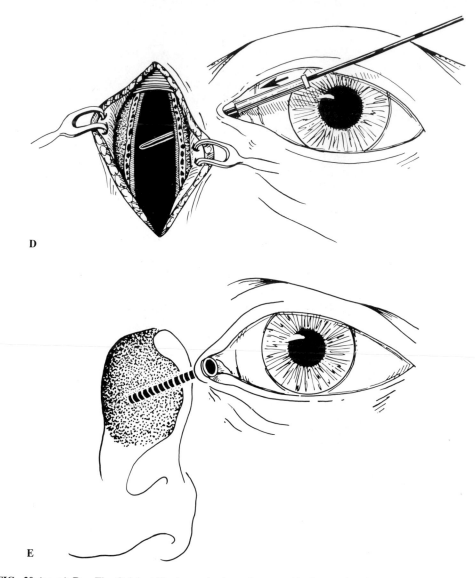

FIG. 20 (cont.) D: The Quickert-Dryden probe is used as a guide for passing the glass Jones tube into the nose. **E:** The tube, properly positioned in the nose, should be suspended within soft tissues.

Dryden probe through the lumen, as a guide to be left in place until the tube is replaced. Topical anesthetic is generally required.

The evaluation of the tube length or position is easier with the fiberoptic principle than with direct illumination in the nose. A sharp focal light source (transluminator) is applied to the collar of the Jones tube while the surgeon looks into the nose with the nasal speculum. The tube tip is brightly illuminated. Intranasal relationships can be well seen.

Most complications of the Jones tubes are preventable or manageable. Complications include failure to drain, migration, loss, and infection. Drainage problems are usually avoided by proper placement of the tube in the nose. The tube should not be against a turbinate, septum, polyp, or the lateral wall of the nose. A tube against solid tissue may migrate or not function. The tube has to be shortened, moved, or given clearance by resecting the offending nasal anatomy. Epistaxis may occur if the tube is too long. Loss is more apt to occur before the tube is seated in scar tissue. A suture around or through the collar is important initially. Similarly, the tube should be protected with gentle finger pressure when sneezing or gentle nose blowing occurs. Tubes are left in place for life. Occasionally patients will have done well with an epithelialized tract without the tube. However, a trial without the tube is not encouraged. Infection of the conjunctiva due to the direct connection with the nose needs treatment as indicated. Tissue infection deep in the medial canthus has not been a problem.

Various alternative tubes have been introduced, but the authors strongly advocate the Jones tube. The Thornton tube is a plastic tube placed down the nasolacrimal duct into the nose. The angled silicone Reineke tube passes from the caruncle into the nose through a dacryocystorhinostomy ostium (35). These tubes are being mentioned only to discourage their use; they are harder to service and lack wettability.

DACRYOCYSTECTOMY

Dacryocystectomy is indicated in patients who usually fall into one of two groups (10). One group are those with acute or subacute dacryocystitis who do not suffer from epiphora. In elderly patients with dacryocystitis without epiphora, the relatively brief dacryocystectomy operation is well tolerated and has a short recovery period. The second group of patients in whom dacryocystectomy is indicated are those with lacrimal sac tumors (36,37). The usual presentation of lacrimal sac tumors is as a lacrimal sac mass above the level of the medial canthal tendon, as chronic dacryocystitis that irrigates freely, or as bloody tears or bloody reflux with irrigation. With epithelial tumors of the lacrimal sac, it is necessary to surgically excise the entire sac and the nasolacrimal duct.

A simple dacryocystectomy may be performed under either local or general anesthesia. Lidocaine with epinephrine will aid hemostasis and is infiltrated around the lacrimal sac. If a tumor is suspected, general anesthesia is preferred. The standard DCR skin incision is made with a #15 blade and the orbicularis muscle is dissected down to the level of periosteum. The periosteum of the anterior lacrimal crest is incised and the periorbita and lacrimal sac are reflected laterally out of the lacrimal sac fossa. The anterior limb of the medial canthal tendon is severed to expose the fundus of the lacrimal sac. Subcutaneous tissue attachments to the sac are dissected, including the fibers of the inferior oblique muscle origin, and the superior and inferior preseptal muscles, so as to mobilize the entire body and fundus of the lacrimal sac. The needle Bovie or Westcott scissors is then used to excise the sac superiorly at the level of the common canaliculus and inferiorly at the nasolacrimal duct as it enters the bony canal. The above procedure is adequate to cure the patient with dacryocystitis without epiphora. A dacryocystectomy is a much shorter operation than the standard DCR, and the recovery period more brief.

If a tumor is suspected, a frozen section biopsy of the lacrimal sac must be submitted. In the presence of an epithelial tumor of the lacrimal sac, the entire lacrimal sac and nasolacrimal duct must be excised. The lacrimal sac is removed as described above. The nasolacrimal duct is best removed from a Caldwell-Luc transantral approach (see Chapter 8 for detailed description of this technique). Transantrally, the bony nasolacrimal canal is visible as a prominence under the sinus mucosa. The bone is chipped away to expose the nasolacrimal duct, which is then removed in its entirety. It is often necessary to excise the tip of the inferior turbinate in order to expose and remove the distal portion of the nasolacrimal duct. An alternate method of removing the nasolacrimal duct is from above via the DCR incision. An external ethmoidectomy is performed to enhance exposure of the nasolacrimal duct. It should be noted that the transantral approach ensures the most complete removal of the entire nasolacrimal duct.

REFERENCES

1. Duke-Elder, S., and MacFaul, P. A. (1974): Diseases of the lacrimal passages. In: *The Ocular Adnexa, Vol. XIII, Part 2: System of Ophthalmology*, edited by S. Duke-Elder, pp. 675–766. Mosby, St. Louis.
2. Bouzas, A. (1973): Virus etiology of certain cases of lacrimal obstruction. *Br. J. Ophthalmol.*, 57:849–851.
3. Flanagan, J., and Stokes, D. P. (1978): Lacrimal sac tumors. *Ophthalmology*, 85:1282–1287.
4. Walter, J. R., Stratford, T., and Harrell, E. R. (1956): Cast-like fungus obstruction of the nasolacrimal duct. *Arch. Ophthalmol.*, 55:320–325.
5. Walter, J. R. (1977): Pityrosporum species associated with dacryoliths in obstructive dacryocystitis. *Am. J. Ophthalmol.*, 84:806–809.
6. Jones, L. T. (1962): The cure of epiphora due to canalicular disorders, trauma, and surgical failures on the lacrimal passages. *Trans. Am. Acad. Ophthalmol. Otolaryngol.*, 66:506–524.
7. Flanagan, J. (1978): Epiphora following rhinoplasty. *Ann. Ophthalmol.*, 10:1239–1242.
8. Newell, F. W., and Ernest, J. T. (1974): The lacrimal apparatus. In: *Ophthalmology Principles and Concepts*. Mosby, St. Louis.
9. Kohn, R., Romano, P. E., and Puklin, J. E. (1976): Lacrimal obstruction after migration of orbital implant. *Am. J. Ophthalmol.*, 82:934–936.
10. Jones, L. T., and Wobig, J. L. (1976): *Surgery of the Eyelids and Lacrimal System*. Aesculapius, Birmingham, Alabama.
11. Hecht, S. D. (1978): Evaluation of the lacrimal drainage system. *Ophthalmology*, 85:1250–1258.
12. Flack, A. (1979): The fluorescein appearance test for lacrimal obstruction. *Ann. Ophthalmol.*, 11:237–242.
13. Hornblass, A. (1973): A simple taste test for lacrimal obstruction. *Arch. Ophthalmol.*, 90:435–436.
14. Hurwitz, J. J., Welham, R. A. N., and Maisey, M. N. (1976): Intubation macrodacryostography and quantitative scintillography: The complete lacrimal assessment. *Trans. Am. Acad. Ophthalmol. Otolaryngol.*, 81:575–582.
15. Milder, B. (1977): Diagnosis and treatment of lacrimal diseases. In: *Ophthalmic Plastic Surgery*, edited by B. Silver et al., pp. 161–173. American Academy of Ophthalmology and Otolaryngology, Rochester, Minnesota.
16. Crigler, L. W. (1923): The treatment of congenital dacryocystitis. *JAMA*, 81:23–24.
17. Price, H. W. (1947): Dacryostenosis. *J. Pediatr.*, 30:302–305.
18. Kusher, B. J. (1982): Congenital nasolacrimal system obstruction. *Arch. Ophthalmol.*, 100:597–600.
19. Nelson, L. B., Calhoun, J. H., and Menduke, H. (1985): Medical management of congenital nasolacrimal duct obstruction. *Ophthalmology*, 92:1187–1190.
20. Quickert, M. H., and Dryden, R. M. (1970): Probes for intubation in the lacrimal drainage system. *Trans. Amer. Acad. Ophthalmol. Otolaryngol.*, 74:431–433.
21. Crawford, J. S. (1977): Intubation of obstructions in the lacrimal system. *Can. J. Ophthalmol.*, 12:289–292.
22. Shore, J. W., and McCord, C. D. (1982): Modified Crawford hook for lacrimal intubation. *Am. J. Ophthalmol.*, 94:255–256.
23. Peterson, R. A., and Robb, R. M. (1978): The natural course of congenital obstruction of the nasolacrimal duct. *J. Pediatr. Ophthalmol. Strabismus*, 15:246–250.
24. Scott, W. E., Fabre, J. A., and Ossoinig, K. C. (1979): Congenital mucocele of the lacrimal sac. *Arch. Ophthalmol.*, 97:1656–1658.
25. Wojno, T. H. (1985): Congenital dacryocystocele in identical twins. *Ophthalmic Plast. Reconstr. Surg.*, 1:263–265.
26. McCord, C. D., Jr. (1985): The lacrimal drainage system. In: *Clinical Ophthalmology*, edited by T. D. Duane and E. A. Jaeger, Vol. 4, Chpt. 13, pp. 1–25. Harper & Row, Philadelphia.
27. Hanselmayer, H. (1973): Prognosis of injured canaliculi in relation to elapsed time until primary operation. *Ophthalmologica*, 166:175–179.
28. Dortzbach, R. K., and Angrist, R. A. (1985): Silicone intubation for lacerated lacrimal canaliculi. *Ophthalmic Surg.*, 16:639–642.
29. Shead, J. W., Rathbun, J. E., and Crawford, J. B. (1980): Effects of the silicone tube on the canaliculus. An animal experiment. *Ophthalmology*, 87:1031–1036.

30. Morrison, F. D. (1973): An aid to repair of lacerated tear ducts. *Arch. Ophthalmol.,* 72:341–342.
31. Saunders, D. H., Shannon, G. M., and Flanagan, J. C. (1978): The effectiveness of the pigtail probe method of repairing canalicular lacerations. *Ophthalmic Surg.,* 9:33–40.
32. McLachlan, D. L., Shannon, G. M., and Flanagan, J. C. (1980): Results of dacryocystorhinostomy: Analysis of reoperations. *Ophthalmic Surg.,* 11:427–430.
33. Zolli, C. L., and Shannon, G. M. (1982): Dacryocystorhinostomy: A review of 119 cases. *Ophthalmic Surg.,* 13:905–910.
34. Jones, L. T. (1965): Conjunctivodacryocystorhinostomy. *Am. J. Ophthalmol.,* 59:773–783.
35. Reinecke, R. D., and Carroll, J. M. (1969): Silicone lacrimal tube implantation. *Trans. Am. Acad. Ophthalmol. Otolaryngol.,* 73:85–90.
36. Ryan, S. J., and Font, R. L. (1973): Primary epithelial neoplasms of the lacrimal sac. *Am. J. Ophthalmol.,* 76:73–88.
37. Stokes, D. P., and Flanagan, J. C. (1977): Dacryocystectomy for tumors of the lacrimal sac. *Ophthalmic Surg.,* 8:85–90.

Oculoplastic Surgery, 2nd edition, edited by
Clinton D. McCord, Jr., and Myron Tanenbaum.
Raven Press, New York © 1987.

Chapter 15

Evisceration, Enucleation, and Exenteration

*Henry Baylis, *Norman Shorr, **Clinton D. McCord, Jr., and
†Myron Tanenbaum

*Division of Ophthalmic Plastic and Reconstructive Surgery, Jules Stein Eye Institute, University of
California at Los Angeles, Los Angeles, California 90024; **Department of Ophthalmology, Emory
University School of Medicine, Atlanta, Georgia 30308; and †Bascom Palmer Eye Institute, Department
of Ophthalmology, University of Miami School of Medicine, Miami, Florida 33101*

ENUCLEATION VERSUS EVISCERATION

General Considerations

Enucleation is the surgical procedure in which the globe and a portion of the optic nerve are removed from the orbit. Evisceration is the surgical procedure in which the intraocular contents, and possibly the cornea, are removed, leaving the sclera intact. The choice between these two operations may be extremely difficult. Many complex factors must be considered before selecting the appropriate technique.

Advantages and Disadvantages

The advantages and disadvantages of these two procedures must be considered relative to the management of intraocular tumors, the surgical treatment of uncontrollable endophthalmitis, the prevention of sympathetic ophthalmia, and the maintenance of maximal anatomic integrity of the orbit.

An enucleation must be performed in cases of suspected malignant intraocular tumor, where the histologic examination, as well as total removal of the tumor, is an absolute necessity. Enucleation provides an intact globe as a pathology specimen for histologic examination. Examination of the globe for extrascleral extension or optic nerve involvement of the tumor can only be performed during or following enucleation. On the other hand, evisceration provides a disrupted pathology specimen and risks leaving residual tumor behind.

The choice between these two procedures is particularly significant relative to enophthalmitis. Evisceration involves the extirpation and drainage of the ocular contents without invading the orbit. This procedure avoids contamination of the orbit and a possible subsequent orbital cellulitis. Enucleation involves severing the optic nerve and cutting across the potential subarachnoid space, which communicates with the same space in the cranial cavity. This procedure risks spread of the ocular infection and possible subsequent meningitis. The use of systemic antibiotics diminishes this potential risk of enucleation for endophthalmitis.

These two procedures have great significance in both the cause and avoidance of sympathetic ophthalmia. The removal of an eye following trauma presents a difficult decision as to the choice of operation. While sympathetic ophthalmia is a rare occurrence, it must be considered in all cases involving injury to the eye with uveal prolapse. The total enucleation of the globe within 10 to 14 days following the injury is considered the most certain way of preventing sympathetic ophthalmia (1,2).

In the authors' experience an evisceration, with special attention to the total removal of any uveal tissue, may also be considered as a way to prevent sympathetic ophthalmia. The evisceration procedure itself has been known to cause sympathetic ophthalmia (3). However, several reports, with a total of approximately 1,000 cases of evisceration, had no incidence of subsequent sympathetic ophthalmia. Unfortunately, there are no firm statistics regarding evisceration and its relationship to sympathetic ophthalmia (3).

A major factor in the selection of the surgical procedure is the markedly different long- and short-term effects of each on the position and appearance of the orbital contents. In this context, enucleation is decidedly inferior to evisceration in every respect.

Evisceration has the distinct cosmetic and functional advantage of leaving the orbital anatomy virtually undisturbed. Motility of the socket and eyelids may be retained indefinitely. Following evisceration, ptosis of the muscle cone and socket may never occur because of the undisturbed suspensory ligaments. Retention of the sclera provides approximately 0.5 cm^3 of retained orbital volume with less subsequent enophthalmos. The simplicity of an evisceration permits the performance of this surgery on even the most debilitated patient. On the other hand, an enucleation is a complex orbital operation. This operation, frequently disdained for its simplicity, is in fact very involved and fraught with difficulties. The orbital anatomy is severely disrupted by this operation, leading to diminished motility of the socket as well as other early and late postoperative cosmetic defects. The removal of the well-suspended, properly located scleral pouch and its replacement by a poorly supported implant may lead to subsequent enophthalmos, migration of the orbital implant, and a ptosis of the muscle cone and entire orbital contents.

Indications

There are some absolute indications for both enucleation and evisceration. However, frequently the choice of one procedure over the other is difficult and must be based on the individual preference of the ophthalmologist and the particular circumstances. This decision must be made on a case-by-case basis with the consent of the fully informed patient. For example, an enucleation should not be performed for the pathology specimen alone without informing the patient of the alternative of evisceration. Conversely, an evisceration should not be performed for its definite cosmetic and functional advantages without informing the patient of the possible associated hazards.

In all cases of removal of the eye for suspected intraocular malignant tumor, enucleation is the procedure of choice. The methods and successes of various treatments for tumors of all types are changing almost daily. Therefore, indications for removal of an eye for a malignancy must be reviewed frequently. The decision as to modality of treatment for various intraocular tumors should be arrived at with the help of specialists in this field.

In cases of ocular injury with prolapsed uvea, the patient must be told of the possible, albeit rare, chance of sympathetic ophthalmia with evisceration. The authors believe that evisceration performed soon after an ocular injury of this type is relatively safe, but there are no statistics available to either substantiate or refute this belief. If the patient wishes to feel as safe as possible, enucleation is the procedure of choice. The patient must be made aware of the cosmetic benefits of evisceration versus the cosmetic difficulties of enucleation in making this choice.

In a blind, painful eye in which a tumor can be ruled out by direct visualization, the authors prefer an evisceration. Pain is relieved by evisceration equally as well as it is by enucleation. In a blind, painful eye in which an intraocular tumor is suspected or cannot be ruled out by ultrasound or a computed tomography (CT) scan, an enucleation is the procedure of choice. If there is no suspicion of an intraocular tumor, and if the patient is aware of the potential problem if there is a tumor, an evisceration may be considered.

An enucleation is the procedure of choice in removal of an eye with a staphyloma or following repeated ocular surgery, such as scleral buckling. An evisceration may be used for removal of an eye during or following enophthalmitis, although there is a potential risk of sympathetic ophthalmia (4).

Typical Clinical Problems

Case #1—Severe Ocular Trauma—Delayed Removal

A 10-year-old child fell from a tree, sustaining an eye injury. Examination revealed a hyphema of the affected eye with prolapse of the uvea through the cornea. Orbital X-rays were normal. Surgical exploration revealed a corneal scleral wound extending 8 mm into the sclera with uveal and retinal prolapse. The prolapsed tissue was excised and reposited and the wound was closed in surgery. Although it was certain that the eye would be blind, the eye was retained in hopes of maintaining a blind, comfortable eye. Over the 6 days following the surgery, the pain and inflammation were constant. The patient and his parents had had time to digest the severity of the injury. On the seventh day, when everyone had accepted the fact that the eye was not salvageable, the patient was returned to surgery. At that time, with fully informed consent, an evisceration was performed.

Case #2—Severe Ocular Trauma—Primary Removal

A 20-year-old man was stuck in the right eye with a broken bottle. In surgery, examination revealed multiple, extremely ragged lacerations of the globe with extensive prolapse of intraocular contents. Surgical exploration revealed posterior extension of these lacerations with fragmented wound edges. Because of the extensive nature of the wound, it was necessary to remove two rectus muscles from the globe in order to visualize the posterior extensions of the laceration. The decision to remove the eye was made at surgery because of the extensive nature of the injury and the unsalvageable status of the globe. It was necessary to remove the sclera in order to remove all the uveal tissue. A 16-mm hollow glass sphere was placed in the orbit and the remainder of the enucleation was performed.

Case #3—A Blind, Painful Eye of Questionable Etiology

A 60-year-old woman complained of a blind, painful right eye. There was history of long-standing inflammation of the eye of unknown etiology. The fundus of that eye could not be visualized and the ultrasound and CT scan were negative. Because of the uncertainty of the etiology and the inflammation, an enucleation was performed.

Case #4—A Blind, Painful Eye—Tumor Extension Discovered at Surgery

A 60-year-old man with a dense cataract of 5 years' duration and a mildly inflamed, blind, painful eye of 6 months' duration had a CT scan and ultrasound findings with posterior pole organized hemorrhage or tumor. At surgery, a pigmented tumor was discovered extending through the sclera. A frozen section pathology report revealed a cellular tumor consistent with melanoma. Additional local excision of all pigmented tumor was carried out and the orbit was patched with Vaseline gauze. Immediately after surgery, consultation was obtained from pathology and oncology. Recommendations for additional tests, additional surgery, or other treatment modalities were presented to the patient.

Case #5—Blind, Painful Eye of Known Etiology

A 55-year-old diabetic man had lost his vision over the past year because of rubeosis and uncontrollable glaucoma. The fundus could be seen and revealed no tumor. Intraocular pressure was 50 mm Hg. Because of the pain, the patient wished to have the eye removed. The patient was concerned with appearance and an evisceration was performed. Contrary to common misconception, evisceration relieves ocular pain as well as enucleation.

Case #6—Blind, Painful Eye in Elderly Debilitated Patient

A 92-year-old woman resident of a nursing home complained of severe pain of the left eye. The patient was debilitated from multiple other medical problems. Previous alcohol injections had not relieved the ocular pain. An evisceration, without an implant, was performed on the patient under local anesthesia.

Case #7—Enophthalmitis—Evisceration with Implant

A 65-year-old woman had been treated for enophthalmitis following cataract extraction. Treatment over the past 3 weeks had quieted the infection, but severe pain was still present. An evisceration was performed on the patient under general anesthesia and, following irrigation of the scleral pouch with the appropriate antibiotic, a 16-mm hollow glass sphere was sutured into position. The patient had been prepared for the possibility of an extrusion. In the event of an extrusion, the patient will be no worse than had the procedure been done without an implant.

In the same situation, but with a more active infection or a patient who is less concerned with cosmetic appearance, a drain of iodoform gauze is placed in the scleral pouch. The drain is gradually removed over a 5-day period and the socket heals by secondary intention. The socket is fully healed and a prosthesis is fitted after 1 month.

ENUCLEATION

Patient Preparation

Prior to enucleation, the patient is prepared for the fitting and wearing of a prosthesis. An appointment with the ocularist is made for approximately 2 weeks following surgery. It is explained to the patient that the prosthesis will look similar to the normal eye with variable loss of movement and some asymmetry. The possibility of extrusion and infection is explained. The incidence of early postoperative extrusion of an orbital implant is low enough that the authors have never knowingly had one. If surgery is to be performed for a severe ocular injury, the possibility of enucleation or evisceration is discussed, as well as the choice between these two procedures.

Removal of the Wrong Eye

Removal of the wrong eye is one of the greatest disasters that can occur to the ophthalmic surgeon and patient. Every ophthalmologist and surgeon must be aware of this possibility, no matter how remote. It is unfortunate that standard textbook chapters on the enucleation technique (5,6) typically fail to even mention this possible tragedy.

Preoperatively, the ophthalmic surgeon may mark the forehead or trim the lashes on the appropriate side. These methods, however, are not failsafe. In the operating room, the surgeon must compulsively review the chart, including the operative permit and examination notes. It is important, then, that the surgeon himself or herself prep and drape the patient. Traquair (7) has suggested the use of local anesthesia as a means of preventing removal of the wrong eye. It must never, never happen that a surgeon hurries into the operating room where the patient is already under general anesthesia and begins the operation without delay. This is not the way to perform an enucleation!

Once a sterile operative field is set up, the surgeon must again verify that the correct eye is about to undergo enucleation. In situations of enucleation following severe trauma, the correct eye is often externally deformed. In cases where the external appearance of both eyes is normal, the surgeon must compulsively reexamine the fundus. Intraoperative, indirect ophthalmoscopy is necessary to confirm that the surgical field has been set up correctly.

The authors stress the finality of the enucleation procedure. No degree of thoroughness is excessive in order to avoid removal of the wrong eye.

Surgical Technique

Anesthesia

An enucleation may be performed under local or general anesthesia. General anesthesia is preferred over local anesthesia by the authors because of the severe emotional impact of the removal of an eye. If enucleation is performed under local anesthesia, at least 5 ml of 2% lidocaine (Xylocaine®) with epinephrine and hyaluronidase (Wydase®) is used in a retrobulbar injection. Additional infiltrative anesthesia with the same solution is used in the eyelids. If general anesthesia is used, 5 ml of 1% lidocaine with epinephrine and hyaluronidase is used in a retrobulbar injection for hemostasis. An additional 2 ml of

0.5% bupivacaine (Marcaine®) with epinephrine and hyaluronidase may be added to the retrobulbar injection to prolong the analgesic effect for several hours following surgery.

Removal of the Globe

A 360° peritomy is performed. The conjunctiva and Tenon's capsule are dissected back to the rectus muscles. Tenon's capsule is further separated from the globe to the equator in the four quadrants between the muscles. Relaxing incisions are made at the 3 o'clock and 9 o'clock positions only if needed. The insertion of the medial rectus muscle is isolated with a muscle hook, but care is taken not to dissect the intermuscular septum along the length of the muscle. The maintenance of the integrity of Tenon's capsule and the intermuscular septum preserves the layers that prevent the later migration of the orbital implant. The medial rectus muscle is divided from the globe, leaving a long stump on the globe to be used for traction. The rectus muscles are then isolated and divided from the globe. The medialrectus, lateral rectus, and inferior rectus muscles are secured with double-armed 6–0 Vicryl sutures (Fig. 1A). The superior rectus muscle is simply detached from the globe and allowed to retract. Manipulation and suturing of the superior rectus muscle is more likely to induce a postoperative ptosis than to enhance motility of a prosthesis. The superior oblique tendon is gathered on a muscle hook and severed. The inferior oblique muscle is similarly identified and detached from the globe.

It should be mentioned at this point that enucleation for a possible melanoma should be treated in a special manner (8). Intraoperative, indirect ophthalmoscopy should be performed on the eye in the sterile operative field to verify that the enucleation is being performed on the correct eye. Additionally, special care should be taken to avoid excess manipulation or pressure on the globe in cases of intraocular tumors. It is thought that the manipulation of the surgery itself may be responsible for metastases (9,10). Fraunfelder et al. have described a "no touch" enucleation technique (11), although its efficacy remains controversial.

The medial rectus stump is grasped with a hemostat. Anterior traction on the stump of the medial rectus stretches the optic nerve and rotates it medially. It should be noted that abduction of the globe, which results from the forward traction on the stump of the medial rectus muscle, accentuates the already nasal position of the optic nerve, thereby making the cutting of the nerve more accessible from the nasal side. Therefore, the enucleation is always performed from the nasal side. A curved hemostat is introduced from a superonasal direction. The closed hemostat is then used to strum the optic nerve. The hemostat is then opened slightly, and with strumming, the optic nerve is straddled by the blades. The partially opened hemostat is worked back along the nerve, and then clamped. With the hemostat in place, a slender Metzenbaum scissors is then used to transect the optic nerve (Fig. 1B). The enucleation specimen is inspected before being passed out of the sterile field for pathologic exam. The needle Bovie is used to cauterize the cut stump of the optic nerve. Following cauterization, the hemostat is removed. The socket is inspected for any evidence of bleeding (Fig. 1C). Hemostasis should be meticulously achieved to avoid postoperative hematoma formation.

In special circumstances, such as enucleations for choroidal melanomas and intraocular retinoblastomas, it is important to remove a long section of optic nerve. The principle of obtaining a long piece of optic nerve is to manipulate the cutting instrument along the optic nerve, behind the normally adherent posterior Tenon's capsule. The posterior Tenon's capsule would otherwise limit the length of optic nerve obtainable to 3 to 4 mm only. A

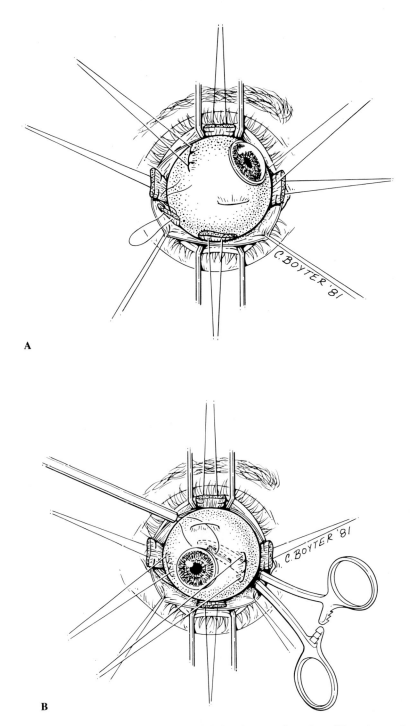

FIG. 1.   Basic steps in enucleation. **A:** A standard limbal peritomy and opening of Tenon's capsule have been performed. In this diagram, the recti muscles are secured with double-armed 6-0 Vicryl sutures. (*NOTE:* In many cases the superior rectus muscle is simply allowed to retract following disinsertion from the globe.) **B:** The globe is abducted via traction on the medial rectus stump and the optic nerve has been clamped with a hemostat. A snare is being introduced over the globe to transect the optic nerve.

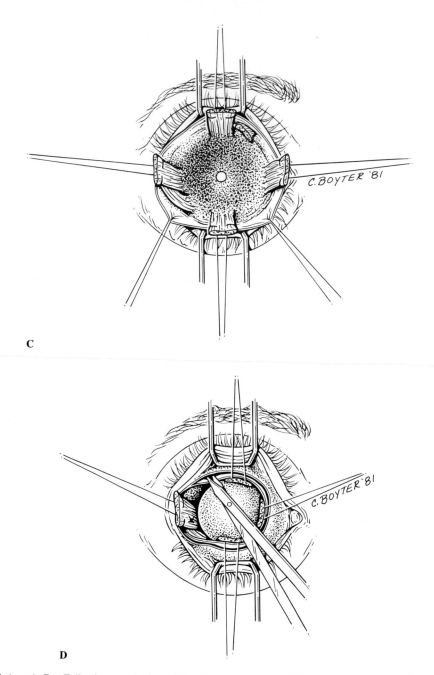

C

D

FIG. 1 (*cont.*) **C:**   Following enucleation of the globe and cautery of the optic nerve stump, the socket is inspected to verify that meticulous hemostasis has been achieved. **D:** An implant sphere is introduced into the socket; Tenon's capsule is brought up around the sphere. **E:** The anterior Tenon's capsule is closed in two layers (criss-cross fashion) with interrupted 4-0 Vicryl sutures. The recti muscles are still secured with double-armed 6-0 Vicryl sutures and will be sewn into the fornices. (Courtesy John Shore, M.D., and William Chen, M.D.)

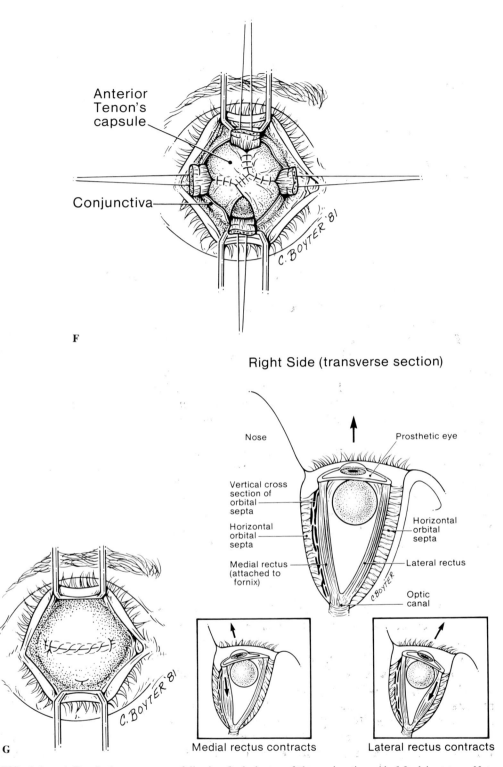

FIG. 1 (*cont.*) F: Socket appearance following final closure of the conjunctiva with 6-0 plain suture. Note that the medial, lateral, and inferior recti muscles have been sewn to the fornices and attached to conjunctiva with the double-armed 6-0 Vicryl sutures, which have been tied and cut. The superior rectus muscle is simply allowed to retract back into the socket. **G:** Cross-sectional view of the anophthalmic socket demonstrating horizontal movement of the prosthetic eye. The recti muscles transmit motility via their attachment to the fornices. (Courtesy John Shore, M.D. and William Chen, M.D.)

snare can be placed over the globe and worked posteriorly along the optic nerve toward the apex of the orbit. When tightened, the snare will thus cut a long section of optic nerve. The slender Metzenbaum scissors can also be maneuvered effectively along the nerve toward the orbital apex to ensure that an adequate optic nerve specimen is obtained. The Metzenbaum scissors otherwise can be used to focally incise the posterior Tenon's capsule to gain access to an apical portion of the optic nerve (12). In cases of retinoblastoma, the optic nerve should be cut without the use of a hemostat. In these cases, pathologic exam of the optic nerve is of critical importance; therefore, crush artifact must not be introduced.

Enucleation Implants

At this point a rent is visible in the posterior layer of Tenon's capsule. The posterior layer of Tenon's capsule is the portion that covers the posterior half of the globe. Posterior to the posterior layer of Tenon's capsule is the fat lying within the muscle cone. Large rents in the posterior Tenon's capsule are closed with interrupted 4–0 Vicryl sutures. A 16-mm (or 18-mm) hollow glass sphere can then be inserted into Tenon's capsule (Fig. 1D). The authors prefer this implant because of its light weight and inert characteristics. The authors' second choice is a hollow or solid 16-mm silicone sphere. The silicone implants have no advantage over the hollow glass sphere. Their disadvantage is their additional weight. The weight of the 16-mm hollow glass sphere is 0.5 g. The weight of the solid silicone 16-mm sphere is 2.0 g. The total volume of an average eye is 7.5 cm^3. A 16-mm sphere is equal to 2 cm^3 in volume. An 18-mm sphere is equal to 3 cm^3 in volume. However, an 18-mm sphere has the disadvantages of too much pressure on the tissue anterior to it, greater pressure on the surgical wound, and an increased tendency to migrate within the orbit. The authors do not use tunnel-type implants for several reasons. These implants require that the rectus muscles be sutured across the anterior surface of the implant. This results in the too-posterior placement of the implant. The irregular anterior surface of the implant causes irregular pressures on the tissues anterior to it, which may lead to late extrusion of the implant. The tantalum mesh implant has an unacceptably high extrusion rate and is no longer recommended as an implant choice (13).

Closure

The 16-mm or 18-mm glass sphere is inserted into Tenon's capsule. Interrupted 4–0 Vicryl sutures are used to close the anterior Tenon's capsule in criss-cross fashion over the implant sphere (Fig. 1E). The double-armed 6–0 Vicryl sutures attached to the recti muscles are brought up through the Tenon's layer closure. The conjunctiva is closed with a running 6–0 plain suture. The 6–0 Vicryl recti muscle sutures are sewn through the medial, lateral, and inferior conjunctival fornices of the socket and tied (Fig. 1F). Prosthetic motility will ultimately reflect the motility of the fornices, which is derived from the attached recti muscles (14) (Fig. 1G). As stated previously, the superior rectus muscle is routinely allowed to retract back into the socket; any advancement of the muscle could lead to a postoperative ptosis. A soft eyelid conformer is placed in the socket to maintain the shape of the fornices. Some surgeons prefer not to use conformers.

Antibiotic-steroid ointment is placed in the cul-de-sac between the lids, after which a moderate pressure dressing is applied. This dressing consists of three eyepads secured with benzoin compound and 1-inch white paper tape.

The authors soak all foreign implant materials in a solution of gentamicin. However, systemic antibiotics are not used in routine enucleations.

Problem Cases

Cases in which Tenon's capsule or the conjunctiva are compromised or inadequate present special problems. These problems predispose to an inability to retain an implant following surgery. Additionally, the vertical shortage of these layers will result in inadequate fornices. Compromise or inadequacy of conjunctiva and Tenon's capsule may be the result of alkali burns, irradiation, multiple retinal surgeries, trauma, burns, and infection. In the situations above, a graft of autogenous material may be used to augment the compromised layers. Autogenous material is much better tolerated and requires less blood supply than homologous material or any preserved graft material. Every free graft must be completely covered with a blood supply. To avoid extrusion the spherical implant may be encapsulated with autogenous fascia lata or temporalis fascia prior to insertion in the orbit. The implant is completely covered by the fascia, which is tailored to form a snug pouch and sutured securely in place. This covered implant is then placed in the orbit with the sutured side posterior. The medial and lateral rectus muscles are sutured to the fascia approximately 10 mm apart. If the Tenon's capsule layer is inadequate and cannot be closed in a normal fashion, its edges may be sutured to the implant cover. The conjunctiva, however, must be closed over the entire graft. A dermis fat graft implant as described in Chapter 16 may be used as a primary implant.

Postoperative Care and Complications

The pressure bandage is removed 48 hr after surgery. If no bleeding is present and the wound is clean and dry, antibiotic steroid ointment is reapplied and a double patch is applied. If there are signs of infection, systemic broad-spectrum antibiotics and frequent hot compresses are initiated. In the routine enucleation patient, hot compresses are initiated on the fourth postoperative day. The patient is sent to the ocularist 4 to 6 weeks following surgery for fitting of a prosthesis.

EVISCERATION

Patient Preparation

Prior to surgery, and following the discussion outlined under enucleation, the patient is told of the fitting and the wearing of a prosthesis.

Surgical Technique

Anesthesia

The same anesthetic considerations as those reviewed under enucleation are considered here. Evisceration, which is a less invasive and shorter procedure, is more commonly performed on the debilitated patient. For these reasons, local anesthesia is more commonly used with evisceration than it is with enucleation. Local or general anesthesia may be used in this technique. In either case, a retrobulbar injection of 5 ml of lidocaine with epinephrine and hyaluronidase is used. An additional 2 ml of 0.5% bupivacaine with epinephrine and hyaluronidase may be added to the retrobulbar injection to extend the period of analgesia for several hours.

Removal of Ocular Contents

The authors prefer the evisceration technique with removal of the cornea. A 360° peritomy is performed and the conjunctiva and Tenon's capsule are dissected to the insertion of the rectus muscles. The anterior chamber is then entered at 12 o'clock with a scalpel, and scissors are used to excise the cornea (Fig. 2). A spatula is used to separate the ciliary body from the sclera. An evisceration spoon is then slipped between the sclera and ciliary body and the contents of the globe are scooped from the scleral pouch. A curette is used to remove all the gross remnants of uveal tissue. A test tube may be inserted in the scleral pouch against the optic nerve. Sites of bleeding may be identified through the test tube and a cautery used to stop the bleeding. The posterior sclera is grasped with Brown-Adson forceps and pulled forward, turning the sclera inside out. The uveal pigment may be curetted using a 4 × 4 or scalpel blade. Every effort is made to remove all pigment from the sclera. Some pigment staining is inevitably left on the sclera. Cotton swabs saturated with 70% ethanol are used to denature any remaining strands of uveal tissue. The opening created by removing the cornea is extended at the 3 and 9 o'clock positions to allow better access to the inner surface of the sclera for cleaning.

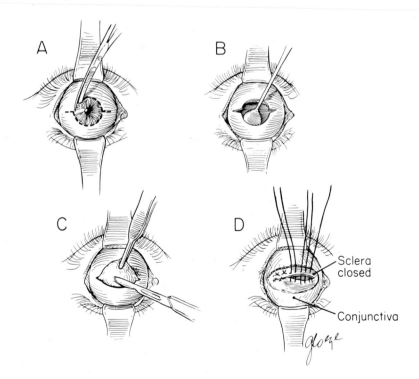

FIG. 2. Basic steps in evisceration. **A:** After a peritomy is made and the conjunctiva reflected, the cornea is excised. **B:** The evisceration spoon is used to separate and remove the ocular contents from the sclera. **C:** The posterior sclera is pulled forward through the wound and curetted to remove all uvea. **D:** The inferior scleral wound edge is brought under the superior scleral wound edge and the superior edge is then imbricated over the inferior sclera.

After all uveal tissue is removed and meticulous hemostasis obtained, a 16-mm hollow glass sphere is placed into the sclera and the scleral edges are trimmed to avoid dog ears. The sclera is then closed in a horizontal fashion by imbricating the wound edges over the surface of the spherical implant. This is accomplished by placing a double-armed 5–0 Dexon or Vicryl suture in a horizontal mattress fashion beginning 1 mm inferior to the inferior scleral wound edge. Each arm of the mattress suture is brought up through the posterior surface of the superior scleral wound 5 mm superior to the cut edge. As many of these horizontal mattress sutures are used as is necessary to close the wound tightly. The superior free edge of the sclera is then sutured down to the sclera inferiorly with simple interrupted sutures, creating a double layer of sclera over the implant. Following this closure, the conjunctiva is approximated with 6–0 plain catgut running or interrupted sutures. The use of a conformer is optional, as explained in the enucleation section. A pressure bandage is then applied over the orbit.

Problem Cases

When evisceration is performed following an ocular injury, a rupture may be found in the scleral wall. If all uveal tissue can be removed with reasonable certainty, the implant may be placed in the scleral pouch with no need to repair the rupture. If the uvea cannot be removed adequately, the evisceration may be converted to an enucleation.

In an evisceration for enophthalmitis, the scleral pouch is copiously irrigated with saline and then irrigated with antibiotics, and an implant is placed in the scleral pouch. The authors have never seen an implant extrude under these circumstances. If the implant does extrude, there is no greater problem than if a drain were placed in the pouch initially.

Postoperative Care and Complications

The pressure dressing is removed 48 hr following surgery. If the socket is clean and without hemorrhage, it is redressed with antibiotic steroid ointment and a double patch. On the fourth postoperative day, hot compresses are initiated. The patient is seen by the ocularist and the prosthesis is fitted 2 weeks following surgery.

Infection may occur following evisceration. Medical management should be attempted first and the implant removed only if this fails. If extrusion of the implant takes place shortly after surgery, an attempt should be made to replace it immediately before the sclera shrinks. It may be necessary to excise the sclera posteriorly to allow the wound to be closed without tension.

EXENTERATION

Indications

Orbital exenteration is a sometimes mutilating procedure involving, in most cases, total removal of the orbital contents and the partial or total removal of the eyelids. This procedure is indicated for malignant orbital tumors that cannot be successfully treated by other modalities. Certain other nonmalignant clinical situations can also utilize exenteration as a means of treatment or palliation. Probably the most common situation for which this operation is indicated is for malignant eyelid tumors that invade the orbit. Many of these malignant eyelid tumors need wide local excision because of potential metastases. The usual tumors are the basal cell carcinomas, particularly the sclerosing or morpheaform type, squamous cell carcinomas invading the fornix, sebaceous carcinomas, particularly those that are recurrent, and certain malignant melanomas. With the advent of CT scanning and Mohs' micrographic surgery, certain tumors that have previously been treated with exenteration are now treated with anterior resection and subtotal exenterations and are looked at more critically preoperatively with radiologic imaging of soft tissue in the orbit. Orbital tumors that are malignant or locally aggressive, such as lacrimal gland tumors, malignant hemangiopericytomas, or fibrous histiocytomas, may also warrant exenteration, since many or most of them are radio-insensitive. Exenteration has been proposed as a treatment for orbital deformities associated with neurofibromatosis, the management of the severely contracted and unreconstructable socket, and end-stage sclerosing orbital pseudotumor in the presence of a blind eye.

Meningiomas of the optic nerve sheath in young patients are considered to behave in a very biologically aggressive manner, and exenteration in these patients combined with a craniotomy has been recommended (15). Metastatic disease to the orbit may even warrant exenteration in some patients for relief of pain if the tumor is not radiosensitive. Controversy exists regarding the need for exenteration with ocular uveal melanomas that extend beyond the boundaries of the sclera. There is no firm evidence to support the fact that exenteration improves the prognosis in these patients, although some form of wide local excision, such as tenonectomy and additional fat removal, is usually recommended. Some diseases that have previously been treated with exenteration, such as rhabdomyosarcoma in children, have been shown to respond better to a combination of radiotherapy and chemotherapy (16,17).

The treatment of choice for all orbital tumors is changing rapidly enough to warrant a review of the subject each time the problem arises.

Patient Preparation

The patient must be told of the multilating nature of this operation and the possible failure to control the type of tumor that would warrant this operation. The patient must be prepared for the prolonged recovery period requiring daily dressing. The patient must have realistic expectations regarding the cosmetic results of a prosthesis. In situations where the patient's only seeing eye will be removed, the patient must have the informed choice among exenteration, allowing the tumor to take its course, and being treated by other means.

Surgical Technique

Anesthesia

General anesthesia must be used for this operation. The patient must be prepared for the possibility of blood loss. However, the authors have yet to have a patient lose enough blood to require a transfusion.

Removal of Eyelids and Orbital Contents

Total or partial excision of the eyelids may be performed in conjunction with the exenteration. This decision is based on the nature of the tumor and the possible involvement of the eyelids. If the operation is performed for a basal cell carcinoma, the uninvolved portion of the eyelids may be retained, provided the incision is made at least 15 mm from the obvious lesion. Salvaging the skin of the eyelids should not be done if there is any question as to the total excision of the tumor.

The best way to avoid excessive blood loss is to proceed with the operation without delay once the incision has been made. For this reason, the proposed incision should be marked with a marking pen initially. The incision is made down to the rim of the orbit and the periosteum is incised (Fig. 3). The incision is started medially. The periosteum is elevated posteriorly toward the apex of the orbit with a periosteal elevator. The lacrimal sac is divided from the nasolacrimal duct. When the orbital contents are attached only at the apex of the orbit, large Mayo scissors are used to divide the contents from the apex. Bleeding is controlled with a unipolar cautery. Once bleeding is controlled, the bony orbit is inspected for possible tumor extensions. Special attention is paid to the nasolacrimal duct and the thin bone over the perinasal sinuses. Care must be taken to avoid penetrating the medial wall of the orbit, because this may lead to the formation of a fistula postoperatively.

After bleeding is controlled, a 0.3-mm (0.012-inch) split-thickness skin graft is taken from the anterior surface of the thigh with a dermatome. The bony orbit is lined with the skin graft, which is sutured anteriorly to the skin edge. If this operation is not performed with a skin graft, healing is delayed and the posterior portion of the orbit is filled in with

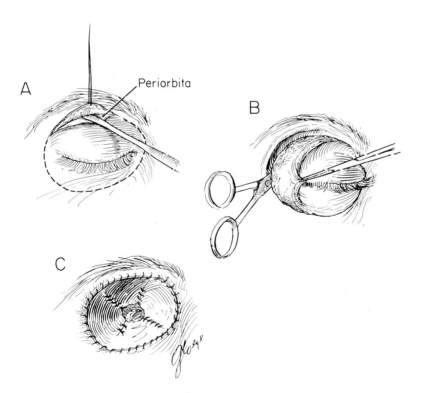

FIG. 3. Basic steps in exenteration. **A:** The incision is extended down to the orbital rim and the periorbita is elevated toward the apex of the orbit. **B:** A large scissors is used to cut off the attachment of the orbital contents near the apex of the orbit. **C:** A split-thickness skin graft from the thigh is placed over the bare bone and fleshy apex of the orbit.

granulation tissue. This thick layer of granulation tissue may obscure a recurrence of the tumor. Even with the skin graft, the healing may be a long, extended process.

Pieces of Telfa are then placed over the skin graft, covering it in at least two layers. Cotton soaked in mineral oil is then stuffed into the orbit, taking care not to wrinkle the graft. After the orbit is filled with cotton, the mineral oil is aspirated with suction, thus creating a mold. A pressure dressing is then placed and secured with a head wrap.

Problem Cases

If, during the operation, the tumor is found to extend into the ethmoid or maxillary sinuses, it is essential to open these sinuses to the extent necessary and to remove the remainder of the tumor. If the sinuses are entered inadvertently, a fistula may form. However, it is not necessary to treat this occurrence at the time of surgery. In the event that the extension of the tumor was through the roof of the orbit, it is then necessary to explore this area either at surgery or at the time of second surgery shortly afterward. If the cranial cavity is entered inadvertently during exenteration, a temporalis muscle flap is brought through the lateral wall of the orbit and used to close the defect. The decision to use a temporalis muscle flap is influenced by the likelihood of tumor recurrence. In fact, Mustarde (18) stated that any tumor dangerous enough to warrant this mutilating removal procedure should not be hidden from view with a muscle flap. The vast majority of patients who have had exenterations subsequently wear a patch, although some do wear a prosthesis.

Postoperative Care and Complications

The pressure bandage is removed on the third postoperative day. Over a period of 1 week, the cotton is removed from the orbit. The Telfa is allowed to fall out by itself. The graft may be viable from the beginning and then become necrotic after several weeks, or the graft may be necrotic from the beginning, in which case a large eschar is formed. This eschar acts as a bandage and should be allowed to fall out spontaneously. After approximately 1 month, the eschar falls out, leaving underlying granulation or epithelium, which has the same appearance as that following a successful graft. It is frequently difficult for the patient to clean the surgical area and apply dressing. Therefore, this procedure is performed by the physician every other day for the first 2 or 3 weeks. The orbit is cleaned using cotton-tipped applicators dipped in a solution of hydrogen peroxide. Care is taken to remove the crusts without disturbing the healing skin grafts. After approximately 1 month, the orbit is usually clean and well healed anteriorly. The central and posterior aspects of the orbit continue to heal slowly. During this period the patient may clean the orbit with warm wet compresses. Total healing may require 3 to 6 months. Once the orbit is fully healed, the patient may be sent for fitting of a prosthesis. The fixed, rigid appearance of a prosthesis may discourage the patient. If a fistula forms in the ethmoid sinuses, it causes the surrounding epithelium to break down periodically. Under these circumstances, it may be difficult to wear a prosthesis. The patient may be advised of the possibility of covering this with a vascular flap from adjacent tissues along with extirpation of the sinus. This operation is only moderately successful and, as mentioned above, may cover a subsequent recurrence of the tumor. The patient must be checked frequently during the first 2 years for the possibility of a tumor recurrence. Breakdown of the epithelium frequently mimics a recurrence of a basal cell epithelioma. Nevertheless, any suspicious lesion should be biopsied.

Modifications of Exenteration Techniques

It has been previously stated that one should not impair the ability to diagnose possible local recurrence of malignant disease. There are some situations, however, that occur in which local recurrence is not the issue and the surgeon does have the option of performing some reconstructive procedures and modifying the exenteration technique to provide a lesser deformity in patients.

Exenteration with Salvage of Eyelid Skin

In certain patients undergoing exenteration in whom the musculocutaneous layer of the eyelid is not involved in the pathologic process, one may dissect the musculocutaneous layer from the lids before the exenteration procedure is carried out, allowing the surgeon to infold the skin around the orbital rim and the orbital cavity. This does give a head start on epithelialization of the orbit and decreases the morbidity of the patient. Malignant disease that does not involve the musculocutaneous layer, such as conjunctival lesions or ocular lesions, can be treated in this manner.

Salvage of the Eyelids and Conjunctiva with Orbital Implant and Temporalis Muscle Flap

This procedure is commonly used in the younger patients who undergo exenteration for orbital meningioma. It allows the patient to wear a prosthetic eye in a normal manner with preservation of the lids. There is no motility of the prosthesis and a ptosis procedure has to be performed postoperatively, but the result is cosmetically superior to the complete exenteration. The technique involves first performing a conjunctival peritomy and dissection of the conjunctiva from the surface of the globe with dissection past the fornices to the orbital rim. The conjunctiva and lids are then retracted away from the orbital rim with rakes or retention sutures and the exenteration proceeds as previously described. Following completion of the removal of the globe and orbital contents, including the apex of the orbit, methyl methacrylate is then used to fill in the apical cone of the orbit. A flap of temporalis muscle, which is dissected from the anterior third of the muscle, can then be brought across the orbital rim, into the orbit, and sutured across the cranioplast implant. Many times, a section of the lateral wall of the orbit must be removed to facilitate the transfer of the flap into the orbital area. Following this, the conjunctiva is then closed in the usual manner over the temporalis muscle and a conformer is inserted. Secondary lid surgery is necessary many times in these patients, but the improved cosmetic appearance is many times worth the effort.

Subtotal Exenteration with Dermis-Fat Grafting

Specific situations may warrant a subtotal exenteration at the time of enucleation, with salvage of the conjunctiva and eyelids. For example, during enucleation for uveal melanoma, if gross amounts of extrascleral tumor are found many experts feel that additional tissue should be removed. This ''extra tissue'' may include Tenon's capsule, orbital fat proximate to the globe, and possibly the extraocular muscles. The authors reiterate, however, that the management of uveal melanoma remains controversial and bears constant review for each individual case.

The best method of restoring volume to the subtotal exenteration socket is to perform a primary dermis-fat graft (19). The reader is referred to Chapter 1 for the standard methods of harvesting dermis-fat grafts. The dermis acts as a platform for conjunctival reepithelialization, thus restoring lost conjunctiva. The subtotal exenteration socket contains viable vascularized tissue and is an excellent recipient bed for a dermis-fat graft. The graft is usually oversized to replace lost orbital volume. If extraocular muscles are present, they may be attached to the edge of the dermis to achieve socket motility.

REFERENCES

1. Marak, G. E. (1979): Recent advances in sympathetic ophthalmia. *Surv. Ophthalmol.,* 24:141–156.
2. Rubin, J. R., Albert, D. M., and Weinstein, M. (1980): Sixty-five years of sympathetic ophthalmia. A clinicopathologic review of 105 cases (1913–1978). *Ophthalmology,* 87:109–121.
3. Green, W. R., Maumenee, A. E., Sanders, T. E., and Smith, M. E. (1972): Sympathetic uveitis following evisceration. *Trans. Am. Acad. Ophthalmol. Otolaryngol.,* 76:625–644.
4. Croxatto, J. O., Galentine, P., Cupples, H. P., et al. (1981): Sympathetic ophthalmia after pars plana vitrectomy-lensectomy for endogenous bacterial endophthalmitis. *Am. J. Ophthalmol.* (1984): 91:342–346.
5. Older, J. J., and Levine, M. R. (1984): Enucleation, evisceration, and exenteration. In: *Ophthalmic Plastic and Reconstructive Surgery,* edited by W. B. Stewart, pp. 329–339. American Academy of Ophthalmology, San Francisco.
6. Raflo, G. T. (1985): Enucleation and evisceration. In: *Clinical Ophthalmology,* edited by T. D. Duane and E. A. Jaeger. Vol. 5, Chpt. 17, pp. 1–16. Harper & Row, Philadelphia.
7. Traquair, H. M. (1916): Local anesthesia in enucleation of the eyeball. *Ophthalmic Rev.,* 35: 75–89.
8. Zimmerman, L. D., and McLean, I. W. (1979): An evaluation of enucleation in the management of uveal melanoma. *Am. J. Ophthalmol.,* 87:741–782.
9. Zimmerman, L. E., McClean, I. W., and Foster, W. D. (1978): Does enucleation of the eye containing a malignant melanoma prevent or accelerate the dissemination of tumor cells? *Br. J. Ophthalmol.,* 62:420–425.
10. Niederkorn, J. Y. (1984): Enucleation-induced metastasis of intraocular melanomas in mice. *Ophthalmology,* 91:692–700.
11. Fraunfelder, F. T., Boozman, F. W., Wilson, R. S., and Thomas, A. H. (1977): No-touch technique for intraocular malignant melanomas. *Arch. Ophthalmol.,* 95:1616–1620.
12. Havre, D. C. (1965): Obtaining long sections of optic nerve at enucleation. A new surgical technique based on the anatomy of the posterior fascia bulbi. *Am. J. Ophthalmol.,* 60:272–277.
13. Przybyla, V. A., and La Piana, F. G. (1982): Complication associated with use of Tantalum-mesh covered implants. *Ophthalmology,* 89:121–123.
14. Nunery, W. R., and Hetzler, K. J. (1983): Improved prosthetic motility following enucleation. *Ophthalmology,* 90:1110–1115.
15. Alper, M. G. (1981): Management of primary optic nerve meningiomas. Current status—therapy in controversy. *J. Clin. Neuro-ophthalmol.,* 1:101–117.
16. Abramson, D. H., Ellsworth, R. M., Tretter, P., et al. (1979): The treatment of orbital rhabdomyosarcoma with irradiation and chemotherapy. *Ophthalmology,* 86:1330–1335.
17. Sutow, W. W., Linberg, R. D., Gehan, E. A., et al. (1982): Three-year relapse-free survival rates in childhood rhabdomyosarcoma of the head and neck: Report from the Intergroup Rhabdomyosarcoma Study. *Cancer,* 49:2217–2221.
18. Mustarde, J. C. (1966): *Repair and Reconstruction in the Orbital Region,* pp. 273–274. Williams & Wilkins, Baltimore.
19. Smith, B., Bosniak, S., Nesi, F., and Lisman, R. (1983): Dermis-fat orbital implantation: 118 cases. *Ophthalmic Surg.,* 14:941–943.

Oculoplastic Surgery, 2nd edition, edited by
Clinton D. McCord, Jr., and Myron Tanenbaum.
Raven Press, New York © 1987.

Chapter 16

The Anophthalmic Socket:
Evaluation and Management of Surgical Problems

*Henry Bayliss, *Norman Shorr, **Myron Tanenbaum, and
†Clinton D. McCord, Jr.

*Division of Ophthalmic Plastic and Reconstructive Surgery, Jules Stein Eye Institute, University of
California at Los Angeles, Los Angeles, California 90024; **Bascom Palmer Eye Institute, Department
of Ophthalmology, University of Miami School of Medicine, Miami, Florida 33101, and †Department
of Ophthalmology, Emory University School of Medicine, Atlanta, Georgia 30308*

The purpose of this chapter is to enable the reader to approach a very complex subject in an analytical and organized manner. The anophthalmic socket is a uniquely complex system of structural and functional elements in which a change in any single element profoundly affects the other elements. Because of this complex circle of relationships, understanding each section of this chapter is dependent on an understanding of the whole chapter. Consequently, the entire chapter must be read before an intensive study of one particular section is undertaken.

This chapter has been organized into three sections, the first of which describes the functional and structural elements of all sockets. This section also defines the three most common general types of socket abnormalities. The second section details the clinical evaluation of the anophthalmic socket. The third section describes concepts for clinical and surgical decision making, arrived at by integrating the information presented in the first and second sections. The six types of surgical problems discussed are:

1. Lower eyelid laxity
2. Inadequate lower fornix
   a. with adequate mucous membrane
   b. with inadequate mucous membrane
3. Enophthalmos
4. Upper eyelid ptosis
5. Extruding orbital implant
6. Contracted socket
   a. moist
   b. dry

Finally congenital anophthalmos and its management are discussed.

THE SOCKET

The proper approach to problems of the anophthalmic socket requires an understanding of the complex interrelationships of its structural and functional elements (1). The structural and functional elements of the socket are: (a) a centrally located orbital implant with adequate total orbital volume to allow for a thin prosthesis to lie in the same frontal plane as the opposite cornea, (b) a mucous membrane–lined pouch of the proper size, shape, and position to hold the prosthesis correctly, (c) a properly fitted ocular prosthesis, (d) a lower eyelid that is at the same level as the opposite lower eyelid and that can support the weight and pressure of the prosthesis, and (e) an upper eyelid that has good levator function, is not ptotic, has a satisfactory lid contour and lid crease, and closes in repose. Each of these structural and functional elements is dependent on each of the other structural and functional elements to fulfill its role properly in the maintenance of a satisfactory socket. An involutional or surgical change in any single element will alter each of the other elements. The normal socket must have all of the structural and functional elements described.

There are three general types of sockets with which one must be familiar. They are the lax socket, the implant problem socket, and the contracted socket (2–4).

Lax Socket

This is the most common and least dramatic socket problem. There is some degree of laxity in every otherwise normal socket. The socket is usually loose from the stretching of all the structural and functional elements because of time and gravity. Often, as the lower eyelid has horizontally loosened and the upper eyelid has become ptotic, a larger and heavier prosthesis has been fitted. This increases pressure on the lower eyelid and the cycle of laxity continues. The globe, weighing 7.5 g and 7.5 cm^3 in volume, is supported by the normal orbital ligament and muscle system. In enucleation this system is disrupted and the globe is replaced by a 16-mm diameter implant weighing 2.5 g and 2 cm^3 in volume. In addition, a prosthesis weighs approximately 3.5 g, has a volume of 3 cm^3, and is not supported by any of the suspensory ligaments of the globe. Therefore, it is supported totally by the lower eyelid. With the passage of time, these factors result in a sagging of the lower eyelid. This is accompanied by a falling of the implant and the muscle cone. Along with the ptosis of the muscle cone, all of the soft tissue contents of the orbit are displaced inferiorly. The levator muscle and upper eyelid move downward, enlarging and deepening the upper eyelid sulcus. At this point in the evolution of the anophthalmic socket, a larger and heavier prosthesis is usually fitted. This results in greater lower eyelid laxity, further downward movement of the prosthesis and implant, and enlargement of the upper eyelid sulcus (Fig. 1).

Frequently there is anophthalmic enophthalmos. The 7.5-cm^3 globe is replaced by a 2-cm^3 orbital implant and a 3-cm^3 prosthesis, leaving a 2.5-cm^3 deficit in orbital volume. This enophthalmos is accentuated over a period of years by gravitational displacement of the muscle cone and orbital contents. A resultant enlargement of the superior sulcus occurs. In addition to the volume loss, there is a redistribution inferiorly and anteriorly of orbital fat. The fat that has been redistributed anteriorly into the lax eyelid represents volume lost from the orbit. In the opinion of the authors, this anteriorly redistributed volume loss represents in large part the volume loss frequently attributed to "fat atrophy."

The surgical approach is to reverse the above sequence by placing volume in the orbit

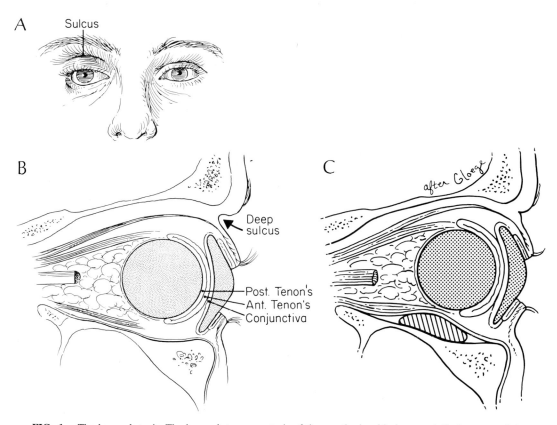

FIG. 1. The lax socket. **A:** The lax socket causes ptosis of the prosthesis with downward displacement of the lower eyelid and a deepened upper eyelid sulcus. **B:** The weight of the prosthesis creates ptosis of the lower eyelid. The ptosis of the orbital implant causes downward displacement of the muscle cone, levator muscle, and orbital fat, causing the upper eyelid sulcus to deepen. **C:** Subperiosteal volume agmentation elevates the orbital implant, which, in turn, raises the socket and prosthesis, filling in the upper eyelid sulcus. The lower eyelid is elevated with a lateral canthal tightening.

in such a way as to elevate the implant and muscle cone (see Fig. 1). The lower eyelid is horizontally shortened and tightened to support the prosthesis, which in turn supports the upper lid and fills in the superior sulcus (5,6).

Implant Problems

An extruding implant may occur in the early postoperative period or may gradually occur many years following surgery (7). The differing types of extruding implants have different pathogenetic mechanisms.

Early postoperative extrusion is characterized by the sudden presentation of the implant through the wound. Early wound separation is generally a result of inadequate wound closure. Early postoperative extrusion is frequently accompanied by inflammation and discharge. This discharge is generally a result of the extrusion and not a manifestation of an infection causing the extrusion.

A late orbital implant extrusion may be either partial or complete. Partial late implant extrusion is generally a gradual process. It may present in two different ways. The process of extrusion may begin in an otherwise normal socket with a tiny, almost invisible, fistula from the implant through the conjunctival surface. This fistula will slowly enlarge without a thinning of the overall covering of the implant. This type of extruding orbital implant lends itself to repair with a patch graft because the implant is generally well supported and encapsulated with adequate anterior tissue and blood supply. The other, and more common, presentation is that of slowly progressive thinning of overlying tissues with eventual exposure of the implant. Often the implant has migrated and an edge or surface (especially if not a sphere) may be presenting. The thin tissues overlying the implant are frequently associated with a progressive cicatricial process. If this process is allowed to proceed, a significant amount of conjunctiva may be lost, leading to a contracted socket. Once the fistula exposing the implant has developed, it will inevitably progress over weeks, months, or years to total extrusion. Therefore, once a late partial extrusion is diagnosed, surgical repair is indicated. When late orbital implant extrusion is complete, there is usually an underlying etiology such as orbital infection or fibrous contraction. Orbital infections may be due to sinus fistulas to the orbit, chronic sinusitis or retained infected foreign body material. This contraction with late implant extrusion is commonly associated with a history of irradiation to the orbits, alkali burns, or previous severe trauma.

Contracted Socket

The most challenging of the anophthalmic socket problems is the contracted socket. There is a spectrum from a modest vertical shortening of the tarsal conjunctiva to vertical shortening of the inferior fornix to a severely contracted socket that is without fornices and both vertically and horizontally shortened.

We classify socket contracture into three levels of severity. The first, mild socket contracture, is characterized by early vertical shortening of the tarsal and palpebral conjunctiva, resulting in cicatricial entropion of the eyelids. The eyelashes are vertically directed and lie against the prosthesis. The fornices are still adequate to retain a prosthesis. The second level of severity, moderate socket contracture, is defined as contracture of the upper and lower fornices, resulting in the inability to retain a properly sized prosthesis. Frequently, as the socket contracts, a progressively smaller prosthesis has been fitted. The third level of severity is severe socket contracture, in which there is horizontal shortening of the lid aperture and mucous membrane as well as vertical contracture of the fornices. The fornices are severely contracted or obliterated such that a prosthesis cannot be retained. The socket is frequently so small as to only admit the tip of the examiner's finger.

Unusual Socket Problems

There are a wide variety of socket problems that do not fit into the previously described categories. These socket problems often are associated with the cause or treatment of the condition that resulted in the loss of the eye.

These unusual socket problems may be divided into those of the bony orbit and those of the soft tissue contents of the orbit. The etiology of these problems may be traumatic or congenital.

EVALUATION OF THE ANOPHTHALMIC SOCKET

A thorough physical examination with evaluation of each functional element must be performed prior to surgical planning:

1. Evaluate the general symmetry compared to the normal side.
2. Evaluate for enophthalmos. Have the patient tilt his or her head back and raise his or her chin. Look along the plane from the chin to the forehead. Is the prosthesis sunken? Note the number of millimeters of enophthalmos according to the exophthalmometer reading.
3. Is the superior sulcus symmetrical with the opposite side? Is the sulcus deep and sunken, indicating a loss of volume and an inferior displacement of the existing orbital volume?
4. Note the lower eyelid position. Is the lower eyelid displaced downward, indicating horizontal laxity? Is the prosthesis displaced downward as well? By pulling the lower eyelid laterally with your fingers (horizontally tightening), are the lower eyelid and prosthesis elevated to the normal position?
5. Elevate the lower eyelid with your fingers. Is there resistance, indicating a vertical shortening of the conjunctiva of the lower fornix?
6. Look at the lid margins and lashes of the upper and lower eyelids. Is there cicatricial entropion with lashes turned against the prosthesis, indicating mild socket contracture?
7. Is the upper eyelid in the proper position? Is there upper eyelid ptosis? Does the eyelid close, indicating a deep upper fornix? Measure levator function. Is levator function normal, indicating a levator that is present and unrestricted?
8. Ask the patient if the prosthesis falls out. If it does, manipulate the prosthesis to observe it falling out. Which fornix appears inadequate to retain the prosthesis?
9. Remove the prosthesis and inspect it. It should be thin (approximately 8 mm thick). If it is thicker, it is being used to provide additional orbital volume, which, as already mentioned, leads to increased vertical pressure on the lid. The prosthesis should be of a large circumference, indicating deep fornices. It should not be built up and thickened superiorly. If it is, this is to support a ptotic lid, and the additional weight and vertical pressure will (while supporting the upper lid) stretch and displace the lower eyelid and cul-de-sac. The prosthesis can be oriented by red vessels painted on the nasal side.
10. Consider if changing the prosthesis could solve the problem.
11. Inspect the socket. Is there vertical shortening of the fornices? Carefully inspect the conjunctiva. It is often bunched up centrally. Are the fornices deep and well formed, or does the conjunctiva seem to be plentiful but lax, without well-defined fornices? Is the implant position visible? Does the tissue covering the implant appear thin? Is there a fistula or an extruding implant?
12. Put your finger in the socket and palpate. Evaluate the size and position (and existence) of the orbital implant. Can you feel more than one implant or more subperiosteal beads? Are the bony walls of the orbit smooth and apparently intact?

With all the above information compiled, one can prepare a plan for surgical rehabilitation of the socket.

EVALUATION OF THE PROSTHESIS IN SURGICAL PLANNING

It is generally taught that the patient must be fitted with the best prosthesis possible before surgery is undertaken. Fitting this ''best possible'' prosthesis is, indeed, appropriate when it will result in a satisfactory socket-prosthesis relationship.

However, in many circumstances fitting the ''best possible'' prosthesis will result in an unsatisfactory prosthesis that does not provide an acceptable socket-prosthesis relationship.

For example, in a socket without an orbital implant, the "best possible" prosthesis will necessarily be extremely large and heavy. The result of this fit may appear acceptable, but this socket-prosthesis relationship is unsatisfactory! Additionally, the oversized prosthesis will undergo the accelerated changes of time and gravity.

Furthermore, in some cases, the "best possible" prosthesis will be inadequate and surgery will be performed. The making of this prosthesis was unnecessary and, in fact, counterproductive for two reasons. First, surgery and surgical planning should not be performed around a "compromise" prosthesis but rather around an "ideal" prosthesis. Second, following the socket reconstruction, a new prosthesis will be required in any case. For example, in the lax socket with enophthalmos, upper eyelid ptosis, and lower eyelid laxity, the "best possible" prosthesis will be unsatisfactory. It will be thick to augment the volume and have a shelf superiorly to support the upper eyelid. Surgical planning will be difficult because the amount of necessary volume augmentation and ptosis correction has been masked by the prosthesis.

Therefore, the "best possible" prosthesis should only be fitted when, in the surgeon's judgment, the result will be a satisfactory prosthesis without surgery. If the surgeon believes socket surgery will be necessary, he or she may choose one of two acceptable courses. The surgery may be performed around the existing prosthesis and the final prosthesis may be fitted postoperatively. Or the "ideal" prosthesis may be made and the socket reconstructed around the "ideal" prosthesis.

PROBLEM CONCEPTS AND GENERAL SURGICAL MANAGEMENT

Volume Considerations

The first consideration must be of total orbital volume and its distribution. Normal orbital volume is 30 cm^3. In the anophthalmic socket, this is made up of orbital soft tissue, orbital implant, and prosthesis. Ideally, the implant should be the size of a 16-mm or 18-mm diameter sphere. Soft tissue volume and orbital implant volume should be adequate, such that with a relatively thin prosthesis there will be no enophthalmos. If this is not the case, the volume must be augmented.

Sphere implants can be augmented by implanting subperiosteal bone cement in the socket. Glass beads can migrate into the lids, sinuses, and other structures and are no longer in common use (8,9). Unlike solid spheres, dermis-fat graft implants are not well supported by subperiosteal, volume-augmentation techniques. In this situation, inserting a solid-sphere implant behind the existing dermis-fat graft is the best option if the graft is healthy. If the existing orbital implant is very small, has significantly migrated, or is thinly covered and at risk for extrusion, then replacement of the implant with a dermis-fat graft is appropriate.

Surgical Procedure for Placement of an Orbital Implant

In a socket that has no orbital implant, the best method of volume augmentation is the placement of a centrally located orbital implant (10). The incision is made through the conjunctiva at the posterior face of the socket and carried posteriorly to the orbital apex. The incision is placed centrally and horizontally to avoid injury to the levator. Meticulous hemostatis is maintained. A sphere is placed in the fat at the apex of the orbit and deep tissues are closed with multiple, interrupted sutures of absorbable material such as 4–0 Vicryl, using a small, half-circle needle. A second layer of Vicryl is placed, again in interrupted sutures, just deep to the conjunctiva. Layers may not be well defined, so these sutures are placed in firm tissue. The conjunctiva is closed with a running 6–0 plain catgut suture. There should be no tension on the wound. It is important to realize that the second (more superficial) layer of sutures must be just immediately subconjunctival and approximate, not bunch up, Tenon's capsule. If they do bunch up Tenon's capsule, they will shorten the vertical tissue between the eyelids and therefore shorten the cul-de-sacs.

Surgical Procedure for Management of Migrated Implant with Dermis–Fat Graft

The location of an extruding implant is usually evident. Palpation of the socket may be useful in locating a migrated implant. In most situations, a horizontal, transconjunctival incision is used. The horizontal approach minimizes the risk of injury to the levator muscle. A needle Bovie is used to make the conjunctival incision. Dissection is continued through the Tenon's fascia and subconjunctival scar tissue. The pseudocapsule around the extruding implant is opened. Solid-sphere implants generally pop out without resistance. Implants that have attached extraocular muscles, such as the tantalum mesh implant, may require extensive dissection in order to remove them (Fig. 2A). With the implant removed, a subtotal excision of the pseudocapsule should be performed (Fig. 2B). Minimal hemostasis efforts, as necessary, are performed with electrocautery. The dermis-fat graft (methods of harvesting dermis-fat grafts are discussed in Chapter 1) is trimmed to the appropriate size to fit the patient's socket (11). Three (or four) 4–0 Vicryl cardinal sutures are used to secure the dermis-fat graft to quadrants of Tenon's fascia or to the recti muscles if identifiable (Fig. 2C). Additional interrupted 4–0 Vicryl sutures are used to further secure the dermis-fat graft in place in the socket. If additional volume is needed, a solid-sphere implant may be inserted behind the dermis-fat graft. When using a sphere implant, it is conveniently inserted after a few cardinal Vicryl sutures have been placed to secure the dermis-fat graft. The ability to vascularize limits the largest dimensions of the dermis to 20 to 25 mm in our graft. The Tenon's layer closure is to the edge of the dermis-fat graft. The conjunctiva, however, should be undermined and then sutured over the anterior surface of the dermis-fat graft. The final central bare area of dermis should not exceed 10 to 15 mm. Using a larger dermis-fat graft would increase the risk of central graft necrosis and sloughing. A lid conformer is placed to maintain the fornices. The dermis will appear white during the immediate postoperative period. In the ensuing weeks, the dermis will assume a healthy, pink color, reflecting successful vascularization. It may take 2 to 4 or more weeks for healthy conjunctiva to cover the initially bare dermis. Pyogenic granulomas can develop along conjunctival healing lines and may be simply excised and cauterized at their base. Fitting the socket with a prosthesis can usually be done by 6 weeks.

Surgical Procedure for Subperiosteal (Subperiorbital) Volume Augmentation

If the implant is relatively central and well covered, it is best to avoid surgery through the soft tissue socket. Volume augmentation can be achieved by implanting alloplastic material in the subperiorbital space (Fig. 1C) (8,12). This approach works very well in volume-deficient sockets that already contain a sphere implant. Subperiorbital augmentation techniques are less effective when a dermis-fat graft is present, the subperiorbital implant tending to compress the graft rather than augmenting socket volume. In placing the subperiorbital material, a rough rule of thumb is that 1 mm of enophthalmos will be resolved with each 1 cm^3 of implant material. Most of the volume should be placed inferiorly, since

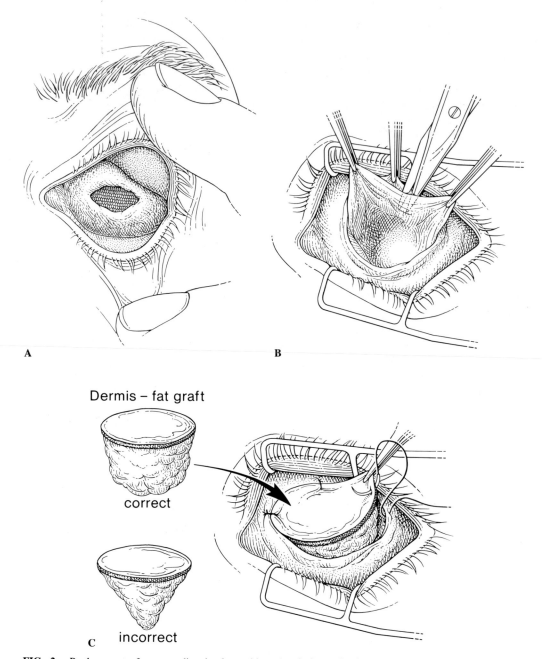

FIG. 2. Replacement of an extruding implant with a dermis-fat graft. **A:** Anophthalmic socket showing an extruding tantalum mesh implant. **B:** Once the implant is removed, the surrounding capsule (pseudocapsule) is resected via sharp dissection. **C:** An autogenous dermis-fat graft is secured to Tenon's capsule and conjunctiva with interrupted 4-0 Vicryl sutures.

superiorly placed volume will press on the levator because of gravity and tends to displace the socket inferiorly. Inferior volume will support the socket and prosthesis. Subperiorbital volume should be as posterior as possible because anteriorly placed volume will encroach on the cul-de-sac and displace the prosthesis. As a general rule, when the inferior orbit is used for volume augmentation, the lower lid should always be horizontally tightened. In some cases, it may be necessary to support the lower eyelid with a fascia sling.

At present, the authors' material of choice for subperiorbital volume augmentation is bone cement. Bone cement is inert, easily molded into the desired shape, and readily available. It does not migrate or resorb with time. Contraindications to using bone cement are an acute socket infection or an exposed sinus, usually present as the sequela of previous trauma.

Excellent exposure of the orbital floor can be achieved by an inferior fornix incision combined with a lateral canthotomy and cantholysis. This surgical approach can be used for subperiosteal volume augmentation, orbital floor fracture repair, or orbital floor decompression. In the anophthalmic socket this approach offers a convenient opportunity to perform horizontal lower lid tightening.

The lower eyelid at the lateral canthus and the conjunctiva of the inferior fornix are infiltrated with lidocaine 2% with epinephrine 1:100,000 and hyaluronidase (Wydase®). The lateral canthotomy is made with the dissection carried down to the periosteum of the lateral orbital rim. A cantholysis is performed, severing the inferior crus of the lateral canthal tendon. Traction sutures are applied to the lower eyelid to reflect it downward. The needle Bovie is used to incise conjunctiva of the inferior fornix down to periosteum. An incision is made in the periosteum and a periosteal elevator is used to reflect periosteum of the inferior orbital rim and periorbita off of the orbital floor. It is important to reflect the periorbita straight back to the inferior apex of the orbit near the inferior orbital fissure. A large malleable retractor is used to elevate the orbital contents to secure excellent visualization of the entire orbital floor. Bone cement is mixed and allowed to set to a doughy consistency. This partially hardened bone cement can be cut with a scissors in order to obtain a proper amount. Saline moistened Q-tips are used to pack the bone cement back into the subperiorbital space of the inferior orbit. The bulk of the bone cement should be situated posteriorly toward the orbital apex so as not to compromise the lower lid fornix. Bone cement edges should be meticulously smoothed over at the level of the inferior orbital rim and the excess bone cement trimmed away. A power-driven polishing burr is useful for sculpting the bone cement, if it becomes too hard to trim with a scissors. The inferior fornix conjunctiva is loosely sutured with a running 6–0 plain suture. It is not necessary to close the periorbital/periosteal layer. A 4–0 nonabsorbable suture is used to horizontally tighten the lower lid, achieving lateral canthal fixation to periosteum inside the lateral orbital rim. Use of a fascia strip to support a lax lower eyelid will be discussed later in this chapter. Skin closure over the lateral canthal tendon is achieved with interrupted 6–0 nylon sutures. A pressure bandage dressing and ice compresses are useful in the first postoperative week toward minimizing swelling.

Surgical Procedure for Volume Augmentation of a Dermis-Fat Graft

As stated in the previous section, a subperiorbital implant is not an effective means of volume augmentation in the presence of a dermis-fat graft. If the dermis is healthy, implantation of a solid sphere behind it is the simplest and most effective means of adding volume to the enophthalmic socket. If there is significant necrosis of the dermis-fat graft, replacing it entirely with a smaller dermis-fat graft and a sphere is a good choice. An alternative to using a smaller dermis-fat graft would be to replace the necrosing graft with a fascia-covered sphere. If there is evidence of socket infection, the infection must be treated medically before any surgical intervention is planned.

The technique of augmentation of dermis-fat graft volume with a sphere is quite simple. The socket conjunctiva and dermis-fat graft are infiltrated with lidocaine 2% and epinephrine and hyaluronidase. The needle Bovie is used to make a central horizontal incision through the conjunctiva. An incision is then made full-thickness through the dermis. At this point, if a pocket of liquified fat is encountered, it should be aspirated. If formed adipose tissue is encountered, it should be bluntly dissected to expose the posterior aspects of the orbit. A sphere implant, usually 12 mm or 14 mm in size, is inserted through the dermal opening and placed back in the posterior orbit. The dermis incision is closed with interrupted 4–0 Vicryl sutures. The conjunctiva is closed with a running 6–0 plain suture. Postoperatively, pressure bandages and ice compresses are used.

Concepts of Lower Lid Laxity and Inadequate Fornix

In the lax socket the most common finding is horizontal laxity of the lower eyelid. The lower eyelid eventually becomes lax because of the weight and pressure of the prosthesis. Additionally, stabilizing factors of the lower eyelid retractors, inferior rectus muscle, and orbicularis are out of balance. Laxity of fixation of the conjunctiva of the lower fornix to the inferior rectus muscle may result in the loss of depth of this fornix. An adequate inferior fornix is one that has sufficient vertical height of conjunctiva on the posterior lid surface to retain a prosthesis. There are two types of inferior fornix problems. The first is an inadequate fornix in the presence of adequate conjunctiva. The second is inadequate fornix with insufficient conjunctiva. This is a result of the shortening of the inferior cul-de-sac due to contracture of the inferior conjunctiva.

In all sockets with inadequate inferior fornix, the lower eyelid must be tightened and resuspended at the lateral canthus (6). Along with this, the inferior fornix must be deepened and re-formed with either refixation or a free mucous membrane graft if the amount of socket conjunctiva is inadequate.

Surgical Procedure for Correction of Lower Eyelid Laxity

The correction of lower eyelid laxity may be achieved by lateral canthal tightening (Fig. 3). The lateral canthal tendon and lower eyelid laterally are infiltrated with lidocaine 2% with epinephrine and hyaluronidase. The lateral canthotomy is performed and the inferior limb of the lateral canthal tendon is separated from the lateral orbital rim. The lower eyelid is grasped with an Adson's forcep and held on stretch in the desired position, with the eyelid passing over the lateral canthus. The point on the lid margin where it crosses the lateral orbital rim is marked. The marked point will be the new lateral extent of the lower eyelid. If horizontal eyelid shortening is necessary, the needle Bovie is used to excise full-thickness portions of the eyelid. To achieve a good tightening effect, it is rarely necessary to excise more than 2 to 4 mm from the lateral portion of the eyelid. A 4–0 nonabsorbable suture is used to fixate the lateral portion of the lower eyelid tarsus to the periosteum just inside the lateral orbital rim. It is important to supraplace the lower eyelid at the time of lateral canthal fixation, because this will generally lower with time. It is

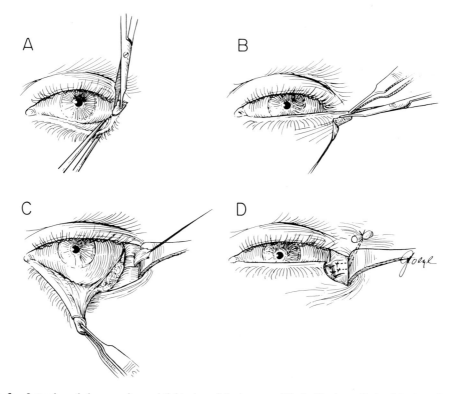

FIG. 3. Lateral canthal suspension and tightening of the lower eyelid. **A:** The lower limb of the lateral canthal tendon is isolated and divided from its insertion. A lateral segment of the eyelid margin is removed in preparation for resection and reattachment of the tongue of tendon. **B:** A tongue of tarsus is developed at the lateral extent of the eyelid by removing the lid margins superiorly, the skin anteriorly, and the conjunctiva posteriorly. **C:** The tongue of tarsus is retracted with forceps. A temporally based periosteal flap has been elevated at the lateral orbital rim. **D:** The shortened tongue of tendon and tarsus is reattached under a temporally based periosteal flap, which is sutured down to the anterior surface of the tarsus.

important to warn patients preoperatively that they will have this temporarily "accentuated" appearance or mongoloid slant to their eyelids.

There are certain cases where lateral canthal tightening alone is insufficient in restoring adequate lower eyelid tone to support the weight of a prosthesis. In this setting, a reinforcing strip of autogenous fascia is the procedure of choice to correct lower lid laxity. In borderline cases or in cases where the surgeon is uncertain regarding eyelid laxity, it is probably best to go ahead and support the lower eyelid with fascia. Lidocaine 2% with epinephrine and hyaluronidase is infiltrated over the medial canthal tendon and lateral canthal tendon, and across the width of the lower eyelid. A skin incision parallel to and over the medial canthal tendon is made (Fig. 4A). Blunt dissection is used to expose the anterior reflection of the medial canthal tendon. A thin strip (approximately 3 mm) is cut from previously harvested autogenous fascia (see Chapter 1 for standard methods of harvesting autogenous fascia.) A curved hemostat is used to thread the fascia strip around the anterior limb of the medial canthal tendon. The fascia is secured with 6–0 silk sutures (Fig. 4B). Before proceeding further, lateral canthal tightening must be performed. A lateral canthotomy and inferior crus cantholysis is done. A 4–0 nonabsorbable suture is used to secure the lower eyelid to the periosteum of the lateral orbital rim in a supraplaced position.

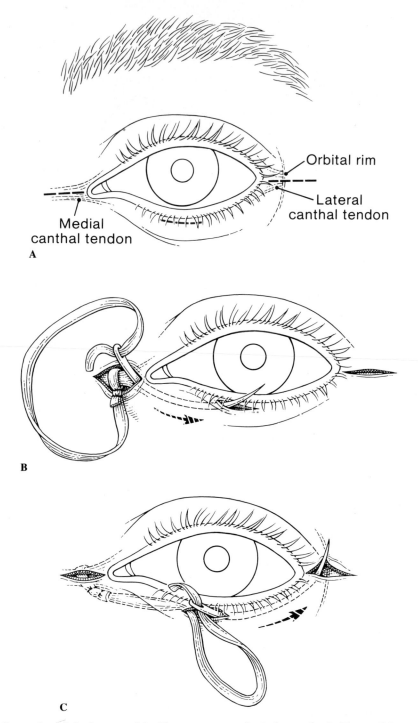

FIG 4. Suspension of the lower eyelid with an autogenous fascia lata graft. **A:** The medial, central, and lateral incision lines (*dashed lines*) are marked with methylene blue. **B:** A fascia lata graft has been wrapped around the medial canthal tendon and secured with 6-0 silk sutures. The fascia strip is then threaded through the lower eyelid with a semicircular general closure needle. **C:** The fascia has been brought out of the central eyelid incision, rethreaded on the semicircular needle, and sewn through to the lateral canthal incision.

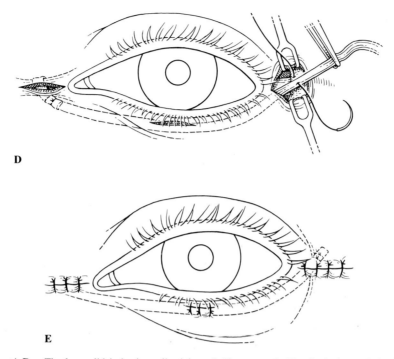

FIG. 4 (*cont.*) D: The lower lid is horizontally tightened (if necessary). The fascia lata strip is then sewn to the periosteum of the lateral orbital rim with a 4-0 nonabsorbable suture. **E:** Final skin closure. The fascia is shown in correct position close to the lid margin.

With the standard lateral canthal tightening completed, the surgeon procedes with the fascia support sling. A small skin incision beneath the lash line is made in the center of the lower eyelid. A hemostat or fascia needle is used to thread the fascia strip from the medial canthal tendon to the nick incision in the center of the eyelid. The fascia is then threaded on through to exit at the lateral canthal angle (Fig. 4C). It is important to have the fascia sling as high as possible on the lower lid tarsal plate. The central eyelid incision adds extra control in ensuring proper threading of the fascia through the lower eyelid, more so than with a single threading maneuver with a fascia needle. Two interrupted 4–0 Prolene sutures are used to tack fascia down to periosteum laterally with appropriate eyelid tension (Fig. 4D). As noted, it is important to have already performed lateral canthal fixation of the lower eyelid itself. The fascia is sewn to the periosteum at the level of the proper lateral canthal angle. The skin is closed with interrupted 6–0 nylon sutures medially, centrally, and laterally (Fig. 4E).

Surgical Procedure for Correction of Inadequate Fornix with Sufficient Mucous Membrane

This is the procedure for refixation of the inferior fornix (Fig. 5) (13). It is always done in conjunction with lateral canthal tightening, as described above. Lidocaine 2% with epinephrine and hyaluronidase is injected over the lateral canthal tendon and subconjunctively in the inferior fornix. A lateral canthotomy and inferior cantholysis are performed. From the lateral canthus, the dissection plane is developed subconjunctively in the area of

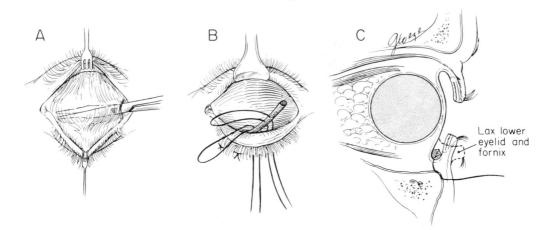

FIG. 5.   Refixation of the inferior fornix with adequate mucous membrane. **A:** A scissors introduced through a lateral canthotomy is used to undermine the conjunctiva and then develop a surgical plane from the inferior fornix to the inferior orbital rim. **B:** A 3-mm diameter retinal sponge is used as a bolster to fixate the inferior fornix to the inferior orbital rim. **C:** A sagittal section demonstrates the change in position of the inferior fornix and lower lid upon completion of this procedure.

the proposed new fornix. This is done with sharp and blunt dissection. The second dissection plane is developed perpendicular to the first, between the proposed new fornix and the inferior orbital rim. Two double-armed 4–0 silk sutures and a large cutting needle are passed in horizontal mattress fashion through a soft silicone eyelid conformer. If a hard methyl methacrylate eyelid conformer is used, it is necessary to drill two holes through the conformer. Each arm of the suture is then passed through the conjunctiva at the proposed new fornix, through the full thickness of the eyelid, picking up periosteum at the inferior orbital rim, and out the skin, where it is tied over cotton bolsters. Great care must be used not to vertically shorten the lower eyelid. Standard lateral canthal tightening is completed, as described in the preceding section. A commonly used splint is a retinal sponge, as shown in Fig. 5.

Surgical Procedure for Correction of Inadequate Inferior Fornix with Insufficient Mucous Membrane

To deepen a contracted lower fornix, the proposed new fornix must be created and lined with a mucous membrane graft from the mouth. This procedure is performed in conjunction with a lateral canthal tightening. After the lateral canthotomy and the creation of the tarsal tongue, the conjunctiva at the apex of the contracted fornix is cut from the lateral to the medial canthus. The proposed new fornix is developed with sharp dissection as a bed for the mucous membrane graft. Meticulous hemostasis is maintained. The size of the necessary mucous membrane graft is estimated. It will be approximately 25 mm horizontally by 15 mm vertically. A full-thickness, millimeter-for-millimeter mucous membrane graft is taken from the mouth (see Chapter 1). The graft is sutured into position with interrupted 6–0 Vicryl sutures (Fig. 6). The prosthetic eye or a conformer that is of the appropriate size to hold the graft against the vascular bed is placed in the socket. A lateral canthal tightening procedure is completed. Two double-armed 4–0 silk sutures are then passed in horizontal mattress fashion through a soft silicone eyelid conformer. Each arm of the 4–0 silk suture is then sewn on a large, semicircular cutting needle through

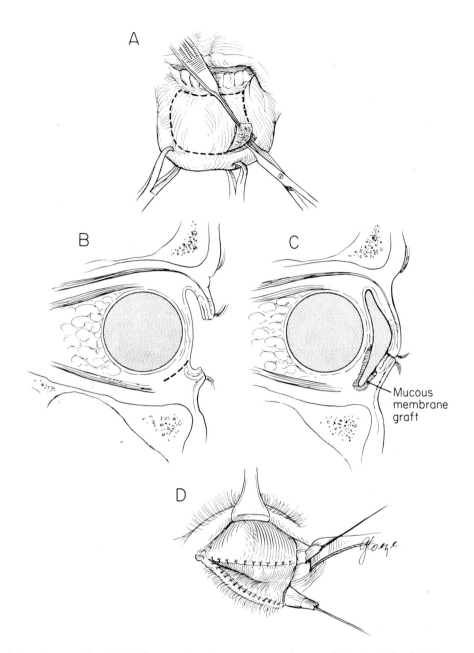

FIG. 6. Reconstruction of the inferior fornix using a mucous membrane graft. **A:** A thin full-thickness mucous membrane graft is undermined and excised from the lower lip. **B:** This sagittal section demonstrates contracture of the inferior fornix. **C:** The mucous membrane graft lining the newly reconstructed inferior cul-de-sac is held in position by the prosthesis. **D:** Inferior cul-de-sac reconstruction is often done in conjunction with a lateral canthal suspension.

the mucous membrane graft, through the full thickness of the eyelids, through the periosteum at the inferior orbital rim, and out the skin. It is important to sew through the mucous membrane graft at the point of the estimated new lower eyelid fornix. The upper and lower eyelids are sewn together with 4–0 silk or Prolene sutures, and the double-armed 4–0 silk sutures are tied snugly over cotton bolsters. A pressure bandage is applied postoperatively. The eyelids remain splinted closed for 1 week with a conformer in place.

Ptosis—Special Considerations (Pseudoptosis Versus True Ptosis)

Upper eyelid ptosis is a common problem in the anophthalmic socket. It may be a true ptosis because of a weak levator muscle or a pseudoptosis because of inadequate support from a prosthesis and orbital implant, which has been inferiorly or posteriorly displaced because of involutional or gravitational forces. This deceptive ptosis can be evaluated by digitally pushing the prosthesis up from below and noticing the effect on the eyelid. The superior sulcus will be filled out by this same maneuver. As a general rule, surgery of the upper eyelid ptosis should be deferred until all other socket problems have been corrected. For example, in a lax socket, the enophthalmos and lower lid laxity should be corrected before upper eyelid ptosis surgery is undertaken.

True ptosis occurs because of: (a) a preexisting condition prior to enucleation, (b) levator damage at enucleation, especially when operating on the adjacent superior rectus muscle, (c) involutional changes, as with levator aponeurosis dehiscence, or (d) scarring of the levator associated with socket surgery, such as superior cul-de-sac deepening surgery or glass beads lying on the levator. The surgeon must determine whether the first step is refitting the prosthesis, surgically correcting the socket problems, or proceeding directly to ptosis surgery.

Modification Procedures for the Prosthesis

The ocularist can build up the prosthesis superiorly to support a mildly ptotic eyelid. It must be kept in mind that there will be increased pressure on the lower eyelid, as described earlier in this chapter.

Surgical Procedures for Ptosis

If good levator function is present, an external levator resection or repair of the aponeurotic defect is the procedure of choice.

If there is no levator function, as is so often the case in a contracted socket, a frontalis muscle suspension procedure, using autogenous fascia lata, will allow for eyelid elevation with some motility. Ptosis repair techniques are described in detail in Chapter 13. Every effort must be made to maintain or create eyelid motility. The fixed, staring prosthetic eye is cosmetically undesirable.

Extruding Orbital Implant Problems

The orbital implant may extrude abruptly in the early postoperative period or gradually do so months or years after the surgery. Early extrusion generally results from inadequate surgical closure. Late extrusion may result from a gradual uneven pressure on the tissues covering the orbital implant. This tissue may gradually thin until the implant is exposed.

In some cases a small fistula may develop through thick tissue from the implant to the conjunctival surface. Once the implant is exposed, the extrusion proceeds with cicatricial changes of the socket. Exposure of the orbital implant inevitably requires surgery, which should be performed before further scarring and contracture develop.

Early extrusion is treated with insertion of a proper-sized sphere implant, usually 16 mm or 18 mm, and meticulous closure of Tenon's capsule. In cases with late extrusion, it must be determined if adequate mucous membrane is present. If adequate mucous membrane is present, either a dermis-fat graft or an implant covered with autogenous fascia lata is used. A fascia-covered implant is a good technique but may shorten the fornices. If the socket contains insufficient mucous membrane, a dermis-fat graft is ideal, acting as a natural socket expander. The implanted dermal surface serves as a platform over which conjunctival mucosa can grow. In settings of inadequate mucous membrane, an alternative to a dermis-fat graft would be to use a sphere implant in the socket and perform a simultaneous free mucous membrane graft to the socket.

Surgical Procedure for Replacement of the Extruding Orbital Implant–Sphere Replacement

The early- and late-extruding orbital implants are managed in different matters (7). In the early-extruding implant, there is dehiscence of the surgical wound. The extruding implant is removed and a new 16-mm hollow glass sphere is placed through the posterior Tenon's capsule deep into the fat of the muscle cone. Firm tissue in the area of the posterior Tenon's capsule is closed horizontally with multiple interrupted 4–0 Vicryl sutures on small half-circle needles. A second horizontal layer of multiple interrupted 4–0 Vicryl sutures is placed in the firm tissue at the level of the anterior Tenon's capsule immediately deep to the conjunctiva. The conjunctiva is closed with interrupted 6–0 plain gut sutures. A loose-fitting eyelid conformer is placed in the socket. An oversized eyelid conformer, which could exert traction on the fornices and create pressure on the wound, is to be avoided. Antibiotic ointment is placed in the cul-de-sac and a firm pressure patch is applied for 48 hr. Systemic antibiotics are not generally used.

The socket with early postoperative orbital implant extrusion frequently presents with inflammation and mucopurulent discharge. Although this may appear to be an infection causing the extrusion, in fact, it usually is an inflammation secondary to the extrusion.

In the repair of the socket with an extruding orbital implant, there may be an insufficient amount of tissue to close the wound without causing a shortage of the cul-de-sac. In such a case, a dermis-fat graft is used for its ability to expand the socket mucosa.

In the late-extruding orbital implant, the tissues around the exposed implant are significantly thinned (Fig. 7). The opening is enlarged with a scissors horizontally and the implant is removed. The incision is then carried through the posterior face of the "capsule," which has surrounded the implant. Next, the incision is carried to the apex of the orbit. Meticulous hemostasis is obtained with the use of pressure, cold packs, hemostats, and Avitine® powder as needed. An implant (our preference is a 16-mm or 18-mm hollow glass sphere) is inserted to the apex. The posterior face of the pseudocapsule is closed with interrupted 4–0 Vicryl sutures on half-circle needles. A second layer of deep interrupted Vicryl may be used if it clearly will not vertically shorten the cul-de-sac. The area about the fistulous opening is excised and the margins freshened. Interrupted Vicryl is used to close the deep layers of Tenon's capsule and scar just below the conjunctiva. This tissue is approximated but not overlapped. Finally, the conjunctiva is closed with interrupted 6–0 plain gut sutures. A firm patch is left in place for 48 hr. After 10 days the patient is sent to the ocularist.

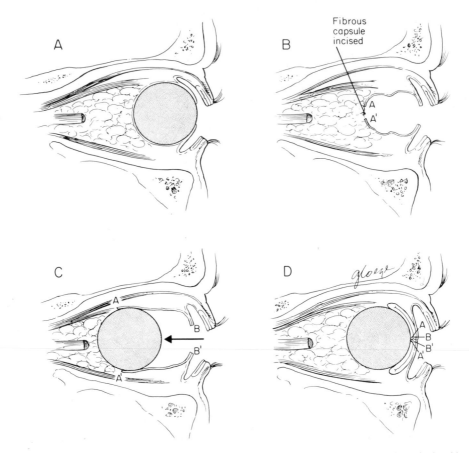

FIG. 7. Replacement of extruding orbital implant. **A:** The extruding implant presents through the thinned tissues of the posterior wall of the socket. **B:** The extruding implant is removed and an incision is made through the posterior aspect of the fibrous capsule. **C:** A 16-mm sphere is passed through the incision in the posterior fibrous capsule into the fat at the apex of the orbit. **D:** The posterior fibrous capsule is closed anterior to the orbital implant. The anterior Tenon's capsule and the conjunctiva are closed in separate layers.

Again, if the tissues cannot be closed without shortening the cul-de-sac, the dermis-fat graft with a sphere implant behind it must be used.

Surgical Procedure using Fascia to Cover Extruding Implant (Patch Graft)

In a socket that has inadequate central tissue, the exposed implant may be covered with autogenous fiscia. In all aspects of oculoplastic surgery, the authors have found autogenous grafts to be far superior to either fresh homologous or preserved homologous grafts. Tissue harvesting techniques for both autogenous fascia lata and temporalis fascia are discussed in Chapter 1. The autogenous graft has the advantage of not inciting an immune reaction or foreign body reaction, not causing inflammation, not shrinking, and predictably surviving, provided there is adequate blood supply. On the other hand, homologous grafts create an immune reaction, cause additional inflammation, and may shrink or even be totally absorbed. In a socket with an extruding implant, socket contracture is already a significant problem. The additional inflammation associated with the use of a fresh homologous graft will worsen

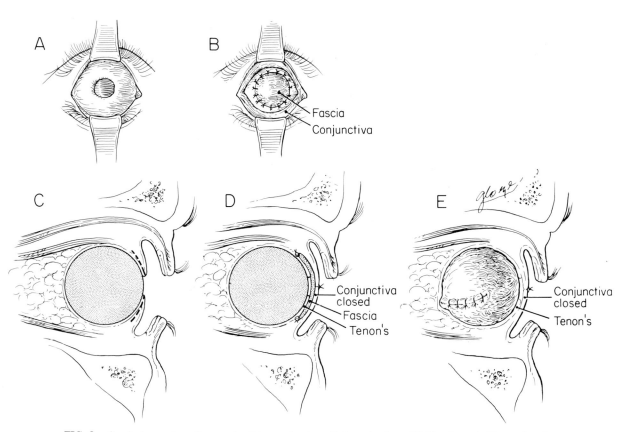

FIG. 8. Surgical procedures for use of autogenous fascia grafts for extruding orbital implants. **A:** The conjunctiva has been undermined and dissected from Tenon's capsule in all meridians. The exposed portion of the extruding orbital implant is visble. **B:** An autogenous fascia patch graft covers the orbital implant and is sutured to the underlying Tenon's capsule. **C:** A sagittal section of an extuding orbital implant shows thinning of the remaining tissue lying anterior to the implant. The *dashed line* is the subconjunctival dissection plane developed prior to the placement of the patch graft. **D:** This sagittal section shows the patch graft covering the extruding orbital implant lying anterior to the remaining Tenon's capsule and posterior to the closed conjunctiva. **E:** A sagittal view of the completed replacement of an extruded orbital implant with an implant fully encapsulated with fascia. This fully encapsulated implant can be sutured to deeper tissues and thus be better stabilized.

this contracture. Preserved homologous grafts, such as preserved sclera, cause an even greater reaction.

When the extruding implant is removed, a horizontal incision is made through the posterior surface of the fibrous pseudocapsule that surrounded it (Fig. 8). A new 16-mm sphere is placed through this incision deep into the fat of the muscle cone. If the incision in the posterior face of the capsule cannot be closed without shortening the fornices, a fascia patch is used to cover the defect. The patch is fashioned to overlap the defect 4 mm in all meridians. It is secured with multiple interrupted 4–0 Vicryl sutures. The conjunctiva is undermined in all meridians so that it will completely cover the patch graft. The conjunctiva is retracted and the existing anterior Tenon's capsule is sutured to the anterior surface of the patch under no traction. The conjunctiva is closed to itself and the patch graft with interrupted 6–0 plain gut suture. Since the conjunctiva provides the major blood supply for the patch graft, it must fully cover the graft. If conjunctival closure produces a shortening of the fornices, a dermis–fat graft should be considered as an alternative.

Surgical Procedure using Fascia to Encapsulate Extruding Implant

When a sphere implant covered with autogenous fascia lata is used to replace a late-extruding implant, it is requisite that adequate healthy Tenon's capsule and conjuctiva be present to fully cover the implant. The socket is infiltrated with lidocaine 2% with epinephrine and hyaluronidase. A horizontal, transconjunctival incision is made to facilitate removal of the extruding implant. The pseudocapsule, which surrounded the implant, should be dissected and removed. A unipolar Bovie unit is useful to achieve hemostasis. The fascia-covered implant is inserted into the socket. The deep layer of Tenon's capsule with the rectus muscles can be sutured directly to the fascia, just anterior to its "equator." Meticulous closure of Tenon's capsule is achieved with interrupted 4–0 Vicryl sutures. It is often necessary to undermine conjunctiva so that closure can be achieved without shortening the fornices. Conjunctival closure is achieved with a running 6–0 plain suture. As has been emphasized, if adequate socket tissues or complete closure are not present, a dermis-fat graft must be used (11).

Socket Contracture

The spectrum of socket contracture has been described in the section on socket types. We classify socket contracture into three levels of severity: mild, moderate, and severe.

Mild Socket Contracture—Cicatricial Entropion

Mild socket contracture may be defined as tarsoconjunctival contracture with cicatricial entropion of the upper and/or lower eyelids. The cicatricial entropion results in a matting of the eyelashes against the prosthesis. Frequently, the cul-de-sac and fornices are still adequate and a prosthesis is well maintained. In such cases, rotation of the lid margins will result in a return of the eyelids to a normal position.

Surgical procedure for lid margin rotation without a graft

In mild cases of upper eyelid entropion and lash ptosis, adequate correction can be achieved with Pang sutures with reformation of the lid crease and tensing of the upper eyelid skin. In this procedure, a lid crease incision is made symmetric to the opposing upper eyelid. A thin ellipse of excess skin and muscle are excised off of the tarsal surface. Four interrupted double-armed 4–0 silk sutures are sewn through the conjunctiva above the tarsus, and then through the levator muscle and skin inferior to the lid crease incision. Tying these sutures firmly will tense the pretarsal skin, evert the lashes, and rotate the upper eyelid margin.

A more involved procedure for effecting marginal rotation is the standard transverse blepharotomy (14). It may be performed on the upper or lower eyelid. Because of the longer and more visible eyelashes on the upper eyelid, this procedure is more commonly performed on the upper eyelid. As in most procedures involving the eyelids, an injection of lidocaine with epinephrine is used for hemostasis. An incision is made using a #15 blade through the full thickness of the upper eyelid 4 mm superior to the lid margin. One blade of a scissors is introduced through this blepharotomy and the incision is extended through the full thickness of the eyelid, nasally and temporally, paralleling the lid margin along the central three-fourths of the upper eyelid (Weis-type procedure). Standard Weis horizontal mattress rotational sutures of 6–0 silk are used. Three such sutures, appropriately spaced, are all that is usually used. The skin is closed with a running 6–0 nylon suture. In the anophthalmic socket, the procedure is never done with a block resection horizontal tightening of the eyelid. This same procedure may be done on the lower eyelid.

Surgical procedure for eyelid margin rotation with a graft

In either the upper or lower eyelids, if the rotation achieved with the above procedure is inadequate, a graft must be used to vertically lengthen the posterior lamella and stabilize the margin rotation. By far, an autogenous cartilage graft is the material of choice. In the anophthalmic socket, an ear cartilage graft can be used without mucous membrane.

This procedure is most commonly performed on the upper eyelid. After injection of the eyelid with lidocaine 2% with epinephrine and hyaluronidase, the upper eyelid is everted over a Desmarres retractor. A #15 blade is used to make an incision in the tarsus 4 mm superior to the eyelid margin. Dissection is carried into the pretarsal space and the scissors are used to extend the incision nasally and temporally along the full extent of the tarsus paralleling the margin. The superior portion of tarsus attached to the levator and Müller's muscles will retract superiorly, creating a bed in the posterior lamella, which is usually 25 mm in horizontal length and at least 5 mm in vertical height. An ear cartilage graft of appropriate size is harvested in the usual fashion (see Chapter 1). Interrupted 6–0 Vicryl sutures are used to secure the cartilage graft to the superior and inferior edges of the eyelid tarsus. In some cases, reconstruction of the posterior eyelid lamella is all that is necessary to stabilize the eyelid and correct entropion. In others, multiple double-armed 4–0 silk rotational sutures are necessary. An eyelid conformer is inserted and antibiotic ointment and a pressure dressing are applied.

Moderate Socket Contracture

Moderate socket contracture is defined as contracture of the upper and lower fornix, resulting in the inability to retain a properly sized prosthesis. Often more than one procedure will be required because of limitations of blood supply when multiple procedures such as subperiorbital volume augmentation, intraorbital implant implantation with autogenous grafting, and mucous membrane grafting procedures are all performed at the same time. Volume augmentation may be done prior to, in conjunction with, or after mucous membrane grafting.

Surgical procedure to enlarge cul-de-sac and deepen fornices

In moderate socket contracture, the inferior fornix is usually foreshortened with inadequate mucous membrane. Additionally, the superior fornix is frequently contracted. Reconstruction of a moderately contracted socket usually requires enlargement of the inferior cul-de-sac with mucous membrane grafting in conjunction with a lateral canthal tightening (see Fig. 6), as described in the section on concepts for lower eyelid laxity and inadequate fornix. That procedure would be performed here. Additionally, a mucous membrane graft from the mouth can be used to reconstruct and deepen the superior fornix. This may be necessary in order to create an upper fornix deep enough to hold the prosthesis superiorly. A deep superior fornix also allows for the movement and closure of the upper eyelid.

Surgery to enlarge the superior fornix is initiated with a horizontal incision through the conjunctiva at the apex of the existing fornix from the medial canthus to the lateral canthus. The dissection plane is carried superiorly and posteriorly, avoiding the levator aponeurosis. In this way, a bed for the mucous membrane graft is created. The graft is sutured into place with interrupted 6–0 plain gut sutures, as described for the lower fornix reconstruction.

A prosthesis or conformer is used as a stent to hold the graft in position. Both superior and inferior fornices can be reconstructed in the same procedure. Additional procedures, such as lid margin rotation, lower eyelid tightening, deep fornix supporting bolsters, or even subperiorbital volume augmentation, can also be performed at the same time. A firm pressure bandage is used to hold the lids closed and press the mucous membrane graft against the vascular bed for 3 days. The lids should easily close, and lid margin sutures could be used to splint the eyelids. In 3 to 4 weeks, the patient is sent to the ocularist to be fitted for a prosthesis.

Severe Socket Contracture

The severely contracted socket is one in which there is horizontal shortening of the lid aperture and mucous membrane as well as vertical contracture of the fornices. The fornices are severely contracted or obliterated such that a prosthesis cannot be retained. Severe socket contracture includes a spectrum from horizontal shortening of the lid apertures with normal lid margins to severe horizontal shortening and corrugation of the lid margins with obliterated fornices or even complete obliteration of lid margins and fornices. In those cases with an active cicatricial process, obliteration of lid margins, and a history of multiple previous failed reconstructive surgeries, the authors feel that additional surgery is unwise. In a socket that has no active cicatricial process, and in which no surgery has been performed for at least 1 year, major surgical reconstruction may be considered only with a major commitment from both the patient and the surgeon (12,15,16).

A key point in evaluating the severely contracted socket is whether it is a ''moist'' socket or a ''dry'' socket. A moist anophthalmic socket can successfully receive free mucous membrane grafts; a dry socket cannot. Mucous membrane grafts in a dry socket will keratinize and rapidly shrink. Typical causes of a dry socket are infection, previous alkali burns or irradiation treatment, and a poorly fitting prosthesis with chronic conjunctivitis. A Schirmer's strip may aid in preoperative decision making by detecting poor tear production in the dry, anophthalmic socket.

Surgical procedure for severe contracture—moist socket

Freshly harvested mucous membrane grafts from the lip or oral cavity are the materials of choice to expand the severely contracted moist socket (Fig. 9). The socket is infiltrated with Lidocaine 2% with epinephrine and hyaluronidase. Relaxing incisions are made at the junction of the palpebral conjunctiva and socket conjunctiva. These upper and lower incisions are made across the entire horizontal width of the socket. In the severely contracted socket, underlying Tenon's fascia and scar tissue must be extensively dissected. Once adequate undermining has been performed, the existing socket conjunctiva (mucosa) will retract back to the apex of the socket. Techniques for harvesting mucous membrane grafts are described in Chapter 1.

It is helpful to harvest the mucous membrane graft at the onset of the procedure so that this tissue, taken from a nonsterile environment, may soak in a gentamicin solution for a period of time. The free mucous membrane graft is then sutured into place with interrupted or running 6–0 Vicryl sutures. It is sewn to preexisting conjunctiva posteriorly in the socket and to palpebral conjunctiva anteriorly. An eyelid conformer is placed in the socket to maintain the expanded fornices. Marginal lid sutures are used to splint the eyelids closed. Antibiotic ointment is applied and a pressure bandage is secured for 1 week.

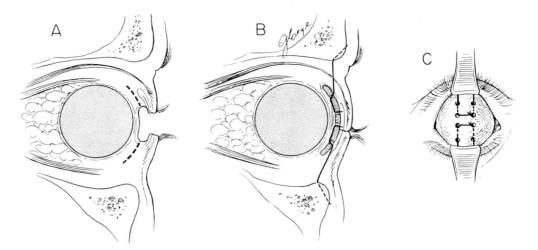

FIG. 9. Total socket reconstruction. **A:** In a severely contracted moist socket, the superior and inferior fornices are developed with sharp and blunt dissection. **B:** The mucous membrane–enveloped "prosthesis stent" is suspended between the orbital rims with wire. **C:** The mucous membrane graft completely envelopes the stent with the epithelial surface against the stent.

Surgical procedure for severe contracture—dry socket

Every experienced oculoplastic surgeon has been frustrated by the dry contracted socket's inability to accept mucous membrane grafts. Reconstruction of these sockets remains a great challenge. The patient must have realistic expectations as to the anticipated result. The goals here are to restore the patient's ability to wear a prosthesis, and to correct an associated eyelid malposition.

Keratinized skin is the only tissue that can be successfully grafted to the dry anophthalmic socket. A Striker keratome is used to harvest split-thickness skin grafts from the anterior surface of the thigh (see Chapter 1). The fornices of the socket are dissected extensively. Scar tissue is dissected and the mucosa undermined such that the existing conjunctiva will migrate back toward the apex of the socket. A round conformer made out of dental wax is molded to the shape of the socket. This wax conformer is then wrapped with the split-thickness skin graft. It is important that the keratinized surface faces inward and is in contact with the wax ball and that the "raw surface" is facing outward. Careful handling of the split-tissue skin graft is important, because it is easy to confuse the keratinized and nonkeratinized surfaces. Double-armed 4–0 silk sutures are then sewn into the wax conformer. The wrapped conformer is placed into the socket and secured into place using double-armed 4–0 silk sutures. Inferiorly, the sutures should be sewn through the lower lid fornix down to the periosteum of the inferior orbital rim and then out through the skin and tied over cotton bolsters. Superiorly the silk sutures are sewn through the upper lid fornix and out through the skin just inferior to the superior orbital rim. The eyelids are sewn closed with marginal 4–0 silk sutures. A pressure bandage is applied.

In 7 to 10 days, the eyelids are opened and the wax is picked out piece by piece. After the split-thickness graft has been exposed to raw socket surfaces, it will have taken as a vascularized graft. In other areas of the socket, such as posteriorly where mucous membrane is present, the split-thickness skin graft will simply have sloughed. The presence of keratinizing skin in the socket presents a hygiene challenge for the patient. Nonetheless, it provides a means of expanding the socket to allow the patient to wear a prosthesis. Associated eyelid deformities or malpositions are treated as described under previous sections.

CONGENITAL ANOPHTHALMOS

True congenital anophthalmos is uncommon, and many cases of "anophthalmos" contain vestigial eye tissue. The manifestations of congenital anophthalmos may include severely small, hypoplastic eyelids with phimosis of the fissure, hypoplasia of the bony orbit with narrowing of the vertical and horizontal dimensions, and deficiency of socket mucous membrane. All of these changes preclude the child from the capability of holding a prosthetic eye in the socket space. Congenital anophthalmos, in most cases, occurs as an isolated entity, although it has been reported from time to time in children with severe chromosomal abnormalities.

Treatment

Expansion Conformers

Congenital anophthalmos has, in the past, been treated primarily with expansion conformers. In this procedure, a conformer is placed in the socket of an infant and periodically changed to a larger size over many years. This procedure is designed to gradually enlarge the socket so that it eventually will retain a prosthesis of satisfactory size. This technique can most certainly obtain some expansion of mucous membrane surface area and enlargement of the socket. However, in most cases, it unfortunately does not produce forniceal enlargement or bony socket enlargement, or correct the eyelid deformities. In most cases, the habit of performing lateral canthotomies to allow one to insert larger conformers has further destroyed the integrity of the lower lid and caused lateral canthal separation and, ultimately, failure to retain any prosthesis at all. The authors feel that socket expansion with enlarging conformers should be looked upon as a temporary procedure until a more definitive surgical correction can be undertaken.

Surgical Enlargement of the Bony Orbit and Socket

When the child has reached an age where he or she will be subjected to peer pressure, consideration should be given to a more adequate correction of the anophthalmos to produce, as much as possible, a matching result compared with the normal eye. It has been the author's experience that surgical enlargement of the bony orbit opening should be undertaken. This can be done in conjunction with reconstruction or expansion of the socket with mucous membrane. The most important dimension to enlarge is the lateral aperture, so that subsequent eyelid reconstruction can be carried out and a proper placement of the lateral canthus can be accomplished. High-speed cutting burrs can be used to sculpt the bone in these areas before the mucous membrane grafts are placed. The mucous membrane is harvested in the manner described in Chapter 1, and is placed into the socket in such a manner as to form an adequate lower fornix and, as much as possible, an upper fornix. This technique has been described in the previous section. Following the expansion of the bony orbit and socket, an attempt at fitting of a standard prosthesis can be undertaken. The problems encountered at this stage are laxity and deficiency of the lower and upper lids.

Eyelid Reconstruction

There is some variation in the amount of hypoplasia in the eyelids in patients with congenital anophthalmos. Some children have extremely deficient lids, which are flabby, contain very little tarsus, and, in the upper lid, have deficiency and deformation. In these patients, a full-scale reconstructive procedure must be considered. In the lower lid, reformation can be obtained with advancement flaps and ear cartilage grafts as described in Chapter 4. Reconstruction in the upper lid generally must be carried out with sharing of adjacent tissue or multiple free grafts, since one is not, in many cases, able to use a lid-sharing procedure. Ear cartilage has been extremely useful in these children since there is generally hypoplasia of the superior tarsal plate. The lower lid is very important for retention of the prosthesis since it is the sole supporting structure, and in many cases an autogenous fascia sling must be used to gain support in these patients. In the upper lid almost all patients have absent levator function, and, following adequate fitting of a prosthesis, if ptosis remains a frontalis suspension procedure must be used.

Congenital Microophthalmos

In mild cases of congenital microophthalmos, the only defect may be an undersized globe. In these cases, a cosmetic shell alone may produce an excellent cosmetic result. If irritation results from wearing a cosmetic shell, the cornea can be desensitized by covering it with a conjunctival flap. In some cases of congenital microophthalmos with no visual potential, which cannot be satisfactorily treated by the above methods, enucleation with a suitable implant should be considered.

REFERENCES

1. Soll, D. B. (1982): The anophthalmic socket. *Ophthalmology*, 89:407–423.
2. Soll, D. B. (1976): The anophthalmic socket. In: *Management of Complications in Ophthalmic Plastic Surgery*. Aesculapius, Birmingham, Alabama.
3. Iliff, C. E., Iliff, W. J., and Iliff, N. T. (1979): *Oculoplastic Surgery*. Saunders, Philadelphia.
4. Callahan, M. A. (1979): *Ophthalmic, Plastic, and Orbital Surgery*. Aesculapius, Birmingham, Alabama.
5. Spivey, B. E., Stewart, W., and Allen, L. (1976): Surgical correction of superior sulcus deformity occurring after enucleation. *Am. J. Ophthalmol.*, 82:365–370.
6. Tenzel, R. R. (1969): Treatment of lagophthalmos in the lower lid. *Arch. Ophthalmol.*, 81:366–368.
7. McCord, C. D. (1976): The extruding implant. *Trans. Am. Acad. Ophthalmol. Otolaryngol.*, 81:587–590.
8. Smith, B., Obear, M., and Leone, C. R., Jr. (1967): The correction of enophthalmos associated with anophthalmos by glass bead implantation. *Am. J. Ophthalmol.*, 64:1088–1093.
9. Walter, W. L. (1977): Complications associated with the orbital bead implant operation. *Ophthalmic Surg.*, 8:68–75.
10. Soll, D. B. (1973): Insertion of secondary intraorbital implants. *Arch. Ophthalmol.*, 89:214–216.
11. Smith, B., and Petrelli, R. (1978): Dermis-fat graft as a moveable implant within the muscle cone. *Am. J. Ophthalmol.*, 85:62–66.
12. Vistnes, L. M., and Paris, F. L. (1977): Uses of RTV silicone in orbital reconstruction. *Am. J. Ophthalmol.*, 83:577–581.
13. Meltzer, M. A. (1977): Reconstruction of lower fornix. *Arch. Ophthalmol.*, 95:1031–1034.
14. Baylis, H. I., and Hamako, C. (1979): Tarsal grafting for correction of cicatricial entropion. *Ophthalmic Surg.*, 10:42.
15. Vistnes, L. M., and Iverson, R. E. (1974): Surgical management of the contracted socket. *Plast. Reconstr. Surg.*, 53:563–567.
16. Putterman, A. M. (1977): Deep ocular socket reconstruction. *Arch. Ophthalmol.*, 95:1221–1228.

Oculoplastic Surgery, 2nd edition, edited by
Clinton D. McCord, Jr., and Myron Tanenbaum.
Raven Press, New York © 1987.

Chapter 17

Blepharoplasty: Cosmetic and Functional

*Robert B. Wilkins, *Gerard J. Hunter, **Clinton D. McCord, Jr., and
†Myron Tanenbaum

*Department of Ophthalmology, University of Texas Medical School, Houston, Texas 77025;
** Department of Ophthalmology, Emory University School of Medicine, Atlanta, Georgia 30308;
and †Bascom Palmer Eye Institute, Department of Ophthalmology, University of Miami School of
Medicine, Miami, Florida 33101*

More ophthalmologists are adding blepharoplasty techniques to their list of surgical procedures, and many more are beginning to do sophisticated blepharoplasty work. This phenomenon has occurred for at least two reasons. The general population in the United States has
doubled since 1900 and the number of people over 65 has increased five times. Approximately
half of our population is now over 45 years of age (1). This increase in longevity requires
continued earning power even during later years of life and usually in competition with
younger people. In addition to the increased longevity, there has been a greatly increased
acceptance of plastic surgical procedures in general. Often the simple desire to look better
has brought about an ever-increasing demand for cosmetic lid and facial procedures (2).
Whereas cosmesis is always strived for, functional blepharoplasty should not be overlooked
as a therapy for those who have ocular fatigue or decreased visual fields as a result of
excessive upper eyelid skin (3).

PATIENT EVALUATION AND WORK-UP

The age of the blepharoplasty patient seen by the ophthalmologist will vary greatly, but
most patients are over 55 years old. In each case the doctor should attempt to determine
the etiology of the patient's complaints. Terminology may be confusing, but the most
commonly used diagnoses are blepharochalasis and dermatochalasis. Dermatochalasis usually
refers to the fine wrinkling and loosening of the eyelid skin, generally as a result of age.
Blepharochalasis is a term describing a syndrome of recurrent edema, usually in young
people over a period of time, producing changes in the eyelid (4,5). The eyelid changes
usually consist of redundant crinkled skin folds, atrophy of the nasal fat pad with ptosis,
and dehiscence of the canthal tendons. A hypertrophic form of blepharochalasis can occur
with protuberant fat pockets as a result of recurrent edema.

At the initial examination the most important consideration in discussing blepharoplasty surgery with the patient is that the patient understands just what the surgeon can and cannot do. We give the patient a mirror and ask him or her to point out the areas that are of particular concern. It is important to ask what the patient believes needs to be corrected and what he or she believes a self-satisfying surgical outcome should be (6). This subjective portion of the examination is important to establish rapport with the patient, and may highlight any unrealistic expectations of the patient. After determining the patient's initial complaints, a good history of current or past medical problems is required. Those patients with concurrent systemic illnesses such as diabetes, renal or circulatory disorders, or thyrotoxicosis should be examined by their internist for stabilization of their disease. A list of the patient's allergies and current medications is obtained. Sodium warfarin (Coumadin®) therapy is an obvious contraindication, but the use of aspirin therapy, usually seen in chronic arthritis or cardiac patients, also predisposes to decreased platelet aggregation and therefore increased bleeding at the time of surgery. We require that aspirin usage be stopped for 2 weeks prior to surgery. Many other agents have an ''aspirin-like'' effect, including antiinflammatory drugs used for arthritis and other related conditions. Cardiac patients are also given drugs that impair platelet aggregation and increase peripheral blood flow; these should be discontinued if possible.

In addition to a general physical examination, a careful ophthalmic examination is mandatory for any surgery on the ocular adnexa. Visual acuity, muscle balance, tonometry with slit-lamp examination, and fundoscopy should all be carried out to rule out any occult eye pathology. Schirmer testing of lacrimal function is useful and should be repeated in any patient with equivocal results or with a history of chronic use of artificial tear substitutes or antihistamines. A basic tear secretion test should be administered to all prospective blepharoplasty patients utilizing topical anesthesia and the Shirmer's strip. Decreased tear production should cause conservativeness in the treatment of the patient.

The Bell's phenomenon is an integral part of protection of the globe, and the small amount of lagophthalmos that can occur following blepharoplasty will result in corneal exposure in the presence of a poor Bell's phenomenon.

External examination of the eyes assumes a special importance when blepharoplasty is contemplated. In addition to the location and extent of excess lid skin, the position and symmetry of the eyebrows in relation to the supraorbital rim should be noted. Elimination of excess eyelid skin in the presence of brow ptosis only accentuates the eyebrow problem by bringing the cilia of the brow into even closer approximation with the lashes. Normally the brow should be firmly attached to the supraorbital rim by heavy fascial bands (7); the loss of this attachment results in a feeling of fatigue from prolonged use of the frontalis muscle in an attempt to restore the superior visual field. Accurate estimation of the amount of excess lid skin can only be made when the brows are restored to the supraorbital rims.

If there is excess orbital fat, gentle pressure on the globe with the lids closed helps to further define the pockets of fat pressing against the orbital septum. Many younger patients do not have excess lid skin in the lower lids, but rather protuberant fat, usually from a familial tendency, that makes the lids appear generally swollen. In older persons, the individual fat pockets are more clearly appreciated, and any asymmetry of the amount or location of the fat should be recorded so that asymmetric removal of the fat can be carried out.

The location of the upper lid in relation to the pupil is noted in all patients, as well as the measurement of the palpebral fissures and the function of the levator muscle in each eye. These measurements combined with the measurement of the lid crease facilitate accurate diagnosis of any co-existent blepharoptosis. The possibility of a disinsertion of the levator aponeurosis from the superior border of the tarsus should be suspected and looked for in elderly patients.

Examination of the lower lid prior to blepharoplasty includes an estimation of the muscular tone of the lower lid to prevent postoperative ectropion (8). In normal individuals, a depression of the lower lid for a few seconds results in an immediate snap of the lid back into close approximation with the globe. If, after depressing the lower lid for a few seconds, it does not spring back but rather sluggishly returns or remains depressed with a frank ectropion, then this patient will have a postoperative ectropion unless a horizontal lid tightening is done at the same time as the blepharoplasty. Additionally, position of the lacrimal punctum should be noted since any postoperative ectropion will be magnified if it is accompanied with epiphora. Periorbital fat and excessive skin are frequently abundant in the lower lid and can be removed by careful blepharoplasty. However, if the patient has the so-called "bags on bags," with edematous skin in folds overlying the zygoma, the patient should be informed that a standard blepharoplasty may not completely eliminate these large bags of skin and that an "extended" lower lid blepharoplasty incision may be necessary.

Finally, the medial canthal area on each side should be examined for the possibility of webbing. Ordinarily the skin is firmly adherent over the medial canthal tendon, but with relaxation of the skin, a definite web extending from the upper to the lower lid may exist in the concavity of the medial canthus. This can be checked preoperatively by putting slight traction over the medial canthal skin and stretching it superiorly and temporally. If a tractional skin web crosses the medial canthus and extends into the lower lid, care should be taken to key the nasal skin incision higher in the canthal region than usual.

During the preoperative discussion, it is mentioned that some problems may not be relieved by the blepharoplasty surgery. Laugh lines or "crow's feet" at the lateral canthus may be minimized but not completely eliminated, since they are lines of dynamic action and will recur postoperatively as soon as muscle tone is restored. Coarse wrinkling of the skin may be markedly relieved, but very thin and fine wrinkles will remain even when the skin is tightened. Likewise, pigmentation of the lids is not eliminated by blepharoplasty except to the extent of excision of pigmented skin. A chemical peel may be necessary for further removal of pigmentation without excision of additional skin.

Documentation of these problems is important for insurance purposes, and visual field tests to determine any visual field loss are being increasingly required. Photographs are especially important in this regard, and they help eliminate any postoperative misunderstandings as well as provide an excellent visual record. Polaroid photographs are taken of both the frontal and lateral views of the full face and are brought to the operating room for reference at the time of surgery. All photographs must be taken in the upright position since the supine position on the operating table camouflages any brow ptosis and minimizes the appearance of any protuberant orbital fat.

At the conclusion of the examination, an attempt is again made to correlate the patient's expectations with the expected surgical outcome. The explanations of the proposed surgery should be repeated or further explained until the patient is able to give a reliable informed consent about the surgery. At this point, the surgeon will know whether the proposed procedure is cosmetic or functional. Whereas superior cosmetic results are always planned, even for the functional problem, if, in the surgeon's estimation, the procedure proposed will be purely cosmetic, the patient should be informed of this also to make appropriate financial arrangements.

Problem Patients

In evaluating patients for blepharoplasty, one must not only meticulously examine each patient, as described in the previous section, but also be aware of and ready to identify the problem patient—the patient who has a much greater chance of developing a complication postoperatively and having an untoward or unsatisfactory result.

Probably the most important category are the patients who have poor eye protective mechanisms. In the presence of a dry eye, a poor Bell's phenomenon, seventh nerve palsy, or any weakness of closure of the eyelids, the stiffness of the lid following the blepharoplasty procedure with minor malposition can produce distressing ocular changes and corneal exposure.

Eyelid disease or systemic disease should be identified and evaluated. Patients with rosacea of the eyelid, early pemphigoid, or any kind of chronic blepharitis will continue to have problems and may have an accentuation of their condition postoperatively. Undiagnosed hyper- or hypothyroidism can lead a patient to request a blepharoplasty, and these conditions should be evaluated.

In evaluating a patient's upper lid complaints, those patients who have brow laxity will have poor results unless specific attention is paid to correcting the laxity (9). Lacrimal gland prolapse (10), true ptosis underlying the dermatochalasis, and a preexisting asymmetry of brows or lid creases will continue postoperatively and cause an unhappy patient unless these are either pointed out to the patient before surgery or corrected during surgery. The most common problem patient with lower lid blepharoplasty is the patient who has lax lower lids, which, if undiagnosed or uncorrected, will lead to lower lid malposition with either inferior scleral show or ectropion (8).

Patients with prominent eyes many times have a stronger tendency for lower lid retraction postoperatively. High cheek bones in patients are an indication for conservative removal of fatty pads. Many times, the fullness of the lower lid is not due to fatty pad herniation but rather to orbicularis hypertrophy. These patients must be identified and specific attention paid to resection of the redundant orbicularis muscle, or they will be dissatisfied with their result postoperatively.

BROW PTOSIS

Complaints of ocular fatigue are common in patients with brow ptosis. The continuous action of the frontalis muscle may produce large furrows in the brow without the patient being aware of the ptosis until asked to relax the frontalis muscle on examination. The brow ptosis can be asymmetrical with the brows being unequal or uneven. The amount of correction is determined preoperatively, since the brows will change position when the patient is on the operating table. To determine the vertical extent of excision, a ruler is held in front of the relaxed brow while the patient is sitting. The brow is then elevated to the desired position and the amount of necessary elevation is recorded. Such measurements are made along the entire width of the brow since areas of uneven ptosis may exist.

On the operating table, the inferior limb of the incision is drawn across the entire width of the brow to be elevated and is placed in the uppermost row of cilia, parallel to their direction of growth. To the vertical measurements determined preoperatively, we add 2 mm of overcorrection to account for the effect of contraction during wound healing and the patient's erect posture postoperatively. The vertical marks are connected to form the superior limb of the incision, and a slight lift at the temporal aspect of the brow is accomplished by upward angulation of the incision at 30° for the lateral few millimeters.

One percent lidocaine (Xylocaine®) with epinephrine and hyaluronidase (Wydase®) is infiltrated beneath the area to be excised and gently massaged in for 3 to 5 min. Excessive amounts of local anesthetic to balloon up the brow tissue are not necessary; they distort the lines of incision. The brow is extremely vascular, and adequate time must be allowed for action of the vasoconstrictors, which will result in less capillary oozing.

The skin is incised with a #15 Bard-Parker blade, and dissection with scissors is carried down until the fibers of the frontalis muscle are encountered. The area under the marks is then excised *en bloc* without interruption of the fibers of the frontalis. Large veins may be encountered in this area, and the bleeding points are sealed with electrocautery.

To prevent excessive scarring, this wound must be carefully reconstructed in layers. The design of the incision may cause some lateral shifting of the tissues on completion of dissection; therefore, the skin edges should be reoriented prior to the beginning of the closure. The deep layers are closed with interrupted 4–0 nylon sutures that engage the subcutaneous tissue and frontalis muscle with each bite. Care is taken not to fixate these tissues to the underlying periosteum, since this will result in a fixed and immobile brow. The more superficial subcutaneous layers are closed with interrupted 5–0 Vicryl sutures that are tied with their knots down to prevent suture reaction beneath the skin (Fig. 1).

At the termination of the subcutaneous closure, there should be no gaping of the skin margins, since this will result in a corresponding postoperative scar of the same width. Skin sutures of 6–0 silk must be used for vertical alignment of the skin only rather than attempting to close any 1- to 2-mm gaps in the skin edges. A small amount of antibiotic ointment is applied to the suture line, and the incisions are covered with Telfa dressings. The skin sutures are removed at 4 to 5 days, and the wound is reinforced with Steri-Strips for the next week.

Two modifications may also be considered for treatment of the ptotic brow. The first

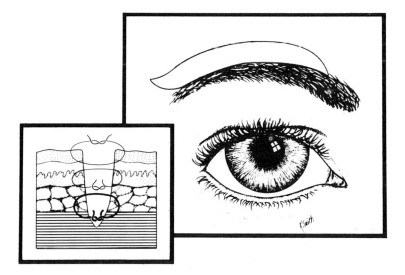

FIG. 1. The incision for a brow elevation is made in a ''lazy S'' fashion. Three sutures are used. One, of 4-0 nylon, fixes the brow to the frontalis muscle. The other two sutures, of 5-0 Vicryl and 6-0 nylon are used for closing the skin and subcutaneous tissue.

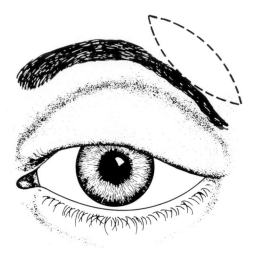

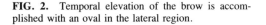

FIG. 2. Temporal elevation of the brow is accomplished with an oval in the lateral region.

uses the same type of incision across the full width of the brow, but in this case the inferior limb of the incision is designed to correspond to a preexisting furrow, usually 2 to 3 mm above the brow. Vertical measurements are identical, but this approach has the advantage of camouflaging the scar in the preexisting furrow and is most applicable in older patients.

The second variation is the "temporal brow lift." This procedure involves the excision of an ellipse of skin and subcutaneous tissue only over the lateral aspect of the brow with similar closure in layers. This has the advantage of being slightly easier technically but does nothing to correct any remaining brow ptosis, especially medially (Fig. 2).

Coronal Forehead Lift Approach to Brow Ptosis

The coronal incision and forehead lift, including brow fixation, is an excellent surgical technique. It is described in detail in Chapter 18, since it is an exposure that is used in many cases to treat essential blepharospasm patients. To supplement an upper lid blepharoplasty, it is an excellent technique and provides not only a brow lift but also additional anatomic corrections such as the smoothing of the glabellar lines, transverse lines of the forehead, and the skin temple to the brow area.

The direct brow fixation with the suprabrow incision is contraindicated in patients who are overly sensitive about visible scars and particularly should be avoided in fair-skinned or reddish-haired women with pale, thin eyebrows. The resulting scar in these patients is unsatisfactory when the direct approach is used and these patients lend themselves well to the coronal approach. Contraindications to the coronal approach are relative but, in general terms, exist in males who would suffer from a receding hairline when the incision is placed within the hair and in any person who is reticent to have any recession of the hair line. Fortunately many women have a fairly low hairline. Those who do get some recession do not mind changing their hairstyle to minimize the appearance of a recession and are quite happy to do so if informed of the possibility ahead of time.

The midline glabellar vertical furrows are quite dramatically improved when the corrugator muscles are removed in a manner similar to that described for the treatment of blepharospasm. It must be noted, however, that much more conservatism is observed in excision of the muscles of this area when doing this procedure for cosmetic purposes. We purposely have not been scoring the frontalis muscle to reduce the transverse furrows of the forehead because of a resulting shiny appearance of the forehead.

The coronal forehead lift does represent the state of the art approach to the correction of brow and forehead laxity.

UPPER LID BLEPHAROPLASTY

Upper lid blepharoplasty takes place after any brow ptosis has been eliminated and is directed at eliminating redundant lid skin and prolapsed orbital fat. If, during the preoperative evaluation, an abnormal lid crease or a blepharoptosis is uncovered, this also may be repaired by careful design of the incision.

On the operating table, the patient is asked to look up and down to determine the natural lid crease in the upper lid. In women this crease is usually 10 mm from the lid margin in the midpupillary line. If the patient has a lid crease lower than 10 mm, slight stretch is put on the skin and the site of the new lid crease is marked 10 mm from the lid margin. With continued slight superior traction on the upper lid skin, the mark is extended medially and inferiorly to a point 4 mm superior to the lacrimal punctum. Similarly, the lateral portion of the incision is formed by extending the mark laterally and inferiorly to the lateral orbital rim. At this point, the proposed site of incision should be not less than 6 mm above the lateral canthal tendon (Fig. 3A). Carrying the incision lower may result in postoperative webbing of the lateral canthus, especially if a lower lid blepharoplasty is also planned. Except for markedly excessive lid skin, usually in older individuals, we prefer to end the lateral extent of the incision at the orbital rim. If there is excessive lid skin, the mark at the lateral point is extended upward and laterally at a 30° angle for a distance of 10 mm, and falling, if possible, into one of the preexisting laugh lines.

After the inferior limb of the incision that will form the new lid crease is marked out, the excess skin to be excised can be determined. Using the inferior limb of the incision as the base, the excess lid skin is grasped with forceps and elevated so that each arm of the forceps grasps an equal amount of skin. Sufficient stretch should be put on this skin to open the palpebral fissure only 1 mm. Similar marking is done across the entire width of the lid to assure that excision in each portion will be adequate but not excessive (Fig. 3B). To form the superior limb of the incision, these marks are connected by a single line starting at the medial canthus and extending laterally to the lateral orbital rim, and again turning up at a 30° angle. This forms the so-called "lazy-S," and the amount of excess skin to be excised should be determined in both lids before any injection of anesthetic. After completion of the marks for incision, two points should be checked: (a) that the lower limbs of the incision are symmetrical and fall either in the natural lid crease or the proposed new lid crease, and (b) that the superior limbs of the incision are symmetrical and both end at the same points on the lateral orbital rim.

One percent lidocaine with epinephrine is infiltrated subcutaneously to only slightly balloon out the tissue. The lids are gently massaged for 3 min to allow for diffusion of the anesthetic and action of the vasoconstrictor and to eliminate any distortion of the lines of the incision caused by the volume of the injected anesthetic. Another technique of injection of the local anesthetic is to use 9 ml of lidocaine with epinephrine mixed with 1 ml of hyaluronidase. The injection is carried out in the eyelids before marking and before the surgeons scrub. The 10 min required for scrubbing and prepping allows the distortion of the tissue to subside when hyaluronidase is used so that bunching of the skin and diagnosis of redundant skin can be made after anesthesia is obtained and after vasoconstriction

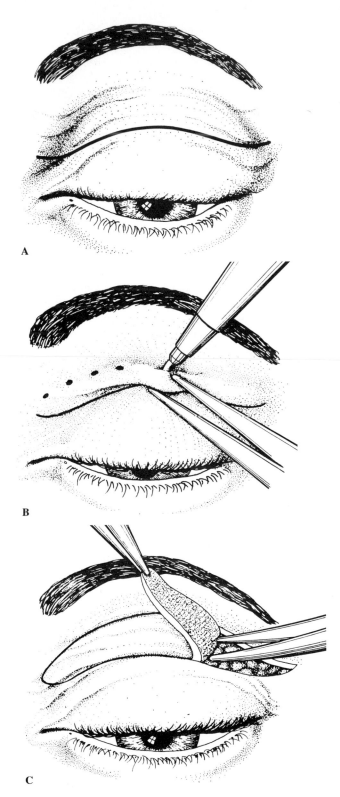

A

B

C

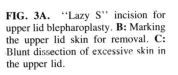

FIG. 3A. ''Lazy S'' incision for upper lid blepharoplasty. **B:** Marking the upper lid skin for removal. **C:** Blunt dissection of excessive skin in the upper lid.

has occurred. A #15 Bard-Parker blade is used to incise only the lid skin over the marks. A skin flap is started at the lateral area using sharp dissection with scissors so as not to damage the lateral points of the incision. After the dissection is started, blunt scissors are used to separate the skin from the underlying orbicularis muscle and the dissection is carried medially across the lid, where the medial point of skin is likewise sharply dissected (Fig. 3C). At this point the scrub nurse should be instructed to separate any excised skin and fat and place them on a small drawing of the lids in their approximate anatomic position. This allows quick estimation of the amount of tissue removed from each lid and prevents asymmetrical excision. Any bleeding points are sealed with gentle electrocautery. If the patient has a normal lid crease and no excess fat, the incision may be closed at this point. Manipulation of the skin at the time of excision will cause shifting of the skin edges, and they should be carefully aligned before insertion of any sutures. The wound is closed with interrupted 6–0 nylon sutures starting centrally to ensure symmetry and then closing the medial and then the lateral canthus. Some surgeons prefer a running subcuticular Prolene suture for this closure.

It is the exceptional blepharoplasty patient in whom skin excision alone will yield a satisfactory result. Most patients will also require an excision of orbital fat. Before closure of the skin incision, gentle pressure is placed on the globe, causing the fat to bulge forward beneath the orbital septum. The septum is grasped with forceps and opened with a scissors across the entire width of the protruding fat pockets. Opening the septum to this extent provides better visualization of the area and prevents injury either to the trochlea or to the levator aponeurosis during fat removal. The medial pocket is evacuated first and can be differentiated from the central pockets by the milky white appearance of the fat rather than the characteristic butter-yellow appearance encountered in the central pocket. The fat is enclosed in a capsule and subdivided by fibrous septa. Pressure on the globe facilitates protrusion of the entire fat capsule, but this structure must be opened to completely expose the orbital fat. After the fat is gently teased from its capsule, the base of the fat pedicle is clamped with a curved hemostat. The distal end of the pedicle is excised, and electrocautery is applied to the jaws of the clamp (Fig. 4). Hemostasis in this area must be meticulous because of the presence of large veins coursing into the bodies of the fat pockets. Before the clamp is released, the base of the fat pedicle is grasped with forceps, and after release of the clamp the stump is examined for any further bleeding sites before being allowed to retract back into the orbit. The fat in the central pocket is similarly excised and given to the scrub nurse for inclusion in the specimens. Care must be taken not to confuse the lacrimal gland and accidentally excise this structure or its ducts.

In many patients who have had long-standing prolapse of orbital fat, the orbital septum and overlying orbicularis muscle may be markedly thinned and atrophic. To eliminate bulging of these subcutaneous tissues during skin closure, a strip of thinned-out orbital septum and orbicularis is excised from the superior and inferior margins of the incision (Fig. 5). No deep sutures are used for closure of the orbital septum or muscular tissues before skin closure. This is contraindicated because it is unnecessary for good results and because poor closure of the septum can result in lagophthalmos or ptosis. Similar procedures are done in each lid, and before suturing the lid incision the excised specimens are examined to ensure that equal amounts of fat, skin, and orbital septum have been excised, unless the patient was asymmetric to begin with and required asymmetric tissue removal. The skin edges are then carefully approximated as previously described and the procedure is terminated. A small amount of antibiotic ointment is put into each eye and over each suture line, and the lids are covered with nonadherent dressings of Telfa and eye pads.

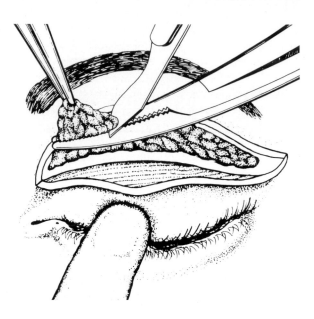

FIG. 4. Gentle pressure on the globe prolapses the fat that is excised after clamping it with the hemostat.

The dressings are not taped in place but are secured with iced saline sponges placed over the dressings before the patient leaves the operating room and are continued for at least the next 24 hr. The sutures are removed at 5 to 7 days and the postoperative swelling and discoloration are usually gone within 2 weeks.

Modifications to this basic blepharoplasty technique may be made to accommodate specific problems noted in the preoperative evaluation. Men normally have a lower lid crease than women and the inferior limb of the incision is placed at 8 mm in the midpupillary line rather than 10 mm. Higher incision will result in a higher lid crease and a "staring" expression postoperatively.

If the patient has a diagnosed preexisting ptosis and one wishes to combine a minimal ptosis procedure with the blepharoplasty, aponeurotic surgery can be performed during the blepharoplasty procedure. After the orbital fat is removed from the preaponeurotic space, the aponeurosis is readily identified. Dissection through the orbital septum into the pretarsal area, exposing the bare tarsal plate, can be carried out. At this point, the aponeurotic

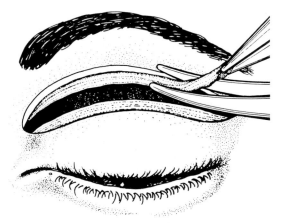

FIG. 5. Redundant, atonic orbicularis muscle and orbital septum are excised when necessary.

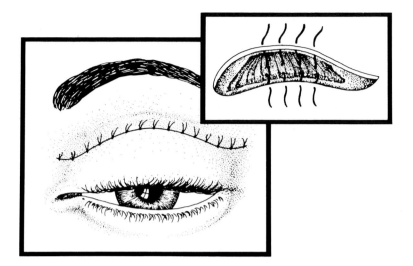

FIG. 6. Sutures from skin to levator aponeurosis to skin for creation of high lid crease. Interrupted 6-0 nylon sutures are used for skin closure.

repair can be performed in the manner described in Chapter 13. After the ptosis has been corrected, the exposure of the aponeurosis facilitates formation of the lid crease by attachment of the aponeurosis to the skin. Lid crease formation is accomplished during the skin closure by passing the skin sutures under the upper wound edge, then through the aponeurosis above the superior border of the tarsus and then out the lower skin edge. Closing the wound thereby attaches the aponeurosis to the skin, creating a new lid crease (Fig. 6).

After excision of all excess upper lid skin, the patient may still have a large amount of heavy "subbrow tissue" that may be corrected with another modification. This modification requires no change in the location of the upper lid incisions but rather additional dissection beneath the superior margin of the upper skin incision. The heavy tissue immediately beneath the brow (usually redundant orbicularis oculi) is excised with heavy scissors and each specimen is removed and labeled as before. After equal amounts of "subbrow tissue" are removed, closure of the skin defect is accomplished in the usual manner.

If lid crease formation is required (with or without a simultaneous ptosis procedure), this is also accomplished after visualization of the levator aponeurosis. Exposure of the levator aponeurosis is accomplished as previously described by removal of a strip of redundant preseptal orbicularis muscle and orbital septum immediately above the tarsal plate area. With this step, the central sutures of 6–0 nylon engage a 1-mm horizontal bite of the levator aponeurosis 1 mm above the superior border of the tarsus. The skin edges only are included in this closure to form a good lid crease (see Fig. 6). Five or six such sutures are placed centrally and the remaining skin defect is closed with additional 6–0 nylon sutures. All sutures are removed 5 to 7 days postoperatively.

Excessive excision of both skin and fat in the medial canthal area (Fig. 7) will result in stretch on the medial line of the incision and the resulting pulling force will be transmitted in the form of a medial canthal web extending past the medial canthal tendon into the lower lid. If a tendency toward this web was noted preoperatively, gentle traction is put on the skin superiorly and temporally to exaggerate this line of stress and the lines of incision are drawn to include an equal amount of skin on either side of this web but not extending further than 4 mm superior to the lateral punctum. If there is a large amount of

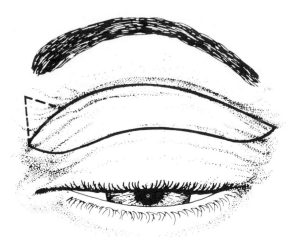

FIG. 7. Extra tissue may be removed in the medial canthus. *Dotted line* marks area for removal of excess skin.

protuberant medial fat, less skin excision is required since the skin edges will fall into the concavity produced by excision of the orbital fat.

Regardless of the modification used, no heavy postoperative dressings are utilized. A thin layer of antibiotic ointment and nonadherent dressing provide protection for the incision and skin while allowing the use of ice packs postoperatively. The patient is sent from the operating room with ice packs in place to eliminate the occasional 2- to 3-hr lag time between the termination of the procedure and the initiation of ice packs on the floor. Iced saline sponges placed in a basin beside the patient's bed are the most comfortable and least bulky and can be renewed by the patient. The ice packs are continued for at least 24 hr, but 48 hr is preferable. Postoperative swelling and discoloration may increase slightly on the second postoperative day as the patient starts to return to his or her normal activities and assumes an erect posture. This is usually not caused by fresh bleeding but rather by forward movement of any extravasated blood that has sunk posteriorly into the orbit at the time of surgery. The patient is instructed to keep the sutures clean with hot tap water and cotton balls. No makeup is used for at least 2 weeks. After suture removal at 5 to 7 days, the lateral edges of the incision are reinforced with Steri-Strips for 1 week. Follow-up examination is scheduled for 1 month and 3 months postoperatively, at which time follow-up photographs are taken for the patient's record.

LOWER LID BLEPHAROPLASTY[1]

Lower lid blepharoplasty, like that in the upper lid, requires excision of excess skin and orbital fat. Lower lid blepharoplasty technique is geared to the prevention of ectropion or lower lid retraction (see Fig. 8 for the steps in lower lid blepharoplasty).

A skin muscle flap is preferred because of its avascular plane. . . . The lower lid is infiltrated with 1:200,000 red label Xylocaine and Wydase and the protective contact lens inserted. It is very helpful to have a 4–0 silk traction suture in the lower lid margin [Fig. 8A]. With the skin under horizontal stretch by the assistant, an incision is made through the skin as high as possible just underneath the cilia in the lower lid. . . . The incision must be carried out in this level to

---

[1] Extracted portions of this section are reprinted with permission from McCord, C. D., Jr. (1985): Surgery of the eyelids. In: Clinical Ophthalmology, edited by T. D. Duane and E. A. Jaeger. Harper & Row, Philadelphia.

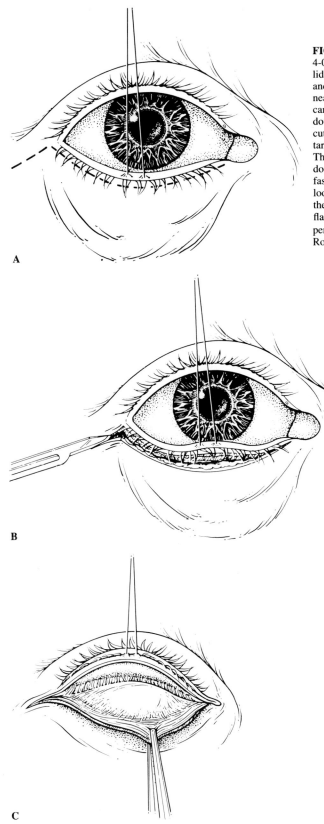

FIG. 8. Lower lid blepharoplasty. **A:** A 4-0 silk traction suture is inserted in the lower lid margin and an incision through the skin and muscle is made as high as possible underneath the lashes carrying the line to the exact canthal angle, and then a dog leg is made downward in a wrinkle line. **B:** The musculo-cutaneous flap is elevated from the anterior tarsal surface and at the canthal angle. **C:** The musculocutaneous flap is dissected downward, exposing the capsulopalepebral fascia, and the orbital septum is seen to balloon forward with pressure on the globe on the inner surface of the musculocutaneous flap. (From McCord and Shore, ref. 8, with permission. © 1983, Lippincott/Harper & Row.)

A

B

C

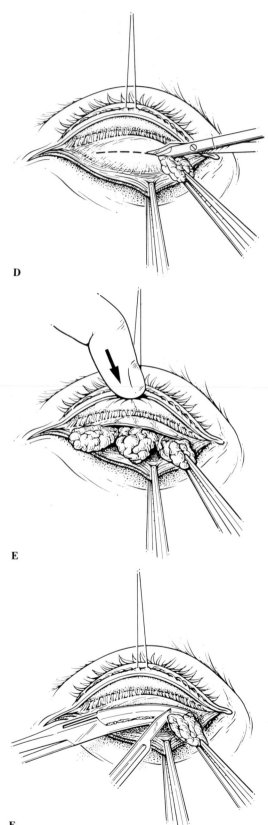

D

E

F

FIG. 8 (*cont.*) **D:** The orbital septum is penetrated with a sharp scissors throughout its entire width. **E:** With pressure on the globe, the three orbital fat pads in the lower lid can be teased forward using traction and dissection with a cotton applicator stick. **F:** The fat pad in the lower lid is clamped with the hemostat and excised. (From McCord and Shore, ref. 8, with permission. © 1983, Lippincott/Harper & Row.)

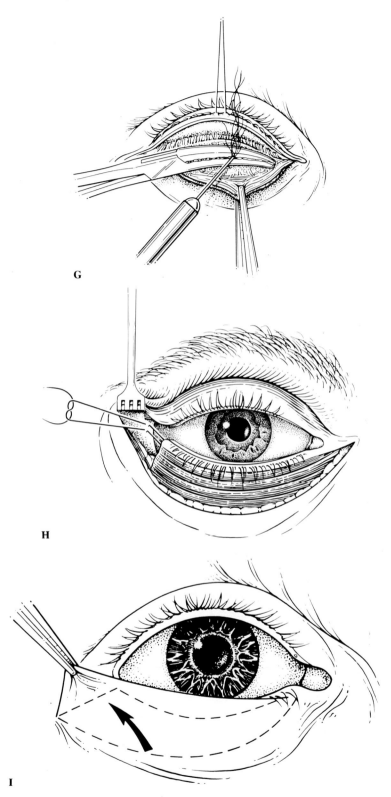

G

H

I

FIG. 8 *(cont.)* **G:** The stump or pedicle of the fatty pad is cauterized with the Bovie before allowing it to retract into the orbit. **H:** After the lower lid is detached from the rim a full-thickness resection of the temporal portion of the eyelid is performed to produce the desired tightening of the lid and a double-armed 4-0 Prolene suture on a half-circle needle is introduced into the edge of the tarsal plate and then introduced inside the periosteal edge of the lateral rim at about the midpupillary level. **I:** Following horizontal tightening, the musculocutaneous flap is then elevated in a rotational manner toward the upper tip of the ear. (From McCord and Shore, ref. 8, with permission. © 1983, Lippincott/Harper & Row.)

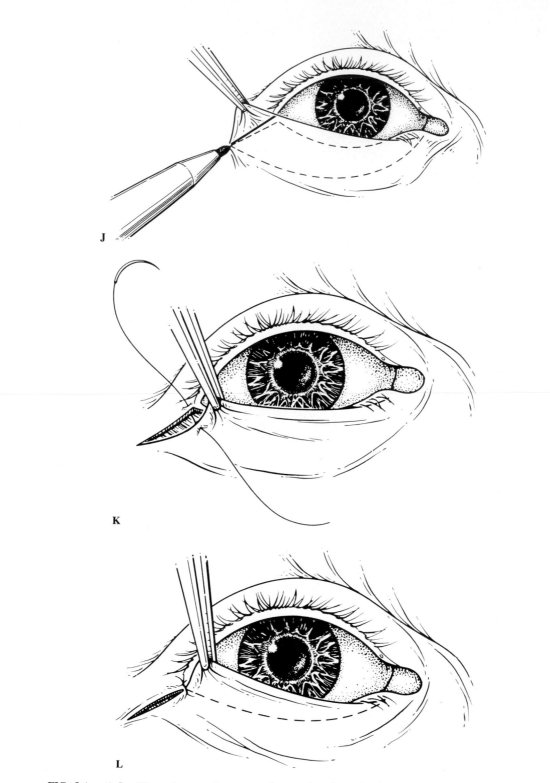

FIG. 8 (*cont.*) J: Where the musculocutaneous flap overlaps the underlying cut edge, methylene blue is used to mark out a triangular excision. **K:** The edge of the musculocutaneous flap is then reapproximated with a 4-0 silk suture and is introduced through the flap in a position to assure an equal-sided wound edge laterally. It is then introduced into the periosteum at about the level that the tightening sutures were introduced, and then brought out through the superior musculocutaneous edge and tied. **L:** The 4-0 silk musculocutaneous flap–fixing suture tied, producing a second triangle of skin and muscle to be excised underneath the lash line margin. (From McCord and Shore, ref. 8, with permission. © 1983, Lippincott/Harper & Row.)

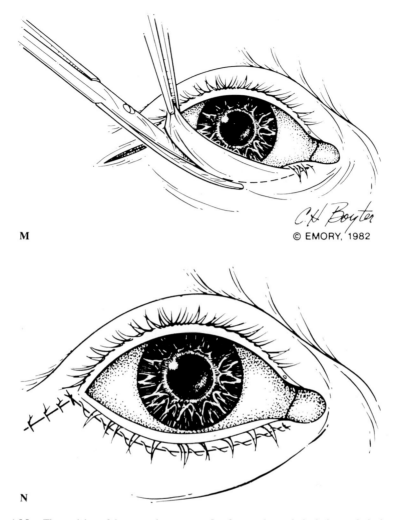

C.H. Boyter

© EMORY, 1982

M

N

FIG. 8 (*cont.*) M: The excision of the musculocutaneous flap from underneath the lash margin is then performed. Conservatism is observed. The skin overlaps the cut edge under gentle traction. **N:** Final closure is obtained with a running suture of 7-0 silk with interrupted sutures temporally. (From McCord and Shore, ref. 8, with permission. © 1983, Lippincott/Harper & Row.)

the exact angle of the lateral canthus. At this point there is a "dog leg" downward, angulating approximately 45° from the horizontal [Fig. 8B]. Through lateral incision the skin muscle is incised and undermined in the submuscular plane anterior to the capsulopalpebral fascia across the lid and anterior surface of the tarsal plate. Once this has been performed, the second incision is made through the muscle fibers at the same level as the subciliary skin excision. With countertraction on the lower lid margin, the skin muscle flap is dissected downward. Hemostasis in several areas must be obtained before exposing the orbital septum and its bulge of fatty pads [Figs. 8C, 8D, and 8E]. Scissors are used to incise the septum throughout its entirety, allowing the fat to prolapse as pressure on the globe is applied. The fat generally presents in three prominent areas in the lower lid: the nasal fat, which is whitish; the middle fat pad, which is more yellowish; and a temporal fat pad. Controversy exists as to the exact number of fatty pads anatomically present in the lower lid because of their interconnections; however, the three areas described above are the usual clinical presentation of the fatty tissue. The fat pads can be made to prolapse further by additional pressure on the globe, mild retraction with forceps, and dissection with a cotton applicator stick. The white nasal fat pocket contains very large veins that are readily visible; it also requires some incision into capsules to allow the fat to prolapse as in the upper lid. The pocket should be clamped with the hemostat before excision, and cautery with the bovie should be performed before allowing the fat to release [Figs. 8F and 8G]. It is important to have photographs of the patient available during surgery to remind the surgeon which fatty pads need to be removed. As the fatty pads are removed, they should be kept on separate 4″ × 4″ gauze pads by the circulating nurse to ensure the symmetry of fat removal on both sides. . . . Following the removal of the fat pads after adequate hemostasis is obtained, sharp scissors are then used to perform a canthotomy and lysis of the lower limb of the canthal tendon at the canthal angle. It is important to detach the lower limb of the canthal tendon and other attachments so that the lower lid swings freely from the canthus. An adequate full-thickness resection of the lower lid can be carried out at this point. . . . After full-thickness lid resection is carried out at the temporal portion of the lid so that stretching the lid temporally produces the desired amount of tension, a double-armed nonabsorbable suture with a half circle needle is introduced at the edge of the tarsal plate. These half circle needles are useful in that one can reach around to the inside rim of the periosteum of the lateral orbital wall easily. The sutures are then placed in the periosteum inside the orbital rim at the mid pupillary level. The upper reflection of the canthal tendon and, perhaps, the lacrimal gland will be encountered when the upper margin is retracted. The sutures are then tied permanently.

Many patients, particularly younger ones, do not require any tarsal resection to ensure against postoperative lower lid malposition. In most patients, however, a plication of the lateral canthal tendon is performed by cantholysis, surgical freshening of the lateral edge of tarsus, and refixation to the lateral orbital rim with a nonabsorbable suture (Fig. 8H). Following the horizontal tightening and removal of fat,

the skin muscle flap is stretched. It is important not to stretch the skin muscle flap straight vertically . . . because it will result in a more vertical skin removal than necessary and result in lower lid retraction or ectropion. It is important not to stretch the flap directly horizontally because that will cause horizontal tension to produce a "clothesline" effect on the lower lid. The proper direction to stretch the skin muscle flap is toward the tip of the upper ear so that it is a rotational flap. Since the corner of the flap overlaps the "dog leg" skin incision, one may outline a triangle of skin to be excised [Figs. 8I and 8J]. After this first triangle of skin muscle is excised, the flap edge is attached to the superior skin edge, at the canthus, first taking a bite of periosteum at the lateral orbital rim [Figs. 8K and 8L]. When this suture is properly placed, it attaches the skin muscle flap to the orbital rim, preventing ectropion. It also closes the incision with equal-sided edges, preventing dog ear formation. The next triangle of skin to be removed is more critical because it is primarily a vertical excision. If the flap is simply draped over the lower lid margin so that it is not under severe tension, a thin triangle of skin and muscle from the subciliary area is incised [Fig. 8M]. If the patient is awake, it is sometimes beneficial to have [the patient] look up, thus allowing [the] lower lid to rise, and the amount that just gently drapes over the wound can be determined. It is wise to excise a portion of this flap in a piecemeal manner to avoid too aggressive an excision. One final step is very important: a strip of orbicularis fibers must be removed from the subciliary horizontal portion of the flap to prevent a ridge of orbicularis underneath the lashes. Patients who suffer from orbicularis hypertrophy can obtain correction by this manner. Edges underneath the lashes and lateral to this point should be fairly well approximated, and a simple closure with running sutures can be accomplished. Multiple interrupted sutures can be used [Fig. 8N].

Modifications of this lower lid technique may be useful in other patients. The amount of lateral extension of the incision beyond the lateral orbital rim is directly proportional to the amount of excessive skin to be removed. With only fat removal, no lateral extension is made. However, when a large amount of skin must be removed, an 8- to 10-mm extension beyond the lateral rim will be necessary. Patients who have extreme redundancy of skin in the malar area ("bag on bag" phenomenon or so-called "malar festoons") will require an extended lateral incision for adequate correction, and must be informed of this modification before surgery because a slightly more conspicuous postoperative scar line will result.

Certain younger patients requesting blepharoplasty have only protuberant fat in the lower lids, usually on a familial basis. In these patients, the evacuation of fat is all that is required, with minimal or no excision of skin. In these patients the skin edge must be handled very carefully during dissection of orbital fat, since almost no skin will be excised and the margins must not be macerated.

It is possible to expose the fatty pads in these patients through a skin muscle flap; however, one must recognize the risk of some contracture of the flap after elevation even though no skin or skin and muscle is excised. Fornix removal of fat in these patients would seem to be the safest way to avoid complications of lower lid malposition.

Technique of Fornix Fat Removal or "Behind the Lid Blepharoplasty"[2]

Infiltration of the lower fornix with red label Xylocaine with 1 cc of Wydase added is performed. It is very important to insert a protective haptic contact lens to prevent corneal injury. The lower lid is then everted with small rake retractors and pressure applied [to the contact lens, causing the fatty pads to bulge in the fornix]. The use of the needle electrode on the bovie unit set to a blend between cutting and coagulation is used to penetrate through the conjunctiva and capsulopalpebral fascia underneath the tarsal plate. This technique is used because of the extreme vascularity of the capsulopalpebral fascia and allows a practically bloodless exposure of the fatty pads in the lower lid. The first fat pad that is exposed is the central fat pad, however, the incision can be extended nasally and until the nasal fatty pad can be identified. . . . The fat pads are then teased into the incision with gentle traction with forceps and dissection with a cotton applicator stick. It should be noted that there are very large blood vessels within the fat pads themselves and even though the capsule is opened they are a source of major bleeding if they are not gently handled. These vessels are noted to be even further engorged in patients who have had thyroid disease. The fatty pads are then clamped, excised, and cauterized. . . . The temporal fatty pad may not be readily seen with downward traction so for adequate exposure the rake retractor must be inserted inside the cut edge of the capsulopalpebral fascia in the lid retracted temporally exposing the temporal pad. One may perform a canthotomy at this point for better exposure if necessary. In most cases this is not needed. After the fatty pads have been excised and any needed hemostasis obtained, closure is accomplished with a running 5–0 [Prolene] suture which is introduced on the external surface of the lid and closes the conjunctiva and capsulopalpebral fascia internally and then is brought out externally and looped for fixation.

COMPLICATIONS OF BLEPHAROPLASTY AND BROW LIFT

Even the most careful lid procedures will have a certain percentage of complications (11,12). The possibility of complications should always be discussed with the patient prior to surgery in an attempt to establish a rapport with the patient. If the patient does not feel that the surgery is worth even the remote possibility of a complication, then he or she feels that the defect is not severe enough to warrant surgery. Discussion of possible complications preoperatively also has the advantage of eliminating many postoperative complaints arising from an unrealistic expectation of the result of the proposed surgery. This is especially true of operations performed strictly for cosmetic reasons (13).

---

[2] Extracted portions of this section are reprinted from ref. 8 with permission © 1983, American Academy of Ophthalmology.

each case the upper lid will appear to have a redundancy of skin that is more apparent than real, and excision of additional skin should take place only after determination of the proper site of the lid crease. If the low lid crease is the result of failure to re-create the attachments of the aponeurosis into the skin, an incision is made at the new site of the lid crease and the levator aponeurosis identified. Very little additional skin excision is required, and the central sutures are used to attach the skin edges to the fibers of the aponeurosis as previously described. In the case of the double lid crease, the apparent redundancy may be excised; the incision is made at the site of the new lid crease with dissection carried beneath the skin to elevate the previously formed scar. Again the lid crease is re-created by attachment of the skin edges to the terminal fibers of the levator aponeurosis.

Frank eversion of the upper lid may result from procedures designed to reform the lid crease. The eversion is usually secondary to attachment of the skin and orbicularis muscle too high on the levator aponeurosis, resulting in stretch on the anterior lamella of the lid. The eversion generally resolves with massage of the lid during maturation of the scar. If this is unsuccessful, the eyelid must be opened over the previous incision, and the abnormal attachments to the levator aponeurosis divided and reattached closer to the margin of the lid.

The most common cause of postoperative ptosis following blepharoplasty is probably unrecognized preoperative ptosis. Postoperative ptosis, however, may also be the result of an injury to the levator aponeurosis during blepharoplasty. The ptosis may result from placement of the sutures too high in the levator aponeurosis, and this type of ptosis usually resolves with removal of the sutures and "tincture of time." As in extraocular muscle palsies, as long as continued improvement is demonstrated, surgical intervention should be deferred. If the ptosis does not respond within 4 to 6 months, surgical exploration is required. In this instance, dehiscence of the levator aponeurosis is a common defect encountered. We have also found traumatized and excised aponeurosis. Repair is facilitated by the use of a local anesthetic and asking the patient to open and close the eyes to further define the area of aponeurosis damage. The edge of the aponeurosis is secured to the superior border of the tarsus or the distal torn segment with 6–0 silk sutures. Repair should be accomplished with approximately 1 mm of overcorrection since the lid will drop slightly postoperatively.

Webbing or pseudoepicanthal folds may result in the medial canthus and are from the excision of too much skin medially or from placement of the incision too far medially and/or too close to the lid margin. Correction is accomplished by using a V-Y-plasty under local anesthetic. The apex of the fold is defined and the skin on either side of the fold is incised with a razor knife with the apex of the V placed inferiorly. The base of the V is extended to the most superior portion of the web over the medial canthal tendon. The skin is dissected from the underlying orbicularis muscle and gently replaced to eliminate the line of tension. At this point, the V of the incision becomes a small Y and the skin edges are approximated with interrupted 6–0 silk sutures. Additional fixation can be carried out by suturing the orbicularis muscle to the medial canthal tendon. Sometimes the use of single or multiple Z-plasties will correct or aid the V-Y correction of this problem.

Complications Involving the Lower Lid

The most frequent complications in the lower lid are increased scleral show and ectropion. Their etiology is similar: excessive excision of skin, increased horizontal lid length, lax lateral canthal tendons, and/or inflammation of the fat pockets in the lid. In patients with mild scleral show without symptoms, treatment is not necessary and the condition will slowly resolve with continued contraction of the orbicularis muscle during blinking. However, patients with a poor precorneal tear film and corneal dehydration become quickly symptomatic with even mild scleral show.

If postoperative lower lid malposition with either ectropion or scleral show does not resolve following the subsiding of edema and the use of massage, tightening of the lower lid must be performed in those cases. The horizontal tightening is best performed at the lateral canthal area, and the method is described in detail in Chapter 12. Postoperative lower lid malposition is certainly a common possibility in any patient with laxity of the lower lid, and this problem is perhaps best avoided by incorporating a tendon tightening with each lower lid blepharoplasty as previously described.

Some patients with postoperative lower lid malposition have a shortage of skin that cannot be overcome by horizontal tightening procedures. A full-thickness skin graft can be used in these patients, but the use of autogenous ear cartilage placed in the posterior lamella of the lid combined with the horizontal tightening procedure can effectively restore lid position. This technique is identical to that used in the treatment of lower lid retraction in Graves' disease, and is described in detail in Chapter 8. The use of ear cartilage in most cases is more cosmetically acceptable in these patients, since the use of full-thickness skin grafts with visible host-graft interfaces is avoided.

A full-thickness skin graft is needed many times in the more severe cases of postoperative lower lid malposition and, if attention to meticulous surgical technique is used (see Chapter 12), the result can be very acceptable cosmetically.

Inflammation of the lower fat pockets as a result of surgery can cause an ectropion from contraction of the anterior lamella and skin of the lower lid. This ectropion is usually not present postoperatively but occurs approximately 2 to 4 days after the surgery and presents as a firm inflammatory mass on palpation of the fat pockets. Treatment consists of taping the lower lid superiorly or securing it with a mattress suture to the brow until the inflammation subsides. Resolution may be accelerated by the injection of 40 mg of triamcinolone into the inflamed fat pockets.

Since the incision for lower lid blepharoplasty is so close to the lash margin, damage to the punctum or canaliculus may occur. Any laceration of the canaliculus or medial canthal tendon should be repaired primarily at the time of surgery to ensure adequate tear drainage. Punctal ectropion is corrected with the application of cautery to the conjunctival surface immediately beneath the punctum, which will result in reapposition of the punctum as healing and contraction progresses. Alternately, a small ellipse of conjunctiva may be removed beneath the punctum and sutured primarily with interrupted sutures of 6–0 chromic to effect immediate inversion of the punctum.

In conclusion, the best method of handling complications of blepharoplasty is to avoid them. Allow plenty of time for surgery, have good lighting, good hemostasis, good instruments, and good nursing help, and all should go well (16,17).

REFERENCES

1. Beyer, C. K. (1978): Symposium: Blepharoplasty procedures. *Trans. Am. Acad. Ophthalmol.*, 85:702.
2. Adler, J., Raine, G., McCormick, J., et al. (1985): New bodies for sale. *Newsweek,* May 27, pp. 64–69.
3. Weinstein, G. W. (1975): Who should perform cosmetic blepharoplasty? *Ophthalmic Surg.*, 6:11.
4. Collin, J. R., Beard, C., Stern, W. H., and Schoengarth, D. (1979): Blepharochalasis. *Br. J. Ophthalmol.*, 63:542–546.

5. Custer, P. L., Tenzel, R. R., and Kowalczyk, A. P. (1985): Blepharochalasis syndrome. *Am. J. Ophthalmol.*, 99:424–428.
6. Wilkins, R. B. (1978): Evaluation of the blepharoplasty patient. *Trans. Am. Acad. Ophthalmol.*, 85:703.
7. Lemke, B. N., and Strasior, O. G. (1982): The anatomy of eyebrow ptosis. *Arch. Ophthalmol.*, 100:981–986.
8. McCord, C. D., and Shore, J. W. (1983): Avoidance of complications in lower lid blepharoplasty. *Ophthalmology*, 90:1039–1046.
9. Brennan, H. G. (1980): Correction of the ptotic brow. *Otolaryngol. Clin. North Am.*, 13:265–273.
10. Smith, B., and Petrelli, R. (1978): Surgical repair of prolapsed lacrimal glands. *Arch. Ophthalmol.*, 96:113–114.
11. Levine, M., Boyton, J., Tenzel, R. R., and Miller, G. R. (1975): Complications of blepharoplasty. *Ophthalmic Surg.*, 6:53–57.
12. Rafaty, F. M. (1983): Complications of cosmetic blepharoplasty. *Cosmetic Surg.*, 2:17–29.
13. Tenzel, R. P. (1978): Surgical treatment of complications of cosmetic blepharoplasty. *Clin. Plast. Surg.*, 5:517–523.
14. Waller, R. R. (1978): Is blindness a realistic complication in blepharoplasty procedures? *Trans. Am. Acad. Ophthalmol.*, 85:730–735.
15. Lloyd, W. C., and Leone, C. R. (1985): Transient bilateral blindness following blepharoplasty. *Ophthalmic Plast. Reconstr. Surg.*, 1:29–34.
16. Tenzel, R. R. (1978): Cosmetic blepharoplasty. *Int. Ophthalmol. Clin.*, 18:87–99.
17. McCord, C. D. (1979): Techniques in blepharoplasty. *Ophthalmic Surg.*, 10:40–55.

Oculoplastic Surgery, 2nd edition, edited by
Clinton D. McCord, Jr., and Myron Tanenbaum.
Raven Press, New York © 1987.

Chapter 18

Essential Blepharospasm

John W. Shore

Department of Ophthalmology, Wilford Hall USAF Medical Center, San Antonio, Texas 78236

Essential blepharospasm is a visually disabling neuroophthalmic disorder characterized by involuntary contractions of the protractor muscles of the eyelids (orbicularis oculi) and the facial muscles in the nasoglabellar area (procerus and corrugator supercilii). The forceful contractions of these eyelids and eyebrow muscles are involuntary and cause functional blindness in affected patients since they cannot open their eyes during periods of muscle spasm. Henderson (1) was the first to emphasize the ophthalmic manifestations of the disease. Subsequent studies have confirmed the natural history and clinical features of the disorder he described so well.

Women are more commonly affected than men at a ratio of 3:1. Symptoms usually begin in the fifth decade of life. The onset of the disease is insidious. Symptoms usually precede clinical signs and many times the diagnosis is not made for 5 or 10 years. A few patients experience an abrupt onset of symptoms with no antecedent signs of the disease, but this is unusual. Frequently patients give a history of having had multiple examinations by a variety of specialists before a correct diagnosis was made.

An increase in the blink rate is one of the first things that patients notice, but they soon begin to complain of asthenopic symptoms such as photophobia, tearing, ocular irritation, and retroorbital discomfort. Eventually the blinks become more forceful and periods of involuntary spasm appear. Gradually eyelid closure cannot be controlled and the patients are unable to keep their eyes open during periods of forceful spasm (Fig. 1). At this stage, patients notice that it is necessary for them to pry their eyelids open in order to see.

The frequency of blinking and the force of muscle spasm is unpredictable and extremely variable. On the worst days, patients are totally incapacitated by the severe spasms and, for all practical purposes, are functionally blind. At other times, spasms may not be evident and the patient is symptom free. This leads to confusion in diagnosis because some patients do not manifest the characteristic muscle spasms during office visits. The history usually

---

The views herein are those of the author and do not necessarily reflect the views of the United States Air Force or the Department of Defense.

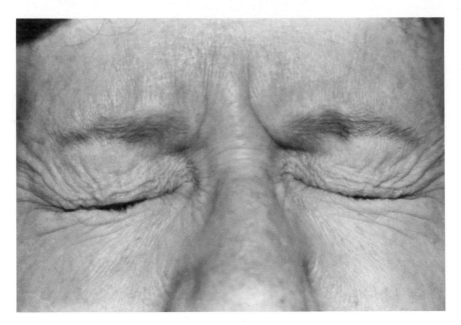

FIG. 1. A 56-year-old female with essential blepharospasm. The characteristic involuntary spasms of the eyelid and eyebrow protractors are clearly evident here. Additionally, the patient has eyebrow ptosis, glabellar furrowing, and dermatochalasis. These anatomic problems are easily managed with the coronal myectomy procedure.

leads one to the diagnosis, however, and even on the best days, and during quiescent periods, one can observe the increased blink rate typically seen in blepharospasm patients. It is interesting that patients do not manifest spasms during periods of sleep or while under anesthesia.

As the disease progresses, spasms may become so severe that patients stop driving, quit their jobs, and withdraw to the confines of their homes, avoiding social contacts and public appearances. At this stage, the diagnosis is not difficult. The patients are agitated, depressed, bewildered, bitter, and anxious for any treatment. These personality changes have been interpreted by some as evidence of a psychological cause for blepharospasm. However, multiple scientific studies have failed to reveal such a cause in the majority of patients, and it is incorrect to consider blepharospasm as a psychiatric disease and deny patients beneficial medical or surgical treatment. It is true that many blepharospasm patients suffer psychological impairment, but it is likely that these psychological disturbances are the result of, not the cause of, blepharospasm.

Some patients with blepharospasm develop other dystonic movements in the head and neck area involving the facial, cervical, pharyngeal, oral, masticatory, labial, and laryngeal muscles. Blepharospasm associated with these movement disorders is termed "Meige's syndrome" or, more properly, "idiopathic craniocervical dystonia." This condition, which has also been termed "blepharospasm plus," will not be discussed in detail in this chapter on surgical management of blepharospasm.

DIFFERENTIAL DIAGNOSIS

As previously mentioned, essential blepharospasm is differentiated from the related condition, idiopathic craniocervical dystonia, by the areas of anatomic involvement. Essential blepharospasm refers to blepharospasm restricted to the eyelids and eyebrows with no facial, oral, or cervical involvement. This isolated condition is rare because the majority of patients with blepharospasm go on to develop idiopathic craniocervical dystonia with involvement of the muscle groups in the head and neck. These patients are more difficult to treat than patients with isolated essential blepharospasm.

The differential diagnosis of blepharospasm is lengthy and includes the following categories of diseases and disorders: reflex blepharospasm associated with intrinsic ocular disease; tardive dystonia; neurodegenerative disorders such as Parkinson's disease, Huntington's disease, Wilson's disease and others; certain seizure disorders; rare movement disorders such as Gilles de la Tourette's syndrome; hemifacial spasm; synkinetic facial spasm following Bell's palsy; facial myokymia; and psychogenic or hysterical blepharospasm (2,3). Detailed explanations of these conditions are available and should be reviewed by those treating blepharospasm patients.

PATHOGENESIS

The pathogenesis of essential blepharospasm is not known. To date it has not been possible to localize a neuroanatomical lesion, but clinical evidence suggests that the basal ganglia are involved. Abnormal blink rates and blepharospasm can be observed in other conditions affecting the basal ganglia. Other possible areas of CNS involvement include diencephalic/mesencephalic dysfunction, the cerebellum, the caudate, and the putamen. Neuroradiologic studies have failed to identify specific lesions in the CNS. For the moment, the pathophysiology and pathogenesis of this condition remain a mystery. Therefore, it has not been possible to develop a "cure" for the disease. Instead, treatment is aimed at alleviating symptoms and restoring functional vision for affected patients.

WORK-UP

The work-up begins with a careful history and a complete ophthalmologic and neuro-ophthalmologic examination. A medication history is particularly important since dopaminergic and antidopaminergic drugs, as well as antipsychotic medications, can cause tardive dystonia, a movement disorder with clinical features indistinguishable from idiopathic craniocervical dystonia (3). The examiner must exclude intrinsic ocular disease and associated reflex blepharospasm as a cause. Keratoconjunctivitis sicca is commonly seen in blepharospasm patients and should be treated before and after surgery. Additionally, it is important to look for bilateral involvement because hemifacial spasm, a unilateral disorder that mimics blepharospasm, has a different cause and can be treated by microsurgical decompression of the facial nerve in the posterior fossa. Patients with essential blepharospasm can have asymmetric involvement and appear to have unilateral disease, but this is unusual. Hemifacial spasm respects the midline and appears clinically like a peripheral neuropathy, which it is.

During the clinical examination it is important to carefully observe the periocular facial movements. Apraxia of eyelid opening and spasms of the frontalis muscle that *raise* the eyebrows during periods of spasm are not characteristic features of blepharospasm, and when seen should caution the examiner to consider another diagnosis. Similarly, a history of a sudden onset of blepharospasm in a patient under 30 years of age suggests the diagnosis of psychogenic blepharospasm. These patients look exactly like typical blepharospasm patients but have a psychological basis for their disease and may respond to psychotherapy, biofeedback, or behavioral therapy. Such patients can spontaneously revert to normal, and aggressive surgical intervention is not indicated.

It is worthwhile asking patients what "tricks" they use to alleviate spasms. Patients can usually perform certain maneuvers such as applying pressure to the temples, thrusting the jaw, or tapping the forehead to reduce the severity of spasms and to get the eyelids open. This characteristic feature of blepharospasm, when present, is helpful in making the diagnosis.

Essential blepharospasm is a clinical diagnosis made by taking a good history, observing the characteristic clinical signs, and excluding other causes of blepharospasm. Neurologic and neuroophthalmologic consultations are helpful and a computed tomography (CT) scan of the brain and posterior fossa is useful in excluding unexpected organic lesions. This is particularly true for patients with hemifacial spasm where a dolechoectatic basilar artery irritating the underlying facial nerve in the posterior fossa can be observed. Other invasive neuroradiologic and laboratory tests are rarely helpful and generally not indicated.

MEDICAL THERAPY

Since the pathogenesis of essential blepharospasm has not been established, specific curative treatment is not available. A host of medical regimens and a variety of neurotropic drugs have been tested to date, but no medical treatment has been shown to have long-term therapeutic efficacy in a substantial number of patients. Some drugs have been effective for a few patients with certain types of blepharospasm and, even though medical therapy has not been effective in the majority of patients, an occasional patient does respond, so it is reasonable to try a variety of medications in the hope of finding one that will work in an individual case. This concept is particularly important in patients with craniocervical dystonia because surgical therapy aimed at restoring functional vision is not always effective in reducing the facial and cervical muscle spasms outside the periorbital area.

The opthalmologist can conduct a short trial of oral medications in selected patients, but prolonged therapy is best managed by neurologists or neuroophthalmologists with experience managing patients on potent neuropharmacologic agents.

Clonazepam, baclofen, trihexyphenidyl, lithium, and tetrabenazine are the agents most commonly used (2). Patients demonstrating a good therapeutic response should be continued on therapy indefinitely; however, in the author's experience, medical therapy loses effectiveness with time and most patients are dissatisfied with their clinical response or drug side effects and discontinue medical therapy on their own.

Other forms of medical therapy excluding drugs have been used with limited success, including hypnosis, biofeedback, behavior modification, and acupuncture. Although these forms of therapy work for an occasional patient, the general experience has been that they have no permanent or long-term effect and are of marginal usefulness. These treatment modalities are best reserved for patients with psychogenic or hysterical blepharospasm and for patients with essential blepharospasm and related secondary or unrelated psychologic disturbances.

Botulinum Toxin

Patients with essential blepharospasm, hemifacial spasm, and blepharospasm associated with idiopathic craniocervical dystonia are excellent candidates for chemodenervation of the eyelid and eyebrow protractor muscles with botulinum toxin (4).

Botulinum A toxin is one of six antigenically distinct neurotoxins produced by the bacteria *Clostridium botulinum.* The exotoxin selectively binds motor end-plates of skeletal muscle and inhibits transmission at the neuromuscular junction. Only minute quantities of toxin are required to give a profound weakening effect. Unfortunately this effect wears off over a period of weeks or months. Thus, patients require reinjections at intervals ranging from 4 weeks to 3 months or more. Nevertheless, this treatment is effective in the short term and many patients have been totally controlled with periodic injections.

The procedure for obtaining, storing, mixing, and administering the toxin are beyond the scope of this chapter, but are available in the literature. In the author's experience, it is best to start with a standard injection of 2.5 units of botulinum toxin (1 ng) in 0.1 ml of diluent (normal saline) administered in five separate injections on each side. Using a 30-gauge needle on a tuberculin syringe, the solution is injected subcutaneously into the affected muscles. The four eyelid sites to be injected are the orbicularis muscle medially and laterally, 2 mm above the lash line in the upper eyelid, and 1 mm below the lash line in the lower eyelid. Injection in the central portion of the upper eyelid should be avoided because the toxin can infiltrate and paralyze the levator palpebrae superiorus muscle, leading to a neuromuscular blepharoptosis. A fifth injection is placed into the corrugator/procerus complex in the nasoglabellar region. Following injection, patients are observed and the clinical response is assessed. In this author's experience, subsequent injections should be tailored to the individual patient. It is important to judge the degree of spasms and the anatomic extent of residual or recurrent clinical involvement. These areas should receive repeat injections while uninvolved areas are spared. Standard treatment regimens have been used by others, but in this author's experience the treatment is more effective if individualized on a case-by-case basis. This principal is very important in patients who have had previous myectomy or neuroectomy, because standard doses of botulinum toxin have a polonged effect in these patients and must be used cautiously.

Side effects of treatment include too much weakening of the eyelid protractors, leading to exposure symptoms; blepharoptosis; eyebrow ptosis, if the frontalis muscle is injected; diplopia, if one or more of the extraocular muscles is affected; and ecchymosis from subcutaneous hemorrhage at the injection site. All of these disappear with time and are easily managed with reassurance and standard therapy for exposure keratitis. It is important to carefully observe patients following injection if prior myectomy or neurectomy has been performed. These patients can have a profound or prolonged drug effect and develop severe exposure problems after treatment. Although it has not been proven, the suggested cause is a reduction in the muscle mass available to bind the botulinum toxin.

One way to maximize the toxin's effect is to perform a myectomy (described below) and plan to use botulinum toxin for office touch-up treatment in postoperative patients with residual spasms. By individualizing treatment for each patient, a good therapeutic response can be achieved in the majority of patients.

Botulinum toxin is excellent for the control of synkinetic blepharospasm seen in patients following Bell's palsy. This annoying tic is disconcerting and responds nicely to small quantities of toxin injected in the areas of clinical involvement.

SURGICAL TREATMENT

Presently there are two basic surgical procedures for patients with essential blepharospasm. Selective seventh cranial nerve ablation, commonly referred to as neurectomy or the Reynold's procedure (5), was designed to selectively resect the temporal and zygomatic branches of the facial nerve innervating the protractor muscles of the eyelid and eyebrow, thus causing a muscle paresis that eliminates or reduces the spasmotic contractions causing functional blindness. This procedure is effective for the treatment of many patients, but has severe and unpleasant side effects that reduce its clinical usefulness (6). These side effects are facial paresis, paralytic ectropion, brow ptosis, epiphora, and synkinetic facial movements associated with recurrent spasms. Recurrence of visually incapacitating spasm following neurectomy approaches 50%, and many of these patients require further surgery for the control of symptoms (7).

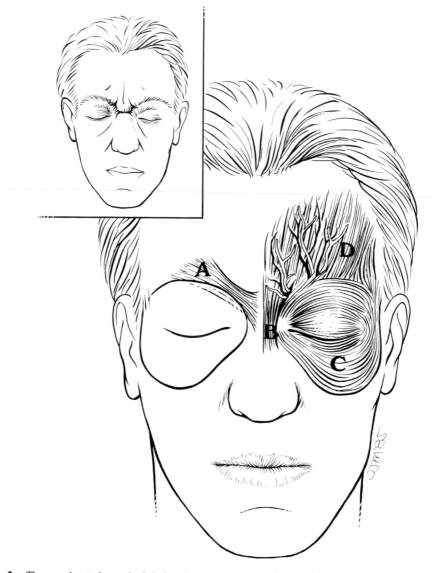

FIG. 2. The muscles to be excised during the myectomy procedure include the corrigator supercilii (A), the proceri (B), and the orbital, preseptal, and part of the pretarsal orbicularis oculi muscles (C). These muscles are responsible for the forced eyelid closure and deep brow furrows (*inset*) seen in blepharospasm patients. The frontalis muscle (D) opposes the eyebrow protractors and does not participate in forced eyelid closure. This muscle should be preserved during surgery. (From Shore, ref. 10, with permission. © 1985, Pergamon Press.)

Selective subtotal excision of the eyelid (orbicularis oculi muscles) and eyebrow (proceri and corrigator supercilii muscles) protractors as popularized recently by Gillum and Anderson (8), now commonly referred to as the Anderson procedure, has been shown to be more efficacious since recurrences are less frequent and side effects less severe (9). Additionally, this procedure gives the surgeon an opportunity to correct underlying anatomic abnormalities present in many patients with long-standing blepharospasm such as brow ptosis and dermatochalasis.

There are many technical variations to both surgical procedures, but the basic goals remain the same: to selectively interrupt the nerve supply to the protractor muscles or to selectively excise the protractor muscles responsible for the incapacitating periocular muscle spasms (Fig. 2).

In recent years there has been a shift away from the Reynold's procedure and today selective myectomy is the surgical procedure of choice for patients requiring surgical correction of blepharospasm.

Myectomy Procedure

Selection of Incision

Protractor myectomy can be performed through a variety of incisions including eyelid only, eyebrow only, combined eyelid and eyebrow, eyebrow incisions connected across the glabella, and combined coronal and blepharoplasty incisions (10). This author recommends the latter because the technique allows direct access to and complete visualization of the muscles to be excised. Also, direct brow incisions, which can cause the dermis to become adherent to the underlying bone or pericranium, are avoided (11). These incisions can result in increased scar formation with persistent eyelid and eyebrow edema, depressed scars, and an immovable, adynamic brow.

Preoperatively the surgeon must decide where to place the forehead incision. An incision in the midforehead can be hidden in a deep furrow and still achieve excellent exposure and a good postoperative lifting affect to correct brow ptosis. Incisions at the hairline or behind the hairline are alternative choices. In making the decision, one should use the same criteria for patients undergoing cosmetic forehead lifts. Since forehead skin or scalp is resected as an integral part of the coronal myectomy with browlift, the hairline will be displaced posteriorly if a scalp incision is used. Therefore, patients with long foreheads, male pattern baldness, receding hairlines, and thinning of the scalp hair are good candidates for the mid-forehead or hairline incision. Patients with low-set brows or normally placed hairlines and thick hair usually choose the scalp incision. If a scalp incision is used, patients should be warned that the forehead will be vertically lengthened and the hairline displaced posteriorly following surgery. The hairline and scalp incisions are easily concealed in most cases by changing the hairstyle slightly.

Preoperative Preparations

The patient is instructed to shampoo the hair with Betadine surgical scrub the evening before surgery. Unlike cosmetic forehead lifts, the myectomy procedure is best performed with the patient under general anesthesia. Local infiltrative anesthesia and regional blocks can be employed if absolutely necessary, but the operation is a long one, tedious for the patient and the surgeon when performed with the patient awake. Patients usually do much better under general anesthesia.

The patient is positioned supine on the operating table in a 15° reverse Trendelenberg (head up) posture. A neurosurgical headrest such as the Mayfield headrest provides the surgeon excellent access to the head and neck region. It is not necessary to shave the hair in the area of the proposed scalp incision for cosmetic cases because the incidence of infection is very low. Shaving the hair does make the scalp excision easier to manage, however, and it is recommended for myectomy cases. Prophylactic antibiotics and perioperative intravenous steroids help reduce postoperative swelling and reduce the incidence of wound infections.

The face and scalp are prepped with Betadine solution and the entire face, both ears, and the scalp 3 cm behind the proposed incision are included in the surgical field. Betadine-soaked cotton balls are placed in the ear canals to prevent blood pooling, which can cause postoperative discomfort and temporary hearing difficulties. If the hair was not shaved, it is parted with a surgical scrub brush along the planned scalp incision. Hand towels are sutured or stapled to the scalp posterior to the proposed incision. The scalp, forehead, and glabella are infiltrated with local anesthetic [lidocaine 2% with epinephrine at a concentration of 1:100,000 and hyaluronidase (Wydase®) 150 U].

Surgical Technique

The midline is marked and a symmetrical incision outlined with a surgical marking pen (Fig. 3). Laterally, the incision should be carried to the anterior and superior reflection of the helix of the ear. One should be prepared to extend the incision inferiorly in front of the root of the ear as a limited rhytidectomy incision if there is a problem "turning down" the flap to expose the superior orbital rim. Initially, the incision should stop at the root of the ear and extended only if adequate exposure cannot be obtained.

The skin incision is made with the surgeon and assistant providing digital pressure to the wound margins for hemostasis. The skin and galea aponeurotica are incised. The incision is beveled and aligned with the hair follicles to minimize postoperative incisional alopecia. Laterally it is important not to incise the temporalis fascia because this causes bleeding from the underlying temporalis muscle, which is a nuisance. Great care should be taken to identify and preserve the superficial temporal vessels on each side. While this is not important in cosmetic forehead lifts, it is important in the myectomy procedure. The anterior forehead, scalp, and frontalis muscle receive blood supply from the superficial temporal arteries, supraorbital and supratrochlear arteries, and anastomotic branches of the angular arteries, which are the terminal branches of the facial artery (see Chapter 2.) Any one of these vessels alone is capable of providing the necessary postoperative blood supply to the coronal flap. During the myectomy procedure, all the vessels except the two superficial temporal arteries are sacrificed during muscle excision. Therefore, the postoperative blood supply to the flap depends on an intact superficial temporal artery and for this reason both should be preserved, if possible.

The galea must be completely incised and retracted to expose the underlying pericranium before hemostatic clamps are applied. It is difficult to place the clips if the galea has not been completely transected.

During cosmetic forehead lifts it is not necessary to apply hemostatic clamps to stop skin edge bleeding or bleeding from the galea because the procedure is short and blood loss is not excessive. The longer myectomy procedure can result in significant blood loss

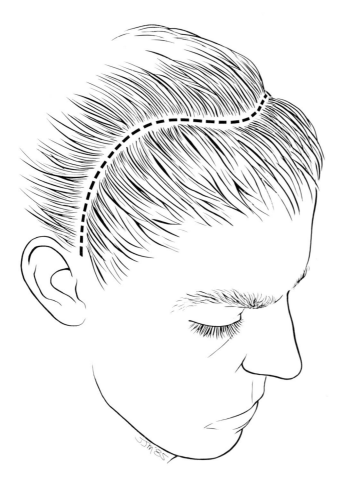

FIG. 3. The coronal incision extends from the root of each ear to the midline of the scalp as depicted. If not shaved, the hair is parted to provide the best possible exposure. When the forehead incision is used, it is made directly in front of the hairline or in a deep midforehead furrow at least 2.5 cm above the orbital rims. (From Shore, ref. 10, with permission. © 1985, Pergamon Press.)

if bleeding is not controlled; therefore hemostatic clamps are recommended. Excellent hemostasis is achieved by applying Raney neurosurgical clips to the scalp and galea on the anterior scalp incision. Dandy hemostatic clamps are placed on the galea posteriorly and allowed to dangle and provide hemostasis. Alternatively, Raney clips may be used on both wound edges. The galea must be incorporated in the clips during application because the vascular supply to the scalp runs with the galea.

Once bleeding has been controlled, the coronal flap is developed with a combination of sharp and blunt (finger) dissection. This dissection is facilitated by vigorous retraction of the flap by the surgeon and assistant using double-pronged skin hooks. These skin hooks must be carefully placed when working superiorly and laterally above the orbital rims to avoid damage to the terminal branches of the facial nerve coursing through this area. These nerves innervate the frontalis muscle and, if transected or stretched, postoperative brow paresis, which is an undesirable complication of cosmetic or functional forehead surgery, may occur.

As the flap is turned down, the dissection proceeds in the subgaleal, avascular plane. Laterally one must develop the plane directly on the fascia of temporalis muscle. This is extremely important as one approaches the temporal fossa, because the frontal branch of the facial nerve runs deep to the superficial musculoaponeurotic system and just superficial

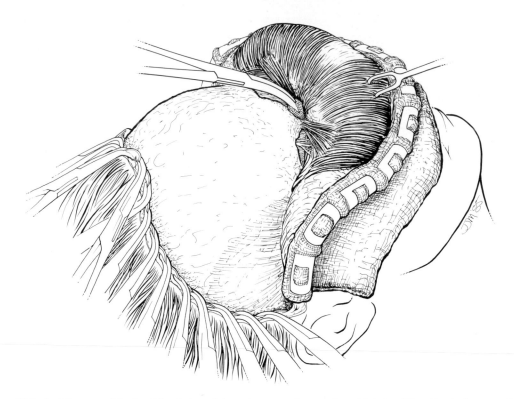

FIG. 4. The coronal forehead flap is turned down to expose the superior orbital rim. Dissection in the area of the glabella and orbital rim is best performed with a "peanut" dissector. (From Shore, ref. 10, with permission. © 1985, Pergamon Press.)

to the temporal fascia enveloping the muscle (12,13). Again, superficial or careless dissection in this area can damage the frontal branch of the facial nerve and lead to postoperative paresis or paralysis of the brow.

As the superior orbital rim is approached, the supraorbital neurovascular bundle is encountered (Fig. 4). A "peanut" dissector is used to expose the neurovascular bundles. Ultimately, the supraorbital and supratrochlear neurovascular bundles are sacrificed, because it is not possible to completely dissect them from the surrounding orbicularis oculi, corrigator supercilii, and proceri muscle fibers. The flap must be "turned down" to completely expose the superior orbital rim, the periosteum over the zygomatic process of the frontal bone laterally, and the superior aspect of the nasal bones in the glabellar region medially. The septum should not be opened since exposure of the preaponeurotic fat is not desired at this time. As the dissection proceeds, the proceri, corrigator supercilii, and orbital orbicularis oculi muscles will be elevated with the forehead skin and frontalis muscle. The fibers of these three muscles are easily identified, blending with vertically oriented fibers of the frontalis muscle (Fig. 5). Once exposed, these three muscles are excised, sparing the frontalis muscle.

Dissection and excision of the proceri and corrigator supercilii muscles begins centrally. The Bovie cautery is used to cut the muscles away from the overlying dermis. The dissection must be meticulous and one must proceed slowly so the dermis will not be injured. The

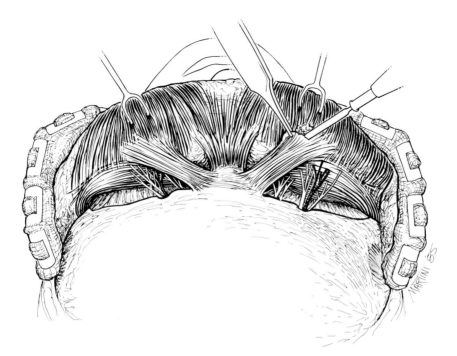

FIG. 5. Bovie cautery is used to excise the corrigator supercilii, the proceri, and the orbital portion of the orbicularis oculi muscles. The supraorbital neurovascular bundles are closely associated with these muscles and must be sacrificed in order to completely remove the eyebrow protractors. The vertically oriented frontalis muscle should not be excised. (From Shore, ref. 10, with permission. © 1985, Pergamon Press.)

Bovie cautery can be used on either the cutting or coagulation mode, but better hemostasis is achieved with coagulation if a fine-needle cautery tip is used. The entire procerus, corrigator superciliaris and the orbital orbicularis oculi muscles are excised bilaterally. As previously mentioned, the supraorbital and supratrochlear neurovascular bundles are sacrificed at this time to ensure total excision of all protractor muscles. Excision of these sensory nerves leads to postoperative cutaneous anesthesia to the level of the vertex of the skull. It is important to warn the patients of this preoperatively. The forehead anesthesia improves with time but full sensory perception never returns. Cutaneous hypesthesia and pruritis are inevitable during convalescence but gradually improve with time.

It is possible to excise the preseptal and pretarsal orbicularis oculi muscle fibers from the brow approach, but it is easier and safer to remove these through a second blepharoplasty incision following completion of the brow procedure.

Once the brow protractors have been excised and hemostasis achieved, the coronal flap is ''turned back'' to the normal anatomic position. The hemostatic clamps are removed and a conservative forehead lift is performed. This is accomplished by pulling the scalp superiorly to overlap the posterior skin edge (Fig. 6). The amount of skin and hair to be resected is estimated and rarely exceeds 2.5 cm. Vertical skin incisions are made anteriorly in the coronal flap corresponding to the amount of scalp to be excised. The apex of each vertical incision is sutured to the posterior skin edge with a 3–0 Prolene suture. The excess skin and galea are excised with a scalpel. The skin and galea are closed in layers. It is possible to merely staple the skin and ignore the galea, but this places excessive tension

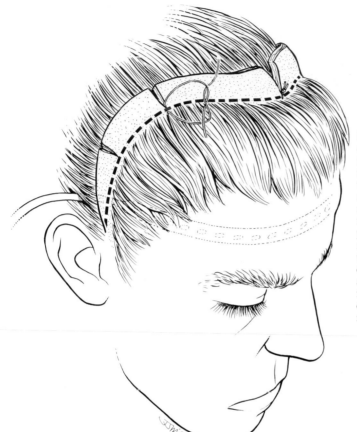

FIG. 6. After the myectomy procedure, a standard forehead lift is performed and the wound is closed. Vertical skin incisions aid in estimating the amount of skin to be excised. A suction drain is placed to prevent hematoma or seroma formation. The forehead lift displaces the hairline posteriorly when a scalp incision is made. Patients should be warned of this preoperatively since they may elect to have the incision placed more anteriorly at the hairline or in the midforehead so scalp hair will not be excised. (From Shore, ref. 10, with permission. © 1985, Pergamon Press.)

on the wound. The best closure is obtained when the galea is closed separately with interrupted sutures of 2–0 Dexon or 3–0 Neurolon on an atraumatic taper needle. The skin is then stapled or sutured in a standard fashion. If a midforehead incision has been used, the transected galea investing the frontalis muscle *must* be approximated prior to skin closure and the skin is meticulously closed in layers. The wound should not be closed under tension, and excessive dermal cautery should not be used or a linear alopecia may result. The skin staples are left in place for 12 to 14 days.

During cosmetic forehead lifts, the wound need not be drained, but drainage is essential following myectomy. If used, a Penrose drain should exit the wound laterally. Suction drainage, such as a TLS drain or a flat, 7-mm Jackson-Pratt drain, can handle more volume and actively remove accumulated serous fluid and blood. When used, the suction drain should be brought out through a separate stab incision posterior and lateral to the scalp wound. The drain is removed on the first or second postoperative day, after the volume of drainage has subsided or stabilized.

Blepharoplasty excision of remaining muscle

Once the coronal flap has been closed, attention is directed to the eyelids, where the remaining preseptal and part of the pretarsal orbicularis oculi muscle is excised through

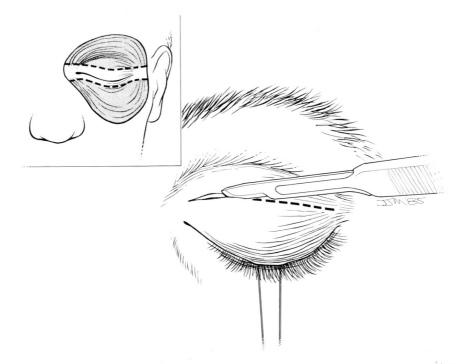

FIG. 7. The preseptal and part of the pretarsal orbicularis oculi muscles are best excised through upper blepharo-plasty incisions (*inset*). A 3-mm strip of pretarsal orbicularis oculi muscle must be left adjacent to the eyelid margins to allow for eyelid closure postoperatively. Eyelid margin traction sutures are placed to aid in the dissection. (From Shore, ref. 10, with permission. © 1985, Pergamon Press.)

blepharoplasty incisions (Fig. 7). One must not excise any upper eyelid skin during this procedure since significant wound contracture does occur. Severe postoperative lagophthalmos can result if skin is excised.

The upper eyelids are infiltrated with more of the same local anesthetic and 4–0 silk traction sutures are placed through the eyelid margins bilaterally to aid in the later dissection. Corneal protective contact lenses are placed and the blepharoplasty incisions are marked on the upper eyelid skin in the lid crease 8 to 10 mm above the lash line. The skin incision is made and a skin flap developed by sharply dissecting the skin off the underlying orbicularis oculi muscle superiorly and inferiorly (Fig. 8). The orbicularis oculi muscle fibers lying directly beneath the skin are not disturbed. One must be careful not to ''button-hole'' or ''tear'' the skin of the eyelids as this dissection proceeds. The dissection is carried superiorly and medially to connect with the space underlying the skin of the glabella and eyebrow where the previous myectomy took place. Inferiorly, the skin is elevated to within 2 mm of the lashes. Once exposed, the preseptal and pretarsal orbicularis oculi muscle fibers are excised with cutting Bovie cautery (Fig. 9). The levator palpebrae superioris muscle and aponeurosis must not be injured during muscle excision. The orbital septum and preaponeurotic fat may be removed if desired, but this is usually not necessary. The preaponeurotic fat provides protection for the underlying levator complex and should be preserved at least initially. A 3-mm strip of pretarsal orbicularis oculi muscle immediately superior to the lashes is left intact to provide postoperative eyelid closure.

When hemostasis has been obtained, the skin is closed loosely, with interrupted sutures.

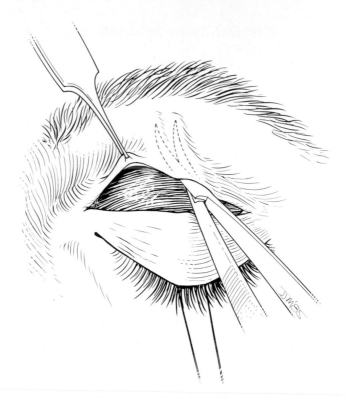

FIG. 8. A skin flap is developed following the skin incision. The underlying orbicularis oculi muscle should not be disturbed. (From Shore, ref. 10, with permission. © 1985, Pergamon Press.)

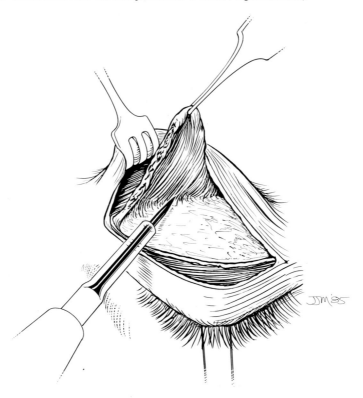

FIG. 9. The orbicularis oculi muscle is excised with a Bovie cautery. Care must be taken not to injure the levator palpabrae superioris muscle or aponeurosis during the myectomy procedure. Preaponeurotic fat may be excised, but this usually is unnecessary. (From Shore, ref. 10, with permission. © 1985, Pergamon Press.)

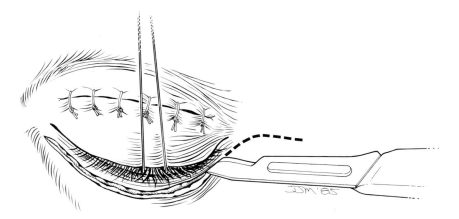

FIG. 10. A lower blepharoplasty incision provides excellent exposure for the lower eyelid myectomy. The incision must be carried laterally at the lateral commissure to aid in developing the skin flap. (From Shore, ref. 10, with permission. © 1985, Pergamon Press.)

The upper eyelid crease is formed with supratarsal fixation sutures placed at the time of wound closure. A tight closure is not desired because there is significant swelling and drainage from the wound and it is important not to trap this fluid behind the skin incision.

Lower eyelid myectomy

The myectomy procedure may include removing the lower eyelid protractors at the time of initial surgery in selected patients, but this is rarely indicated since most patients do not have significant disability from lower eyelid spasms. Additionally, for reasons not well understood, lower eyelid spasms, and to some extent lower facial spasms, decrease significantly following the upper eyelid and eyebrow myectomy. Patients with incapacitating residual lower eyelid spasm usually respond well to botulinum toxin injections. Those few patients not responding to this treatment can be surgically managed by lower eyelid myectomy as described below.

Traction sutures of 4–0 silk are placed in the margin of the lower eyelid to aid the dissection. A modified lower eyelid blepharoplasty incision is made with slight lateral extension over the orbital rim and zygoma at the lateral commissure (Fig. 10). A skin flap is elevated inferiorly to the level of the inferior orbital rim. Again, care is taken not to ''buttonhole'' the skin. The muscle fibers of the underlying orbicularis oculi are not disturbed during this dissection. All of the orbital and preseptal orbicularis oculi muscle fibers are excised, and only 3 mm of pretarsal orbicularis oculi muscle is left for eyelid closure postoperatively (Fig. 11). It is not necessary to open the orbital septum and remove orbital fat, but this can be done, if desired. When indicated, horizontal eyelid laxity is corrected at this time by horizontally tightening the lower eyelid. The wound is closed with interrupted sutures of 7–0 silk (Fig. 12). Eyelid skin should not be excised unless present in excessive amounts. Wound contracture does occur and postoperative ectropion may result if skin is excised.

Postoperative Care

At the completion of the case, a loose turban dressing is placed over the forehead and scalp. Excessive pressure on the forehead flap must be avoided and care should be taken

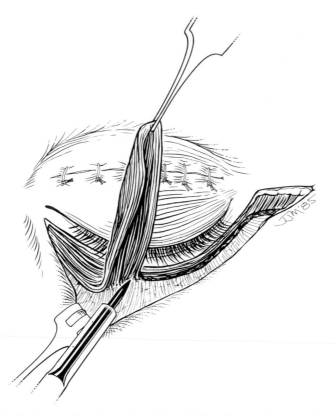

FIG. 11. After the skin flap has been elevated to the level of the inferior orbital rim, the preseptal and orbital portions of the orbicularis oculi muscle are excised with Bovie cautery. A 3-mm strip of pretarsal orbicularis oculi muscle is left near the eyelid margin to allow for postoperative eyelid closure. (From Shore, ref. 10, with permission. © 1985, Pergamon Press.)

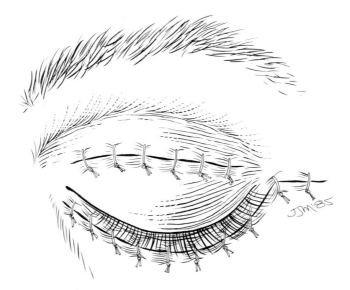

FIG. 12. Excess lower eyelid skin is excised with great caution. The skin is closed loosely with interrupted sutures. (From Shore, ref. 10, with permission. © 1985, Pergamon Press.)

to minimize pressure over the area of the superficial temporal vessels for reasons previously stated. The orbits must remain visible for nursing observation. The head of the bed is elevated 20° to reduce swelling and ice is applied to the eyelids intermittently for 48 hr. The patient is observed carefully on the ward to look for hematoma formation under the coronal flap. The drains are removed on the first or second postoperative day. Ocular lubricants are used to protect the cornea and provide comfort. An ophthalmic antibiotic ointment is placed on the eyelid wounds twice daily until the sutures are removed. Ecchymosis is prominent, but resolves over 2 to 3 weeks. Eyelid swelling may persist for up to 12 weeks. Initially, the brow feels "tight" and appears paretic, but this gradually improves within 2 weeks.

Complications

Complications of the coronal forehead flap include hematoma or seroma formation, flap necrosis, infection, linear or segmental alopecia, brow paresis, forehead anesthesia, "button-hole" formation during myectomy, and eyebrow asymmetry. The incidence of complications is very low and can be further minimized by careful patient selection, meticulous surgical technique, use of suction drainage, and close observation in the postoperative period.

Patient Response

Patient acceptance of the coronal approach to periorbital myectomy for blepharospasm is high. Most patients feel their cosmetic appearance has been enhanced by the forehead lift and are happy to avoid the placement of surgical scars directly above the eyebrows.

Combined Therapy

Recently Perman and Baylis (14) described combining neurectomy with selective myectomy by excising the temporal and zygomatic branches of the facial nerve and performing a myectomy procedure through extended coronal and rhytidectomy incisions in one operation. The idea is an excellent one, but as yet results of combined neurectomy and myectomy have not been compared with myectomy alone, and it is impossible to state that the combined procedure offers significant advantages over myectomy alone.

Combined myectomy and adjunctive chemodenervation with botulinum A toxin is the approach this author advocates. Patients are initially started on botulinum toxin injections and the results are assessed. If the patient tires of the injections, a therapeutic response is not achieved, or injections are required too frequently, myectomy is performed. Botulinum toxin is then used for office touch-up treatment if residual spasms are present. Once the muscle mass has been reduced, standard quantities of botulinum toxin have a profound weakening effect and must be used cautiously to avoid complications related to corneal exposure. It is not unusual for the time between required injections to double or triple following myectomy. The number of injections required during each treatment session is also reduced because the toxin appears to have a better effect in terms of reducing the severity of muscle spasms.

REFERENCES

1. Henderson, J. W. (1956): Essential blepharospasm. *Trans. Am. Ophthalmol. Soc.*, 54:453–468.
2. Jankovic, J., and Ford, J. (1983): Blepharospasm and orofacial-cervical dystonia: Clinical and pharmacological findings in 100 patients. *Ann. Neurol.*, 13:402–411.

3. Jankovic, J. (1985): Clinical features, differential diagnosis, and pathogenesis of blepharospasm and cranio-cervical dystonia. *Adv. Ophthalmic Plast. Reconstruct. Surg.,* 4:67–82.

4. Shore, J. W., Leone, C. R., O'Connor, P. S., Neuhaus, R. W., and Arnold, A. C. (1986): Botulinum toxin for the treatment of essential blepharospasm. *Ophthalmic Surg., (in press).*

5. Reynolds, D. H., Smith, J. L., and Walsh, T. J. (1967): Differential section of the facial nerve for blepharospasm. *Trans. Am. Acad. Ophthalmol. Otolaryngol.,* 71:656–664.

6. Dortzbach, R. K. (1973): Complications in surgery for blepharospasm. *Am. J. Ophthalmol.,* 75:142–147.

7. Frueh, B. R., Callahan, A., Dortzbach, R. K., Wilkins, R. B., Beale, H. L., Reitman, H. S., and Watson, F. R. (1976): The effects of differential section of the VIIth nerve on patients with intractable blepharospasm. *Trans. Am. Acad. Ophthalmol. Otolaryngol.,* 81:595–602.

8. Gillum, W. N., and Anderson, R. L. (1981): Blepharospasm surgery: An anatomical approach. *Arch. Ophthalmol.,* 99:1056–1062.

9. McCord, C. D., Coles, W. H., Shore, J. W., Spector, R., and Putnam, J. R. (1984): Treatment of essential blepharospasm: A comparison of facial nerve avulsion and eyebrow-eyelid muscle stripping procedure. *Arch. Ophthalmol.,* 102:266–268.

10. Shore, J. W. (1985): Coronal approach to protractor myectomy. *Adv. Ophthalmic Plast. Reconstr. Surg.,* 4:333–347.

11. McCord, C. D., Shore, J. W., and Putnam, J. R. (1984): Treatment of essential blepharospasm: A modification of exposure for the muscle stripping technique. *Arch. Ophthalmol.,* 102:269–273.

12. Mitz, V., and Peyronie, M. (1976): The superficial musculo-aponeurotic system (SMAS) in the parotid and cheek areal. *Plast. Reconstr. Surg.,* 58:80–88.

13. Liebman, E. P., Webster, R. C., Berger, A. S., and DellaVecchia, M. (1982): The frontalis nerve in the temporal brow lift. *Arch. Otolaryngol.,* 108:232–235.

14. Perman, K. I., and Baylis, H. I. (1985): Facelift and coronal approach to blepharospasm surgery. *Adv. Ophthalmic Plast. Reconstruct. Surg.,* 4:397–405.

Subject Index